Independent Living for Physically Disabled People

Developing, Implementing, and Evaluating Self-Help Rehabilitation Programs

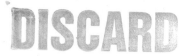

Nancy M. Crewe,
Irving Kenneth Zola,
and Associates

Independent Living
for Physically
Disabled People

People with Disabilities Press

Stanley D. Klein, Ph.D., Series Editor

iUniverse.com, Inc.

San Jose New York Lincoln Shanghai

3/6 n. t

Independent Living for Physically Disabled People

Published by People With Disabilities Press,
an imprint of iUniverse.com.
Stanley D. Klein, Ph.D, Series Editor.

For information address:
iUniverse.com, Inc.
5220 S 16th, Ste. 200
Lincoln, NE 68512
www.iuniverse.com

Originally published by Jossey-Bass

ISBN: 0-595-17797-2

Printed in the United States of America

Preface

Independent living (IL) has been called a social movement, a service paradigm, a research model, a new discipline, a source of hope, and an idea whose time has come. Whatever the descriptor, independent living is a focus of major interest for disabled people and rehabilitation specialists across America.

In essence, IL means allowing people with disabilities to live as they choose in their communities rather than confining them in institutions. But this straightforward concept is not simple in its implementation. For the disabled person, it involves exchanging the safety of custodial care for the risk, stress, and effort involved in making the innumerable large and small decisions that shape one's life. It means finding and maintaining the network of support services that are required just to survive and then reaching for the kind of involvement with other people that gives life meaning.

For the public, the IL movement means a commitment to bringing down the environmental barriers that have so long kept disabled people out of sight and away from our streets and public buildings. It also means supporting essential services, including attendant care and accessible transportation. In some respects, these tenets may seem almost revolutionary because for at least a century we have preferred to pay the high cost of institutionalizing disabled people rather than deal with the complexities of meeting individual needs on the outside.

Directly or indirectly, the IL movement affects all of us, and this book is one example of its growing visibility. It has been written with three major audiences in mind: people who are already working in the field of IL, professionals in the closely related fields of vocational and medical rehabilitation, and students who are preparing for careers that will bring them into contact with disabled persons. Although it is intended primarily for a professional audience, disabled consumers in general will also find this volume enlightening.

Professionals in health care and vocational rehabilitation will be able to use this book to understand and work more effectively with their disabled clients. Because they are aware of and concerned about their rights for self-determination, disabled people are no longer likely to be passive recipients of care. They will expect to be involved to a greater degree in decisions about their treatment, about institutional policies that affect them, and about their future. Furthermore, the day is past when, once medical care has been provided, people can merely be discharged into the community with inadequate living arrangements and support services. Better patient education, increased family involvement, and more effective liaisons with consumer groups and community agencies are all required to make successful the transition from institutionalization to independent living. Physicians, nurses, public health workers, physical and occupational therapists, speech pathologists, therapeutic recreation personnel, psychologists, and social workers all have a stake in the issues covered by this book.

Counselors and administrators in vocational rehabilitation (VR) are also directly affected by the IL movement. The federal legislation passed in 1978 gave the VR system primary responsibility for IL rehabilitation. Although funding to support that mandate has been tragically small, the intimate relationship between the two programs remains. It is only a matter of time before VR counselors will be providing IL services right along with their traditional activities.

Researchers and teachers will find this book a substantial

new resource. Up to now, in large part, IL literature has appeared in the form of monographs or unpublished papers, and these are exceedingly difficult to retrieve. To our knowledge, this book represents the first comprehensive documentation of the IL movement. In writing it we have aimed to create a lasting tool that will contribute to the development of the field.

This book addresses both the philosophy of independent living and its implementation. It contains practical discussions of key services and evaluation strategies that make it directly applicable for personnel in IL programs. The historical and theoretical information encompassed in it is equally important as a basis for making present-day decisions and anticipating future developments.

The significance of this book extends beyond the immediate areas of health care and services. Architects, for example, need to become increasingly aware of barrier-free design, not only in terms of the mechanics of accessibility but also in terms of IL's broader goals. City planners and real estate developers with a knowledge of IL principles would be able to avoid the construction of inaccessible public projects that later require costly retrofitting. Legislators, too, need information to effectively serve their disabled constituents and to make wise decisions about bills related to attendant care and other IL concerns. Service providers in many fields, for example, clergy and teachers, will find themselves working with increasing numbers of disabled individuals who have moved into the mainstream of community life. Knowledge can increase personal comfort as well as professional effectiveness.

Although the book focuses on people with physical disabilities, much of it is equally applicable to IL for the mentally retarded, the mentally ill, and the elderly. We hope that it will serve to identify areas of common interest and thus help unify these groups in pursuit of opportunities for self-determination and a place in the community.

The Genesis of This Book

The plan for this volume originated with the decision by the American Congress of Rehabilitation Medicine to devote the October 1979 issue of its journal, *Archives of Physical Medicine and Rehabilitation,* to the topic of IL. That special issue, which was received with tremendous interest, was notable both for the new information it contained and for the recognition it was awarded as scientific literature. Some of those early articles, updated and expanded, appear as chapters in this book; the bulk of the chapters are original treatments of new topics. Thus this book presents broad, intensified coverage of independent living as it has emerged into the present day.

The authors represented in this volume are a diverse and notable collection of individuals, many of whom are consumers of IL services as well as professional service providers. They represent a variety of academic fields, including sociology, psychology, anthropology, economics, architecture, business, and future studies—and a variety of geographic locations including, within the United States, Massachusetts, California, Texas, Minnesota, and Florida, and also Canada and Ireland.

Organization and Content

Like any major social phenomenon, independent living is a product of its culture and of its time. By understanding its historical roots, one can develop a better appreciation for its goals and methods. Part One of this book attempts to provide such a foundation. It discusses the main factors that have converged to supply the energy, vision, and resources that have created and motivated the IL movement. Unlike earlier vocational and medical rehabilitation efforts, independent living was substantially the product of organized, vocal consumers rather than of service providers and other advocates. Coming as it did from a new perspective, the IL movement offers a new framework or paradigm upon which to structure services and raise researchable questions. This new paradigm is developed in Chapter One.

Legislation is a key topic because of its importance both in reflecting and shaping societal attitudes toward disability. Furthermore, it is legislation that enables the actual delivery of services supporting IL for the severely disabled person. Chapter Two documents disabled citizens' commitment to joining the mainstream of society from the drive for institutionalization a century ago to the passage of the 1978 Amendments to the Rehabilitation Act. The active role of disabled persons is a theme that appears repeatedly in Part One, particularly in Chapter Three, which describes the evolution of IL as a self-help movement. Self-help groups were surprisingly slow to develop in America, but they have flourished and have become a powerful source of mutual support, education, and action among people affected by particular health concerns or disabilities.

Part Two describes the different kinds of IL programs that have arisen in the United States and abroad. It also examines how the accessibility of the environment affects the lives of disabled people. Research conducted by the Independent Living Research Utilization Project in Houston provided the foundation for Chapter Four, which contrasts the goals and activities of community-based centers with those offering residential facilities on a brief transitional or more extended basis. The author also describes an "ideal" IL center model that may be created in the future.

So far, most IL centers have been developed in urban areas in response to a concentration of need and also of services. In individual terms, however, the needs of people in rural areas are no less urgent. Drawing heavily on more than fifteen years of experience logged by the state of Nebraska, Chapter Five describes some strategies that have been used successfully to serve widely dispersed constituencies.

Just as IL programs differ from one part of the United States to another, many distinctive features are evident in the programs of other countries. The use of family support systems and low-cost technology are among the valuable lessons that can be learned from the report in Chapter Six about independent living in Sweden, the Netherlands, Denmark, Great Britain, Canada, and Australia.

The remaining chapters in Part Two examine the effect of environmental factors on independent living. Chapter Seven describes rational planning techniques that can be used to locate residences and facilities so as to eliminate excessive distances between places frequently used by disabled people. People can be limited not only by distance but also by structure. The primary purpose of architecture is to facilitate the activities of daily life. The more conducive the environment, the wider the range of behaviors that can occur. Conversely, quality of living is curtailed by inadequate architecture. The special implications of these truisms for people with disabilities are explored in Chapter Eight.

Part Three is devoted to a description of the various services that have been deemed most important to the achievement of independent living. Attendant care, discussed in Chapter Nine, is a critical issue because it is one of the most essential services for individuals with severe physical disabilities—its availability can literally mean the difference between life and death. The way in which attendant care is delivered can profoundly affect the extent to which the spirit of IL is met for the consumer.

Peer counseling and IL skills training, discussed in Chapters Ten and Eleven, respectively, are also crucial services. Central to self-help efforts, they provide means for people with disabilities to share experiences with one another. Rather than avoid the risk of learning survival techniques by staying in a total care institution, and instead of having to learn them through painful trial, people who desire to live independently can turn to others with personal experience for suggestions, shortcuts, and caveats. Furthermore, while learning and working together, disabled people can combine their power to influence social and political decisions that affect their lives.

The road to accessible transportation has been anything but smooth, as described in Chapter Twelve. Considerable progress has been made in opening some forms of transportation, such as airlines, to disabled persons, but the prospect of widespread urban bus transit seems to be receding at an alarming rate, with serious personal and economic consequences.

No single answer exists to the question of housing for people with mobility impairments. Chapter Thirteen discusses a variety of options that are necessary to meet individual needs and preferences, and provides a detailed introduction to the design, development, financing, and marketing of specialized housing that integrates personal care services with accessible shelter.

No discussion of IL services would be complete without examining the implications of new technology for communication, activities of daily living, education, and employment. Chapter Fourteen describes recent advances in these areas along with problems in the development and delivery of technology. It also offers possibilities for making technological advances more readily available to people who need them.

Part Four assesses present accomplishments and future prospects of the IL movement. Continuing support for IL activities will undoubtedly depend on the accumulation of evidence concerning how such activities affect people's lives. Two distinctly different approaches to evaluation are presented in Chapters Fifteen and Sixteen. Chapter Fifteen details a multivariate survey of the activities and outcomes of eleven centers in California. Chapter Sixteen describes field research, a method that uses direct observation to tap the subjective insights of consumer-participants in IL centers. Both kinds of research contributed to the content of Chapter Seventeen, which addresses the topic of organization and advocacy. This chapter presents an insider's perspective on the development of the disability rights movement in four key states and also draws on interviews with and surveys of rehabilitation officials who were often the target of actions taken by the consumer groups.

Turning from the past and present of IL to its future, Chapters Eighteen and Nineteen and the Epilogue explore the short- and long-range changes that may confront the movement. Just as the technological revolution is altering the lives of citizens throughout America, it promises to modify housing, attendant care, peer counseling, education, and transportation services for people with disabilities. But even the most advanced technology will not eliminate negative attitudes in many sectors that lie at the heart of most problems faced by disabled people. Even among rehabilitation consumers and service providers, more open dialogue on independence, coping, risk taking, and care are necessary if we are to avoid working at cross-purposes in pursuit of IL goals.

A multitude of unanswered questions remain about IL services, delivery systems, funding, and evaluation. Many more years may pass before they can be resolved definitively. Nevertheless, a body of knowledge is emerging that can contribute to the orderly growth of the field. The purpose of this volume is to bring together a substantial part of that knowledge and provide a forum through which some of the IL leaders can communicate the challenge and promise of the future. The message is intended for those who are already a part of the movement, as consumers and/or as providers of services, as well as for those who will join the effort. To those with an "old" disability who see in the movement a reason to live, to students and teachers, to rehabilitators and researchers, to politicians, and to the American public that has supported the movement, this book is dedicated.

January 1983   Nancy M. Crewe
                                                 Minneapolis, Minnesota

                                                  Irving Kenneth Zola
                                                Waltham, Massachusetts

Contents

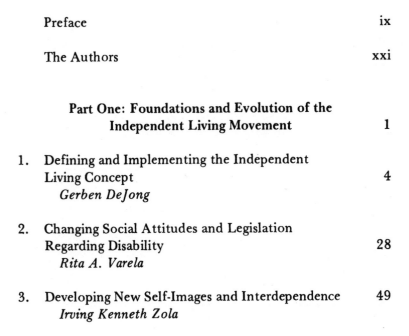

The Authors

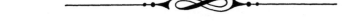

Nancy M. Crewe is a rehabilitation psychologist and associate professor in the Department of Physical Medicine and Rehabilitation at the University of Minnesota. She was trained in psychology at the University of Minnesota, receiving the B.A. degree in 1961, the M.A. degree in 1964, and the Ph.D. degree in 1967.

Crewe became involved with the Independent Living Movement when she chaired the Social and Environmental Aspects of Rehabilitation Committee for the American Congress of Rehabilitation Medicine, 1974–1979. She presently works with two Minneapolis independent living organizations, Comprehensive Services for Disabled Citizens and Accessible Space. Her research and publications have dealt with psychology of disability, creativity, goal setting and outcome measurement, and functional assessment in vocational rehabilitation. In 1978, with Gary Athelstan and Ames Bower, she authored *Employment after Spinal Cord Injury: A Handbook for Counselors.*

Irving Kenneth Zola is professor and chair, Department of Sociology, Brandeis University. He is also a founding member and counselor at the Boston Self Help Center, an organization staffed by and serving people with chronic diseases and disabilities. He was trained in social relations at Harvard University, receiving his B.A. degree in 1956 and his Ph.D. degree in 1962.

Zola is the author of many books and articles on delinquency, social problems, and health care. His most recent works include *Missing Pieces: A Chronicle of Living with a Disability* (1982) and *Ordinary Lives: Voices of Disability and Disease* (1982). He has written numerous scholarly articles on disability and health policy. Zola also contributes to magazines as a restaurant, movie, and book reviewer, as well as a short story writer, frequently providing unique insights into the experiences of disabled people through these varied forums.

Frank Bowe, formerly director of the American Coalition of Citizens with Disabilities, is president of FBA Inc., a management consulting firm in Woodmere, New York.

Nancy A. Brooks is assistant professor, Department of Sociology, Wichita State University.

Jean A. Cole is assistant professor, Department of Rehabilitation, Baylor College of Medicine, and director, Division of Education, the Institute for Rehabilitation and Research in Houston.

Gerben DeJong is senior research associate and assistant professor, Department of Rehabilitation Medicine, Tufts University School of Medicine.

Lex Frieden is assistant professor, Department of Rehabilitation, Baylor College of Medicine, and director, Independent Living Research Utilization Project, the Institute for Rehabilitation and Research, Houston.

Arthur Harkins is associate professor of education and sociology and director of the Graduate Concentration in Future Cultural and Educational Systems, University of Minnesota.

Thomas A. Lee is youth employment adviser on the National Rehabilitation Board, Dublin, Ireland.

Raymond Lifchez is associate professor, Department of Architecture, University of California, Berkeley.

Shelia Stephens Newman is senior research associate, Institute for Information Studies, Falls Church, Virginia.

John Malcolm Phillips is an independent architect and planner in Victoria, British Columbia.

Marsha Saxton is director of consultation and training, Boston Self Help Center.

John E. Schatzlein is a consultant with the Academic/Employment Preparation Division, Control Data Corporation, Minneapolis.

Lois O. Schwab is professor of human development and the family, University of Nebraska, Lincoln.

Rayelenn Sparks is a research associate, Institute for Information Studies, Falls Church, Virginia.

Susan Stoddard is a vice-president, Berkeley Planning Associates, Berkeley, California.

Denise Galluf Tate is assistant professor of rehabilitation, Michigan State University, and senior research associate at the University Center for International Rehabilitation.

Rita A. Varela is director of ALCANZA Research, a Florida consulting firm specializing in disability rights.

Teg Wenker is a self-employed independent living consultant in Seattle and Everett, Washington.

Stephen F. Wiggins, formerly executive director of Accessible Space, Inc., of Minneapolis, is currently a graduate student at the Harvard Business School.

Independent Living
for Physically
Disabled People

Developing, Implementing,
and Evaluating
Self-Help Rehabilitation Programs

Part One

Foundations and Evolution
of the
Independent Living Movement

During the colonial period, before almshouses, asylums, and long-term hospitals were constructed, individuals who could not support themselves were aided by a system that had descended from the English poor laws. Townships were responsible for sustaining the "indigent" (which included many of the disabled), but they did so less out of charity than to prevent them from becoming a public nuisance. Most of the settlers were struggling to eke out a marginal living, so there were few excess resources to provide for dependents.

Assistance provided to the poor in their own homes, known as "outdoor relief," was typical during colonial times. Families usually provided physical care for their disabled members, and some received money from the government for doing

1

so. Those whose families could not help were kept in private homes at public expense. To keep such expense to a minimum, however, they were "auctioned off." The bidder who demanded the least amount of subsidy won the contract and thus acquired an indentured servant. Those who were too disabled to attract any bidders were sometimes cared for in jails or workhouses. The mentally ill or retarded were often kept in tiny, unheated cells, more like kennels than human living quarters (Oberman, 1965).

As the population grew and the number of disabled was augmented by the Revolutionary War, the need for a more organized system of aid was recognized. Townships could no longer manage the responsibility alone, so county and state governments became involved in providing relief. To an even greater extent, voluntary charitable societies assumed the task of caring for the poor. Outdoor relief was substantially replaced by the development of almshouses, institutions that housed all kinds of people, including criminals as well as the able-bodied and disabled poor.

Undoubtedly, the almshouses varied somewhat in the quality of existence they provided to residents, but in general they were rather miserable human storage facilities. By the middle of the nineteenth century the appalling conditions in these almshouses were publicized by such reformers as Dorothea Dix. Change, however, was impeded by the fear that improved conditions or a return to outdoor relief would reduce people's motivation to work. America was viewed as a land of boundless opportunity, and it was commonly believed that anyone who really worked hard could succeed. Therefore, almshouses seemed the most suitable as well as the most economical way to provide for those who were dependent.

The gradual development of specialized institutions provided an escape from almshouses for some groups of disabled persons. In Europe, schools for the deaf were among the first, followed soon after by experimental schools for the mentally retarded, the blind, and the crippled. Hospitals and asylums were also created, and for all of their limitations, at least they had some productive purpose that was missing from the almshouses.

After the Civil War, with the creation of modern social welfare programs and the ascendance of the progressive movement, almshouses were replaced by other forms of assistance. For the severely disabled who needed physical care in order to survive, however, the only public solution continued to be institutionalization. Nursing homes eventually provided an alternative to hospitals, but it remained for the Independent Living Movement to suggest options that offered real autonomy.

Although original references to independent living rehabilitation go back more than twenty years, legislative, social, and philosophical forces finally converged to create the Independent Living Movement in the early 1970s. Throughout the previous decade this country had experienced a growing sensitivity toward the civil rights of minority groups, and people with disabilities began to realize the ways in which they shared a minority status. They also began to recognize themselves as consumers—not merely recipients—of health and rehabilitation services. Furthermore, they began to see more clearly their power to help themselves and each other instead of relying exclusively on professional caregivers.

Understanding the foundations of the movement is essential to grasping the methods and aspirations that characterize its evolution. The authors of chapters in this part, all of whom personally took part in shaping the growth of the independent living concept, not only recount events but also spell out their implications for everyone involved—for disabled persons, professionals in medical and vocational rehabilitation, researchers, and teachers. They show how the movement is changing the way we view ourselves and each other as well as the problems that we seek to solve through our work. Implications for society at large are also explored. No longer can we be satisfied with helping the disabled individual adjust and adapt in isolation. We must also work for changes in society and in the larger environment.

1

Defining and Implementing the Independent Living Concept

Gerben DeJong

Future historians of American social policy will look back to 1973 as a year which separates one epoch of disability policy from another. In that year Congress passed a new rehabilitation act which launched a whole set of initiatives affecting the nation's disabled population, particularly its most severely disabled citizens.

The most visible feature of the 1973 Rehabilitation Act is section 504, a one sentence statement prohibiting discrimination against "otherwise qualified handicapped" individuals "under any program or activity receiving Federal financial assistance." Because of this section's far-reaching implications, the 1973 Rehabilitation Act has sometimes been called "the Civil Rights Act of the handicapped."

Note: This chapter is a revised and updated version of an article that appeared in the October 1979 issue of *Archives of Physical Medicine and Rehabilitation.*

4

The 1973 act cannot be fully understood apart from an emerging social movement: the Independent Living (IL) Movement.

As Turner (1969) notes, "A significant social movement becomes possible when there is a revision in the manner in which a substantial group of people, looking at some misfortune, see it no longer as a misfortune warranting charitable consideration but as an injustice which is intolerable in society" (p. 321). Inspired by strong indigenous leadership from among the disabled population, the movement seeks a better quality of life for all disabled persons.

The IL movement is more than a grass-roots effort on the part of the disabled to acquire new rights; it is also intent on reshaping the thinking of disability professionals and researchers, on promoting new forms of service-delivery, and on encouraging new directions in research.

This chapter evaluates independent living as a social movement and as an analytic paradigm which aims to redirect the course of disability policy, practice, and research. As a paradigm, independent living offers a marked contrast to the definitions and interventions provided by its predecessor, the rehabilitation paradigm. To gain an appreciation of the IL paradigm, it is necessary to understand independent living as a social movement with a distinct constituency and history. The movement is heavily indebted to other contemporary social movements, such as civil rights, consumerism, self-help, demedicalization/self-care, and deinstitutionalization. The significance of independent living for the future of disability practice and research cannot be understood apart from the contributions of these other movements.

The Constituency of the IL Movement

The IL movement has always counted the "severely disabled" as its primary constituency. But who are the severely disabled? How many of them are there? One common criterion used to measure severe disability is the capacity to work or to carry on one's major activity. Based on results from its 1974

Health Interview Survey, the National Center for Health Statistics (1976) estimates that 3.3 percent of the nation's population —about 6.8 million people—are unable to carry on their major activity. This figure represents .2 percent of all children, 2.6 percent of all working-age adults, and 17.1 percent of all the elderly.

However, the movement's core constituency is more limited than these data suggest. The movement has concentrated its energies on a relatively few major disability groups: those with spinal cord injury, muscular dystrophy, cerebral palsy, multiple sclerosis, and postpolio disablement. Moreover, the IL movement has concentrated its energies on a selected age group: the older adolescent and younger working-age adult. The emphasis on this narrow age range is, in part, a function of the disabling conditions mentioned above. Spinal cord injury, for example, is most common among males during their late teens and early twenties because that is when they are most likely to participate in disability-prone activities. Multiple sclerosis generally becomes evident during one's twenties, while cerebral palsy and muscular dystrophy are developmental disabilities and thus are already evident during childhood. Those persons with a postpolio disablement are the senior members of the movement.

The emphasis on the younger adult is also a function of those communities where the movement has taken root. The IL movement has been most active in large academic communities containing critical numbers of university-age persons. Free from some of the more demanding familial and economic responsibilities, this age group is often better able to organize around major social issues.

Notably absent from the movement's constituency are older persons with severe physical impairments resulting from stroke or other degenerative conditions. While the movement's philosophy may have direct relevance to older disabled persons, the movement has focused its concern elsewhere. However, the movement's present age bias is one that cannot last indefinitely. Medical science is not only enabling severely disabled persons to survive initial trauma but is also enabling them to live longer. Thus, as the movement's initial adherents grow older we can expect the movement to enlarge its present focus.

Also absent from the movement's constituency and leadership are racial minorities. This is noteworthy, since disability statistics indicate that blacks have a higher incidence of disability than do their white counterparts. The absence of racial minorities deserves special analysis. Given the similarities of philosophy in the civil rights movement, the black movement, and the IL movement, one would expect the IL movement to attract disabled persons from racial minorities.

Disability professionals and special interest organizations are also part of the movement's constituency. Disability professionals include physicians in physical medicine and rehabilitation, physical therapists, occupational therapists, nurses, rehabilitation counselors, and disability researchers. While the commitment of these professionals to the movement varies widely, the number of such adherents is increasing. Special interest groups include organizations such as the National Spinal Cord Injury Foundation, the Easter Seal Society, and various professional associations. Again, the commitment of these organizations varies widely from chapter to chapter.

In defining the movement's constituency, we should not ignore the overlap between disabled consumers and disability professionals. Many disabled persons are themselves disability professionals. The participation of able-bodied professionals in the movement can be explained to some degree by the influence of their disabled professional peers.

The movement gains strength from the fact that it links the interests of its primary disability groups with the interests of other disability groups on issues of common concern. The issue of architectural barriers, for example, is one that unites other mobility-impaired groups, even though it is of most importance to the core disability groups in the IL movement. Coalition building through organizations such as the American Coalition of Citizens with Disabilities (ACCD) has enabled the movement to enlarge its constituency around specific issues.

It should be noted that the movement's constituency is defined not only by *who* participates but also by *what* it advocates. The constituency, in some respects, extends to those who do not actively participate but who nonetheless come under its consciousness-raising spell and thus become informal advocates of its philosophy and ideology.

Origins and Legislative Background

It is difficult to pinpoint the origin of the Independent Living Movement. The movement springs from two main sources: the efforts of disabled persons to seek a more fulfilling life in an able-bodied world, and the efforts of rehabilitation professionals to reach disabled persons for whom a vocational goal was, until recently, unthinkable. While the efforts of both groups often converge on specific legislation, their interests and origins are sufficiently different to warrant separate consideration.

The disabled students program at the University of Illinois at Champaign-Urbana was among the first to facilitate community living for persons with severe physical disabilities. In 1962, four severely disabled students were transferred from a campus-isolated nursing home to a modified home close to campus. The disabled students program has since emerged as a significant self-help effort, and has helped to make the university one of the most architecturally accessible institutions of its kind.

In the early 1970s, the IL movement gained greater visibility and momentum with the creation of the Center for Independent Living (CIL) in Berkeley, California. The Berkeley CIL incorporated itself in 1972 as a self-help group to be managed primarily by persons who were themselves disabled. The center provides a wide range of services, including peer counseling, advocacy services, van transportation, training in independent living skills, attendant care referral, health maintenance, housing referral, and wheelchair repair (Brown, 1978; Stoddard, 1978). Unlike other centers that have since emerged, the Berkeley CIL has no residential program and serves persons with a greater variety of disabling conditions than do many other existing centers.

On the East Coast, the Boston Center for Independent Living (BCIL) began its activities in 1974. BCIL emphasizes transitional housing and attendant care services (Corcoran and others, 1977). Similar centers and organizations have since sprung up throughout the nation. Each center offers its own unique blend of advocacy and consumer services; together, the various centers have given the IL movement both an organizational focus and a vehicle for realizing some of the movement's more important goals.

The movement's organizational efforts have not been limited to centers for independent living. Allied organizations such as the ACCD have been instrumental in monitoring federal legislation affecting disabled persons. The ACCD also helped to organize the coast-to-coast demonstrations that prompted the United States Department of Health, Education and Welfare (HEW) to issue regulations implementing section 504 of the 1973 Rehabilitation Act.

Developing concurrently with the organizational initiatives of disabled persons were the efforts of rehabilitation professionals to encourage national legislation. In 1959, a bill (HR361) was introduced which contained provisions extending IL services to individuals for whom employment was not an obtainable objective (Urban Institute, 1975; Parsons and Counts, 1978). That bill failed to pass, and in 1961 a new bill, written largely by the National Rehabilitation Association, was introduced. The new bill contained a separate title on IL services. That bill also failed.

In 1972, Congress passed HR8395 amending the Vocational Rehabilitation Act to provide IL services to those individuals "for whom a vocational goal is not possible or feasible." The bill was twice vetoed by President Nixon on the grounds that it "would divert the (vocational rehabilitation) program from its basic vocational objectives" toward more ill-defined medical and welfare goals (Urban Institute, 1975). Eventually the President did sign what became known as the 1973 Rehabilitation Act, albeit with the IL provisions deleted.

Nonetheless, the 1973 Rehabilitation Act contained breakthroughs important to the IL movement. First, it mandated that those who were most severely handicapped were to receive first priority for services under the act. Second, under Title V, it extended new statutory rights to handicapped persons. In particular, sections 501 and 503 of Title V mandated affirmative action programs for the employment of disabled persons within the federal government and by organizations contracting with the federal government. Section 502 created the Architectural and Transportation Barriers Compliance Board. And section 504 banned discrimination on the basis of handicap in any program or activity receiving or benefiting from federal financial assistance.

A statutory authorization for IL services finally came into being when President Carter signed PL95-602 in 1978. This law created a new Title VII, called Comprehensive Services for Independent Living. Title VII established a four-part program: (1) an IL services program to be administered by the state vocational rehabilitation agencies; (2) a grant program for IL centers; (3) an IL program for older blind persons; and (4) a protection and advocacy program to safeguard the rights of severely disabled persons. Title VII authorized $80 million for fiscal year 1979; $150 million for 1980; $200 million for 1981; and "such sums" for 1982. To date, however, Congress has appropriated only a fraction of the amounts authorized—$18 million in fiscal year 1981, for example.

Two things need to be said, in conclusion, about the concept of IL services as advocated by vocational rehabilitation professionals.

First, the concept of IL rehabilitation has changed since it was originally introduced to Congress almost two decades ago. Since then, medical and rehabilitation technology has advanced so significantly that many who would have been targeted for IL-type services are now routinely prepared for gainful employment by state vocational rehabilitation agencies.

Second, vocational rehabilitation professionals have a different conception of independent living than do their consumer counterparts in the IL movement. Many vocational rehabilitation professionals hold that IL services are best suited to those for whom a vocational goal is thought to be impossible. IL rehabilitation, in their terminology, refers solely to those medical and social services that enable a disabled person to live in the community short of being gainfully employed. From this perspective, independent living and rehabilitation are seen as alternative and competing policy goals. Throughout the legislative debate on independent living, professionals and legislators have voiced their fear that independent living would dilute the specificity of the vocational outcome. Some professionals feared that IL services would prompt the same charge of nonaccountability often levied against more ill-defined social services, such as those administered under Title XX of the Social Security Act.

Others in the IL movement, whose involvement does not originate in the vocational rehabilitation tradition, reject the idea that independent living and employment are competing goals. To them, such a conception is potentially sinister in that it implicitly places an arbitrary upper limit to the goals a disabled person might set for himself. In their view, vocational objectives should be seen as an *integral part* of the IL goal, not as a competing goal.

Relation to Other Social Movements

The IL movement has flourished concurrently with several other complementary social movements, including civil rights, consumerism, self-help, demedicalization/self-care, and deinstitutionalization/normalization/mainstreaming. While these movements share common values and assumptions, they arise from differing sources in response to different social problems. Each has influenced the IL movement in its own unique way. The origins and ideology of the IL movement cannot be fully appreciated without noting their contributions.

Civil Rights. The civil rights movement of the 1960s has had an impact far beyond the racial minorities it sought to benefit. The movement made other disadvantaged groups aware of their rights and of the denial of those rights. During its initial stages, the movement was primarily concerned with *civil* rights, as opposed to *benefit* rights. Civil rights are exemplified by the right to vote, the right to hold elective office, and the right to be tried by a jury of one's peers. Benefit rights are exemplified by the entitlement to educational, income, and medical assistance benefits. The benefit rights issue was taken up late in the civil rights movement by the Poor Peoples' Campaign and by spin-offs such as the National Welfare Rights Organization.

The concern for both civil rights and benefits rights has spilled over to other vulnerable groups. In the area of mental health, patients have, in some instances, acquired the right to refuse treatment and to expect quality care. In the area of child welfare, children have acquired new procedural rights, which are slowly replacing the best-interest-of-the-child rule as the legal standard for adjudicating abuse and delinquency cases. Moreover, children now receive rights to treatment and education under special education statutes.

The IL movement has been similarly concerned with both civil and benefit rights. The movement's interest in civil rights is reflected in Title V of the 1973 Rehabilitation Act, which prohibits various forms of discrimination, particularly in the area of employment. However, the concern for civil rights does not stop there. Persons with severe mobility impairments argue that architectural barriers deprive them of their civil rights when these barriers prevent them from participating in the political life of the community. In like fashion, disabled persons have become aware that benefit rights are prerequisites to living in a community setting. Without income assistance benefits or attendant care benefits, many disabled persons would be involuntarily confined to long-term care facilities.

The civil rights movement has had an effect not only on the securing of certain rights but also on the *manner* in which those rights have been secured. When traditional legal channels have been exhausted, disabled persons have learned to employ other techniques of social protest, such as demonstrations and sit-ins.

The black movement that grew out of the civil rights movement has had its own effect on the IL movement. According to the critique offered by the civil rights movement, racial discrimination was an American anomaly that could be largely removed through the enactment of new legal protections. The black movement, however, argued that the main issue was a racism central to the definition of white America and beyond the scope of simple legal remedies. Similarly the IL movement has come to recognize that prejudice against disability is rooted in our culture's attitudes about youth and beauty, and in the able-bodied person's fear of vulnerability to physical disability.

Consumerism. The effects of the consumer movement are harder to define. The movement embraces nearly all social classes and groups. Although personified by Ralph Nader, its membership includes the public interest lawyer representing various disadvantaged groups, the devoted reader of *Consumer Reports,* and the person who campaigns for new consumer protection legislation.

Here I shall evaluate consumerism in terms of its ideology and the expression of that ideology in disability policy. Basic to consumerism is a distrust of seller or service provider. It is up to the consumer to become informed about reliability of products or adequacy of services. Consumer sovereignty has always been the hallmark of free-market economic theory. In practice, however, it is often the professional who has been sovereign.

The rise of consumer sovereignty directly challenges professional dominance in rehabilitation and disability policy. In vocational rehabilitation, for example, the professional counselor no longer necessarily has the final word in case planning. Instead, the Rehabilitation Act of 1973 provides for an *individualized written rehabilitation plan* (IWRP), to be drawn up jointly by client and counselor. Advocacy centers to advise disabled persons of their legal rights and benefits are another product of the IL movement. Because of the awareness generated by the movement, many disabled persons are better informed about governmental benefits and regulations than are their professional counterparts in the human services system.

The doctrine of consumer sovereignty, sometimes referred to as consumer involvement, is now very much a fixture within the IL movement. The doctrine asserts that because disabled persons are the best judges of their own interests, they should have the larger voice in determining what services are provided in the disability services market.

Self-Help. The self-help movement also embraces a large variety of groups, from the Female Improvement Society to Alcoholics Anonymous (Withorn, 1977). There now appears to be a self-help group for every conceivable human condition or problem—drugs, gambling, death, homosexuality, child abuse, women's health, old age, sex, neighborhood crime, cigarette smoking, childbirth, and, of prime interest here, physical disability (Withorn, 1977; Back and Taylor, 1976; Hurvitz, 1976; Levy, 1976; Riessman, 1976). Such organizations view themselves as mutual aid groups that serve either as adjuncts or as valid alternatives to established human service agencies. They usually address problems and needs not dealt with by other institutions in society.

Among disabled persons, the IL center has become the primary self-help unit; they seek to serve both as an adjunct to the present human service system and as an alternative service provider. As an adjunct, the center serves as a conduit for funding human services such as attendant care. As an alternative, the center provides peer counseling and advocacy services not available through mainline human service organizations.

The self-help movement is fueled by the same distrust of professionally dominated services as exists in consumerism. Self-help organizations are intended to give people the opportunity exercise control over their own lives and the services they use. As knowledge-giving organizations, they help to confer sovereignty on the consumer.

Demedicalization/Self-Care. Well-known critics of the medical profession, such as Ivan Illich (1976), have expressed the concern that too many social problems and life conditions are being unnecessarily "medicalized." "Demedicalization" challenges the dominance of medical professionals in these spheres.

Over the last several decades, a number of behaviors once considered sinful or criminal have been reclassified as illnesses (Conrad and Schneider, 1980; Fox, 1968, 1977; Freidson, 1970; Mechanic, 1973; Pitts, 1968; Twaddle, 1973; Zola, 1972). Alcoholism and mental disorders, for example, have been removed from the categories of sin or crime and are labeled illnesses. Some have begun to call child abuse a "disease." Similarly, such life events as birth and death now almost always entail a considerable degree of medical intervention.

Many consumers have begun to react to the excesses of medicalization and to urge that certain conditions and life events be demedicalized. For example, many advocates hold that pregnancy should be removed from the category of illness and that childbirth should be supervised by a midwife rather than a physician (Boston Women's Health Book Collective, 1979; Blauner, 1966; Kalish, 1965). Again, the term *death with dignity* has gained currency with the belief that the terminally ill should be allowed to die at home rather than in a hospital, wired to the latest array of monitoring devices.

Implicit in the argument for demedicalization is the assumption that individuals can and should take greater responsibility for their own health and medical care. In many ways, demedicalization is simply an extension of the self-help movement to the fields of health and medical care, and is so referred to in some quarters. The movement goes beyond the keep-fit, watch-your-weight, stop-smoking, and drink-less campaigns of the recent past. The self-care movement encourages people to administer their own treatment for minor health problems and to avert potential complications arising from chronic health conditions.

The IL movement is very much a partisan in the medicalization/self-care debate. At issue is the extent to which the management of disability should remain under the aegis of the medical care system, once medical stability has been substantially obtained. Today, most public policies respecting disability require some type of professional medical presence, whether in the acute stages of disability, in the determination of eligibility for income maintenance benefits, or in long-term institutional care. The IL movement asserts that much of this medical presence is both unnecessary and counterproductive.

Central to the IL movement is the belief that the management of medically stabilized disabilities is primarily a personal matter and only secondarily a medical matter. A constant medical presence in the life of a disabled person gives rise to behavior on the part of both practitioner and patient that induces dependency and thus hinders achievement of rehabilitation and IL goals.

To understand how such behavior arises, it is helpful to turn to the *medical model,* a loosely used concept that varies with the context in which it is discussed. As used here, the medical model consists of the following assumptions and role expectations in the provision of medical care:

- The physician is the technically competent expert.
- Medical care should be administered through a chain of authority wherein the physician is the principal decision maker; accountability for the care of the patient centers on the attending physician.
- The "patient" is expected to assume a "sick role" that requires him or her to cooperate with the attending medical practitioners.
- The main purpose of medicine is the provision of acute and restorative care.
- Illness is best handled through the use of clinical procedures such as surgery, drug therapy, and the "laying on of hands."
- Illness can be diagnosed and treated only by trained practitioners.

Like most models, this version of the medical model gives a rather rigid description of what the provision of medical care is supposed to entail. The model is not exhaustive; it focuses primarily on those elements that can help us to understand what is meant by the demedicalization of disability.

Before evaluating the role expectations of the medical model, it is worth noting that some of the model's other features have also proved unpalatable to the IL movement. One important reason for demedicalizing disability, the movement argues, is that many of the assumptions of the medical model do not apply to the needs of disabled persons. For example, the model's emphasis on acute and restorative care is not in keeping with the needs of long-term disabled persons who are beyond the acute phase. Likewise, once beyond the acute phase and living independently, many disabled persons are not in need of surgery, drugs, or the laying on of hands that characterizes clinical medicine. Moreover, experienced disabled persons often do not need diagnosis or treatment by medical professionals, since they will have developed sufficient familiarity with the idiosyncrasies of their own condition to be able to do much of their own medical monitoring and treatment.

The IL movement has been particularly critical of the behavioral expectations of the medical model, as expressed in the *sick role.* Originally formulated by Talcott Parsons (1951), the sick role is considered the single most important concept in medical sociology. By understanding it we can gain a better insight into the position advocated by the IL movement.

The sick role consists of two interrelated sets of exemptions and obligations:

- A sick person is exempted from "normal" social activities and responsibilities, depending on the nature and severity of the illness.
- A sick person is exempted from any responsibility for his or her illness, is not morally accountable for the condition, and is not expected to become better by sheer will.

These exemptions are granted conditionally. In exchange:

- A sick person is obligated to define the state of being sick as aberrant and undesirable, and to do everything possible to facilitate his or her recovery.
- A sick person is obligated to seek technically competent help and to cooperate with the physician in getting well.

The sick role is intended to be a temporary one. But for the long-term or permanently disabled person, there is no possibility of immediate recovery, in the sense of being restored to one's original physical condition. Because disability is often an irrevocable part of their existence, disabled people, as a result of the sick role, begin to accept not only their condition but also their very personhood as "aberrant" and "undesirable." Moreover, they begin to accept the dependency prescribed under the sick role as normative for the duration of the disability. Thus, the sick role cancels the disabled person's obligation to take charge of his or her own affairs.

Gordon (1966) and Siegler and Osmond (1973) echo this critique of the sick role in their discussions of the *impaired role.* The impaired role is ascribed to an individual whose condition is not likely to improve, and who is unable to meet the first requirement of the sick role, the duty to try to get well as soon as possible. Persons assuming the impaired role have abandoned the idea of recovery altogether and have come to accept both their condition and their dependency as permanent. Siegler and Osmond argue that the impaired role "carries with it a loss of full human status." The impaired role, they point out, "does not require the exertions of cooperating with medical treatment and trying to regain one's health, but the price of this idleness is a kind of second-class citizenship" (1973, p. 56). The impaired role is not a normative one or one prescribed by the medical model, but is a role the disabled person is allowed to slip into as the passage of time weakens the assumptions of the sick role.

The impaired role is fictionalized in Thomas Mann's Nobel Prize-winning *The Magic Mountain* (1927), a novel about patients living at the Berghof, an international tuberculosis sanitarium for the well-to-do. Here patients abandon the sick role for the impaired role. Siegler and Osmond's description of the impaired role at the Berghof is informative: "The impaired role has a lower status than the sick role, but in return for this childlike status, they are allowed to spend their days as children do, playing card games, taking up hobbies, having meals served to them, "playing" with each other, or, most often, doing nothing at all" (1973, p. 56). Mann's fictionalized account of the Berghof presents us with one variant of the impaired role as it occurs in a particular institutional setting. His account underlines the role's inherent bias toward childlike dependency.

The IL movement rejects the behavioral expectations created by both the sick role and its derivative, the impaired role, asserting that the disabled do not want to be relieved of their familial, occupational, and civic responsibilities in exchange for childlike dependency. In fact, the movement considers any such "relief" tantamount to denying the disabled both their right to participate in the life of the community and their right to full personhood.

The dependency-creating features of the medical model and the impaired role are most pronounced in institutional settings. Institutions are self-contained social systems that allow house staff and various practitioners to exercise a substantial measure of social control with little outside interference.

Prolonged institutionalization is known to have harmful effects:

Patients are encouraged to follow instructions, rules and regulations. Compliance is highly valued, and individualistic behavior is discouraged. The "good" patient is the individual who respectfully follows instructions and does not disagree with staff. On the other hand, the patient who constantly asks for a dime for the pay phone, a postage stamp, or a pass to leave the institution on personal business, tends to be treated as a nuisance or labeled "manipulative." Patients do not make their own appointments, keep their own medical charts, or take their own medications. Responsibility for these things is legally vested in the institution. Yet on the day of discharge, the patient is expected suddenly to assume control of his own health care and life decision making [Corcoran, 1978, p. 63].

The trend to deinstitutionalize is one that cuts across many disabling conditions. The best known deinstitutionalization effort is the community mental health movement, which has allowed many individuals (often with the help of psychotropic drugs) to leave institutional confinement or remain in the community. Similar examples can be found in other fields such as geriatric care and juvenile correction.

Severely physically disabled persons and their advocates are, understandably, latecomers to the deinstitutionalization movement. Unlike mentally impaired persons or ex-offenders, their disabilities are difficult to conceal and thus they could not blend into the mainstream upon their release. Moreover, the deinstitutionalization of severely physically impaired persons usually requires substantial environmental or architectural modifications.

The deinstitutionalization movement has received some impetus from the political argument that institutional care is expensive and that community care will save taxpayer money. Proof of this argument is often hard to establish, however, especially when studies overlook the ever-present tendency of institutions to increase utilization simply to meet capacity. In addition, the argument has begun to wear thin with the taxpaying public, which has not witnessed any significant decreases in hu-

man service expenditures. As latecomers to the deinstitutionalization thrust, severely physically disabled persons are least likely of all to benefit from the money-saving argument. More importantly, public cynicism about deinstitutionalization may
prove yet another barrier to independent living.

Closely related to deinstitutionalization are the concepts
of normalization and mainstreaming. These two issues primarily
concern developmentally disabled children and young adults. At
one time, it was thought that the interests of disabled children
were best served by confining them to institutions or segregat-
ing them in special education classes. It is now accepted that a
disabled child or young adult develops more normally when
"mainstreamed" with his or her able-bodied peers. However,
normalization goes beyond mere deinstitutionalization. As Dybwad explains, "normal on our earth is trouble and strife, trial
and tribulation and the handicapped person has the right to be
exposed to it. Normalization . . . includes the dignity of risk"
(1973, p. 57). Normalization, in other words, takes deinstitutionalization a step further to include the possibility of failure—
a fact which the deinstitutionalization movement has not always been prepared to accept.

The dignity of risk is the heart of the IL movement. Without the possibility of failure, the disabled person lacks true
independence and the ultimate mark of humanity, the right to
choose for good or evil.

Independent Living as an Analytic Paradigm

Social movements eventually find expression in both public policy and professional practice. The IL movement is no different. We began our discussion by saying that the Independent
Living Movement goes beyond the attempt to secure new rights
and entitlements for disabled persons. It also represents an attempt to reshape the manner in which the problem of disability
is defined and to encourage new interventions. We are witnessing the emergence of a new paradigm designed to redirect the
thinking of disability professionals and researchers alike.

As a historian of the natural sciences, Kuhn (1970) observed that scientific facts did not emerge by simple accumula-

tion or evolution, but were the products of new ways of thinking, that is, of new scientific paradigms. Paradigms define reality for the scientist. They provide a framework for identifying and solving problems. A paradigm also prescribes the technology needed to solve a given problem.

Two special concepts are important to Kuhn's analysis. First is the concept of an *anomaly*: an event or observation that cannot be adequately explained by the dominant paradigm of the time. When a sufficient number of anomalies appear, a crisis is precipitated, and disaffected individuals begin to search for an alternative explanation or paradigm. Second is the concept of *paradigm shift*: the moment when one paradigm is discarded for another. Anomalies do not automatically cause individuals to renounce one paradigm for another: "[a] scientific theory is declared invalid only if an alternate candidate is available to take its place" (1970, p. 77). Both these concepts are useful to our inquiry.

The rehabilitation paradigm is currently the dominant paradigm in disability policy regarding both medical and vocational rehabilitation. It could be argued that there are sufficient differences between medical and vocational rehabilitation to speak of two paradigms, but there are also a sufficient number of similarities to consider them as one. Since my main purpose is to contrast rehabilitation and independent living as paradigms, the differences between medical and vocational rehabilitation are less important than the similarities.

In the rehabilitation paradigm, problems are generally defined in terms of inadequate performance in Activities of Daily Living (ADL) or in terms of inadequate preparation for gainful employment. In both instances, the problem is assumed to reside in the individual. Therefore, it is the individual who needs to be changed. To overcome his or her problem, the disabled individual is expected to yield to the instruction of a physician, physical therapist, occupational therapist, or vocational rehabilitation counselor. The disabled individual is expected to assume the patient role. In this view, success in rehabilitation is largely determined by the degree to which the patient or client has complied with the prescribed therapeutic regime.

In recent years, anomalies have appeared that cannot be

explained by this paradigm. The most important anomaly is the fact that very severely physically disabled persons have achieved independence without the benefit of, or in spite of, professional rehabilitation. Their number includes some persons who were considered too disabled to benefit significantly from rehabilitation services. It has become evident that cooperation with professional rehabilitation is not necessarily a prerequisite for independent living. As a result, an increasing number of individuals, particularly the most severely disabled, have become disaffected and have sought an alternative paradigm.

The IL paradigm has emerged, in part, as a response to the anomaly represented by the severely physically disabled person. According to the IL paradigm, the problem resides seldom in the individual, but often in the solution offered by the rehabilitation paradigm, and most notably in the dependency-inducing features of the relationship between professional and client. More particularly, the problem resides in an environment that includes the rehabilitation process, the physical environment, and the social control mechanisms of society-at-large. To cope with these environmental barriers, the disabled person must shed the patient or client role for the consumer role. Advocacy, peer counseling, self-help, consumer control, and barrier removal are the trademarks of the IL paradigm (see Table 1).

Although the IL paradigm is now well beyond the embryonic stage of development, the rehabilitation paradigm remains strong. We can expect the IL paradigm to strengthen as movement leaders continue to refine its basic principles. In this period of paradigm shift, we find individuals with loyalties to both paradigms. Some rehabilitation professionals who have introduced IL concepts into their practice have not yet totally abandoned the rehabilitation paradigm for the IL paradigm. This view of paradigm shift departs somewhat from Kuhn's. Where Kuhn (1970, p. 77) argues that "[the] decision to reject one paradigm is always simultaneously the decision to accept another," the IL example suggests that the transition from one paradigm to another is not necessarily an abrupt one.

Paradigms do not only define problems and the range of appropriate interventions; they also determine what is relevant

Table 1. A Comparison of the Rehabilitation and Independent
Living Paradigm.

Item	Rehabilitation Paradigm	Independent Living Paradigm
Definition of problem	Physical impairment; lack of vocational skill; psychological maladjustment; lack of motivation & cooperation	Dependence on professionals, relatives, and others; inadequate support services; architectural barriers; economic barriers
Locus of problem	In individual	In environment; in the rehabilitation process
Social role	Patient/client	Consumer
Solution to problem	Professional intervention by physician, physical therapist, occupational therapist, vocational counselor, and others	Peer counseling; advocacy; self-help; consumer control; removal of barriers and disincentives
Who controls	Professional	Consumer
Desired outcomes	Maximum ADL; gainful employment; psychological adjustment; improved motivation; completed treatment	Self-direction; least restrictive environment; social and economic productivity

for the purposes of research. Kuhn holds that there is no such thing as research in the absence of any paradigm.

In traditional rehabilitation research, the emphasis has been on gains in carrying out ADL, mobility, and employment. Client characteristics and various kinds of rehabilitation therapy have generally been considered critical in achieving such ends. Such characteristics typically include age, sex, physical impairment, and the psychological makeup of the individual. The focus on these characteristics reflects the assumption that the problem to be addressed resides in the individual. The issue in rehabilitation research is not whether rehabilitation works, but which therapy or intervention works best for which groups of clients.

Independent living as a paradigm of research has just begun to emerge. Much of the research incorporating IL concepts has yet to find its way into the published literature. Nonetheless, given the values and assumptions of the IL movement, we can determine which are relevant to research.

The theory of causation implicit in the IL paradigm asserts that environmental barriers are at least as critical as personal characteristics in determining disability outcomes. A review of the IL literature suggests several key environmental variables: unmet attendant care needs, architectural barriers, transportation barriers, potential loss of public benefits, and the degree to which a person must assume the patient role.

Moreover, the IL paradigm differs from its rehabilitation counterpart in defining desired outcomes. Where rehabilitation has stressed the importance of self-care, mobility, and employment, independent living has emphasized a larger constellation of outcomes. In addition to the three outcomes just mentioned, independent living emphasizes the importance of living arrangements, consumer assertiveness, outdoor mobility, and out-of-home activity. In some instances, the IL paradigm would reject the significance of self-care as an outcome. The fact that a disabled person needs more assistance from a human helper does not necessarily imply that he or she is more dependent. A person who can get dressed in fifteen minutes with human assistance and then be off for a day of work is more independent than the person who takes two hours to dress and then remains homebound.

The challenge for disability researchers is to make the concepts introduced by the IL paradigm operational. Moreover, there is a distinct need to identify outcomes that are consistent with the decision-making needs of policy makers. In the case of environmental barriers, for example, we need to identify meaningful predictors of outcome. Consideration of environmental variables might seem to belabor the obvious. "Ask any disabled person," one might say. At the same time, we are not certain about the relative contribution of individual variables in explaining IL outcomes. Nor do we know the collective importance of environmental variables relative to individual characteristics. We need to go beyond mere statistical significance to show what percentage of the variance in outcome can be explained by variables considered important by the IL paradigm.

But a more important reason exists to consider the impact of environmental variables. There is a growing public debate over the extent to which society should subsidize the removal of environmental barriers. If it can be demonstrated empirically that these barriers are predictive of disability outcome, then the IL movement will have considerably strengthened its case.

Environmental variables, unlike individual characteristics, can be rectified through legislative and administrative action. In his follow-up study of veterans with spinal cord injuries, Eggert makes this observation: "Environmental and individual characteristics . . . have qualitatively different degrees of potential manipulation. Demographic characteristics such as age, sex, and race cannot be altered. Other individual characteristics, such as degree of independence in ADL are subject to slight modification through a program of physical therapy. The nature and level of veterans benefits, an environmental variable, is subject to drastic alteration by the stroke of a pen on a piece of federal legislation" (1973, p. 51). Traditional rehabilitation research that belabors the significance or insignificance of personal characteristics has little policy relevance and, in many instances, has little clinical relevance as well. As a paradigm of research, independent living offers us an opportunity to overcome the myopic preoccupation with unalterable individual characteristics that diverts our attention from the larger institutional and environmental context in which disabled people live. This context has been ignored for too long.

The Future

In a mere ten years, the Independent Living Movement has grown from a small band of disabled persons struggling for simple rights to a significant political force shaping the course of disability policy. It is time now to ask: How is the movement likely to shape the future of disability policy? What will the movement look like in another decade? While these questions cannot be answered directly, certain trends are evident.

The concept of paradigm can be useful in predicting how

the IL movement is likely to affect disability policy. Paradigms are more than analytic frames of reference; they also serve important social functions. They prepare students, scholars, and practitioners for membership in a particular discipline, help to define the boundaries of professional practice, and help to confer legitimacy upon professional groups.

In the case of physically impaired persons, disability policy has until recently been subject to the rehabilitation paradigm and to rehabilitation professionals whose limited frame of reference narrowed the options available to disabled persons. The emphasis on one-to-one clinical practice often excluded the contributions of other disciplines. By broadening the issue of disability to include a wide variety of environmental variables, the IL paradigm has succeeded in opening the field of disability policy to other disciplines. The issue of rights and entitlements has encouraged the participation of legal professionals; the issue of architectural barriers has stimulated interest on the part of architects; and the issue of work disincentives arising from public assistance programs is sure to prove inviting to economists who have already covered similar ground in connection with income transfer programs geared to nondisabled groups.

Furthermore, this infusion of new perspectives will undoubtedly invigorate the field of rehabilitation and enlarge its awareness of related areas. For example, it may lead vocational rehabilitation counselors to learn more about the rest of the human service system, with resulting benefit to their clientele.

One of the most vexing issues in the future will be the role of able-bodied persons in the movement. In some quarters, it is strongly felt that only disabled consumers should hold significant leadership positions. The issue finds a parallel in the civil rights movement, at the stage when whites were asked to relinquish their leadership roles in black advocacy organizations. The debate on this issue is likely to intensify over the next few years. In the long run, however, it should generate less controversy as able-bodied persons accept the significant role they can play outside of movement organizations, especially in the development of public policy affecting disabled persons.

On another front, the authorization for IL services under

PL95-602 presents both opportunities and risks for the movement. The law represents an opportunity to strengthen existing IL programs and to extend IL services to parts of the nation where none exist. The law also affirms the political credibility of the movement. At the same time, there is a danger that new funding may blunt the cutting edge of the movement, involving it in bureaucracy at the expense of advocacy. Moreover, IL funds may be diverted into activities that are only marginally associated with independent living, thus diluting the central meaning of independent living. Finally, since funds must be channeled through state rehabilitation agencies, there is the danger that the movement may yet become a captive of the rehabilitation establishment.

The IL movement represents a new chapter in American disability policy. Considering its brief history, its accomplishments in legislation, services, and raising of consciousness have been truly remarkable. But the movement is still young. We can expect it to reach out to new disability groups and to enlarge its age base as its initial adherents grow older. We can also expect it to produce an increasingly sophisticated disability literature as it continues to redefine its concepts, programs, and services.

Above all, the movement has given disabled persons a voice in their own future, and has fostered the dignity and pride that have for too long been denied them. In the years to come, this will be seen to have been its most important contribution.

2

Changing Social Attitudes and Legislation Regarding Disability

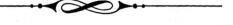

Rita A. Varela

In the spring of 1977, Robert Williams spent a day stalking the halls of Congress. He argued for improvements in government-funded rehabilitation programs and for an end to discrimination against disabled people. Williams, then a student, had cerebral palsy. He walked relatively well, using neither crutches nor canes, but he relied on a word board to communicate. He would point to the letters on the board to spell out sentences explaining his views or to ask guards for directions to his next appointment. Williams was not the only person with cerebral palsy on the Hill that day. He was one of many who formed a nascent self-advocacy movement seeking more direct representation within the board of directors and standing committees of the United Cerebral Palsy Associations (UCPA). His appointments . . those of many other unpaid lobbyists that day had been arranged by UCPA's Governmental Activities Office in preparation for the organization's annual conference.

Had he been born eighty years earlier, instead of walking freely through Washington, Williams might have been standing

before a judge, listening to prosecutors explain why he should
be subjected to medical sterilization. Nonetheless, the impression Williams made on Capitol Hill challenged long-entrenched
attitudes and conventional wisdom about disabled people. That
impression was, in turn, shaped by what congressional representatives had seen on television news shows that morning: hundreds of disabled people demonstrating in front of the Capitol
and sitting in at the office of Joseph Califano, Secretary of
Health, Education and Welfare (HEW). The day's demonstrations were not limited to Washington. Disability rights activists
were sitting in at government offices across the country. They
wanted Secretary Califano to sign the regulations that would implement section 504 of the Rehabilitation Act of 1973, and
said they were not going to leave until he did (Bowe, Jacobi,
and Wiseman, 1978). Section 504 stated that a qualified disabled person could not, solely by virtue of his or her handicap,
be denied the benefits of any program or activity that received
federal funds. The demonstrations were coordinated through
the Washington office of the American Coalition of Citizens
with Disabilities (ACCD), a new organization that in the next
three years would have a significant influence on disability related legislation.

    Though disability has never taken top priority on the na-
tion's social agenda, the issues have always been with us. In ad-
dressing these issues, specialists and interest groups have engaged
the legislative, judicial, and executive branches of government.
No single piece of legislation has ever earned unanimous endorsement or led to a fault-free remedy. Still, the legislative history of rehabilitation is integral to the story of disability in
America. It is from the legislative arena that we issue imprima-
turs on what we can and cannot do to other people, and it is in
this arena that we decide when to apply money, and when to
apply force. We have not always been benevolent.

Roots of Large-Scale Institutionalization

    Attitudes toward disability have changed through the
centuries. To appreciate the range of responses, we need go
back only so far as the 1800s. In his well-known history on the

rise of custodial care institutions in America, Wolfensberger (1969) shows how the concept of deviance has shaped the way society handles certain groups of people.

Wolfensberger believed that the roots of our policies toward mentally retarded persons lay in the institutional models that evolved in the nineteenth century. His treatise focused entirely on how institutional models developed in this country, and did not look into the intellectual baggage that may have been coming from abroad. His survey examined such trends as the social reform efforts of the 1850s to establish special schools for those youngsters who were considered trainable; the move in the 1880s to switch from small centers to large, more economical institutions which could house an ever greater number of people; and the subsequent legislative drives (1880-1925) to enforce involuntary confinement and sterilization.

Obviously, something happened between the 1850s and ι e 1920s. The institutions for retarded persons established in the 1850s were not designed as permanent facilities. They represented a sincere attempt to provide training to those retarded people who were considered to be, in the parlance of the day, "improvable." They were also intended as experiments that would, if successful, be replicated. Some were successful. Wolfensberger notes that 26 percent of the residents who were discharged from one institution in Connecticut became self-supporting. Community integration was not always a matter of course, however, and critics soon began calling for different measures.

The National Conference on Charities and Correction played a major role in shaping this debate. Its membership represented a wide range of professions, from education and social work to medicine and law. Reviewing documents issued by the Conference between 1875 and 1920, Wolfensberger found that they tended to group persons with varying degrees of retardation, mental illness, deafness, visual impairment, and epilepsy into the general class "defective" (p. 66). In fact, other categories, such as legal offenders, vagabonds, and loafers were also routinely classed under that label.

Although today we may cringe at the term "defectives," it serves to remind us that the prestigious Conference was far more concerned with deviance as a concept than with mental retardation as an etiology. The alarmist rhetoric of the early 1900s reveals a strong social Darwinist motif in its insistence on protecting society from people who were seen as different. W. E. Fernald, for example, speaking before the National Conference in 1904, reflected the beliefs of the day: "It is well known that feeble-minded women and girls are very liable to become sources of unspeakable debauchery and licentiousness which pollutes the whole life of the young boys and youth of the community. They frequently disseminate in a wholesale way the most loathsome and deadly diseases, permanently poisoning the minds and bodies of thoughtless youth at the very threshold of manhood" (quoted in Wolfensberger, 1969, p. 102).

The Conference urged states to enact laws preventing "defective" persons from marrying. Many states did. Later, a number of states also enacted sterilization laws. According to Wolfensberger, these remedies lacked the impact their supporters anticipated. The laws were hard to enforce; most parents ignored them and many judges found them distasteful. It was then, argues Wolfensberger, that the real drive for institutionalization began.

What followed was a large-scale push for custodial segregation. Institutions built after 1900 were larger and far removed from the cities. Yet, the social Darwinist presumption that the world could be divided into two classes, those who were fit and those who were defective, was challenged by World War I. When Johnny came marching home without an arm, without a leg, without an eye, people started looking around for other solutions to the problems of disability.

As we shall see, by 1920, *while the push for large-scale institutionalization was in full swing,* the country was also charting another course.

The Development of the Rehabilitation System

As veterans returned from World War I, Congress addressed the problem of helping soldiers get back to work. The National Defense Act of 1916 authorized vocational training for veterans. A year later, the government extended training services to disabled veterans. Congress passed the first Vocational Rehabilitation Act in 1918, and subsequently expanded the program through the National Rehabilitation Act of 1920. With these legislative landmarks, the federal-state rehabilitation services program was established.

More initiatives followed. In 1936, for example, the Rehabilitation Act was amended to include services for blind persons. The attitudes toward disability which prompted this program were far different from those we examined earlier. Whereas proponents of large-scale institutionalization assumed that defective persons should be removed from the mainstream of society, proponents of vocational rehabilitation assumed that people with defects could overcome them and become wage earners if given training.

Certain characteristics of the early federal-state rehabilitation program changed the nature of the debate over what to do about disabled people in a number of very significant ways. In fact, some aspects of the program supplied arguments to its critics as well as its backers.

• First, because the program was supported from the public till through legislative appropriations, its administrators were accountable only to Congress.

Since the program was supported through legislative appropriations, Congress became an important center for debating issues about disability. Congress, having the power of the purse, became a place to bring complaints.

Previously, disability issues were debated in state legislatures, the courts, and the pulpit.

• Second, the program was small: the number of disabled Americans was far larger than the number of clients it could serve.

This aspect of the program could not help but pave the way for competition among different disability groups.

• Third, the program was strongly biased toward the labor market. It did not propose to offer generalized assistance; rather it was geared to vocational readiness and to helping those people who might make a return on the government's investment.

Presumably other institutions, such as families, charities, and state hospitals would care for the rest.

As a result, the program encouraged creaming; that is, it served only those most likely to find a job.

Despite these built-in restrictions, the program struck a popular chord and successive waves of advocates worked to expand its coverage to ever larger segments of the disabled community.

Important legislative initiatives were launched in the 1940s. Congress increased veterans' benefits several times during the decade. The Rehabilitation Act was amended in 1943 to provide some medical services for clients of vocational rehabilitation. Most importantly, the President's Committee on the Employment of the Handicapped (PCEH) was established in 1947.

New advocacy organizations emerged in the 1940s and, together with the older ones, initiated campaigns to rouse Americans, weary of war, to attend to the home front. One of the organizations established in the 1940s was the United Cerebral Palsy Associations (UCPA).

Whether or not the parents who started UCPA thought of themselves as community organizers, that is what they were. As parents, they felt they were not getting the services they needed for their children. They decided to band together and mount an assault on the public conscience to raise money to purchase the kind of medical skills, research, and schooling their children needed. UCPA affiliates were organized in cities around the country. The objectives of these community-based agencies were more generalized than those of the vocational rehabilitation program. The rehabilitation program was set up to promote employment, and its funding was contingent on that premise. The mission of UCPA affiliates was to help parents, and its main objectives were to generate public support, raise money, and provide at least some of the services that cerebral palsy youngsters could not get elsewhere.

UCPA has grown and changed. Today, depending on the affiliate you visit, programs can range from pre-natal care and physical therapy to career counseling, group homes, and assertiveness training. The actual mix of services is shaped by community needs and community involvement. Each affiliate has a board of directors. Some boards take an activist approach to disability rights issues, others do not. Some board members are closely involved in the planning and management of affiliates, others are not. Some board members and staffers have close ties to state and local government—and therefore to funding sources —and others do not. These observations are not only true of UCPA affiliates: they are characteristic of all private community-based organizations. As we shall see later, this motif of local autonomy became a characteristic of the independent living programs that emerged in Berkeley, Houston, and Boston. Independent living in America, however, was never an orchestrated campaign. It was a movement. To understand that difference is to understand the differences between the 1950s, in which organizations such as UCPA took their cues from market research mavens who promised manipulation through media, and the 1970s, in which echos of *We Shall Overcome* still lingered.

Access as a Seminal Concept

The development of the atomic and hydrogen bombs in the middle decades of this century served notice that we could not know what to expect from the white-coated men in the laboratories. Science was a treacherous sorcerer, but never, apparently, an idle one, and never one without bidders for its magic. The American commitment to science became an issue in the passage of the Vocational Rehabilitation Amendments of 1954. Critics charged that the vocational training program was underfunded and served only a fraction of the disabled people who needed vocational assistance. Moreover, they charged that the program did not reflect the times, in that it failed to take advantage of recent medical and scientific advances in solving the rehabilitation problems of hard-to-serve clients. As finally passed, the 1954 amendments expanded the scope of rehabilitation services, authorized research and training of personnel, and established a modest extension and improvement grant program allowing states to study special service problems. This program was the forerunner of what we know today as the innovation and expansion (I and E) grants, which were to have such a dramatic impact on the Independent Living Movement.

The discovery of the Salk vaccine was a triumph of the American belief in medical science. Polio epidemics had brought many families, virtually overnight, into an unknown world. Publicity surrounding the epidemics made Dr. Jonas Salk's 1954 discovery of a vaccine against polio seem all the more remarkable. Since market research and Madison Avenue hype became the state-of-the-art of public relations campaigns of the 1950s, it is not surprising to find that charities eagerly embraced them. However, the images of disabled people promoted through these campaigns proved passive and sterile (Varela, 1978).

Nonetheless, we can trace the tenacity of today's disability rights movement directly to the 1950s. We owe that legacy to disabled veterans and their discontent. In 1951, for example, paralyzed veterans were fighting for more parking spaces, and for accessible commodes, at the Bronx Hospital, which was then in the process of expanding its facilities ("PV Archives," 1981). *Paraplegia News*, the journal of the Paralyzed Veterans of America, tirelessly argued that these seemingly isolated battles required coordinated, nationwide, and aggressive action.

Disabled people fought for local and state accessibility laws throughout the 1950s. The issue gained some attention in the national media in 1956 when President Eisenhower was asked to present the handicapped person of the year award to Hugo Deffner, a well-known civic leader from Oklahoma who used a wheelchair. The first problem to emerge involved the airlines: "For Mr. Deffner to receive his award, the Eisenhower administration secured a special compensation enabling him to fly to Washington. He was then unable to gain access to the Labor

Department Building, so military personnel carried him inside. He was unable to find access to the stage and he was carried on to the stage. We were told that President Eisenhower initiated some architectural barrier removal action in federal buildings following this ceremony" (Hostetter, 1978, p. 18).

In 1959 PCEH, the National Easter Seal Society, the Veterans Administration, and other groups met with the American Standards Association (ASA). The ensuing discussions began the process which led, in October 1961, to agreement on a set of standards for architectural accessibility. The name of ASA was subsequently changed to the American National Standards Institute (ANSI), and the recommendations formed the basis of what are now referred to as the ANSI standards.

When Congress passed the Vocational Rehabilitation Amendments of 1965, it created a National Commission on Architectural Barriers to the Rehabilitation of the Handicapped. The Commission was asked to study the problems involved in making all federal buildings accessible to disabled citizens. As a result of the work of the Commission, and, more importantly, of disabled activists across the country, attitudes toward disability began to change again. The exclusive emphasis on services (that is, on doing something about "those people") began to give way to an emphasis on civil rights (that is, the notion that once certain obstacles were removed, disabled people would be able to do a lot more for themselves than society had imagined).

The next vital piece of legislation was the Architectural Barriers Act of 1968, which stipulated that facilities built with, or receiving, federal funds had to be accessible. It also ordered the various government agencies to issue regulations describing the measures each would take to promote accessibility. The government adopted the ANSI standards. Although the Act also said that the government was to sponsor studies, investigations, and other compliance activities, enforcement was minimal. Congress later established the Architectural and Transportation Barriers Compliance Board (A&TBCB) under section 502 of the Rehabilitation Act of 1973. The job of the A&TBCB was to investigate and enforce federal compliance with the ANSI standards. Later amendments (1974 and 1978) broadened the authority and responsibilities of the Board. However, the Board never received the funding it needed to enforce the law or even to investigate all of the violations that were being reported by disabled consumers around the country (Cleland and Elisburg, 1981).

The struggle for a barrier-free environment was just one of the currents that shaped the Rehabilitation Act of 1973. Later in this chapter I will review others. Before we leave this topic, however, it is important to underscore the fact that the fight for accessibility added a singular perspective to the debate on disability rights. It made clear the fact that "people are handicapped by a poorly designed environment that fails to meet their varying needs" (Mace, 1977, p. 171). Barriers, specifically, were identified as social, political, and intellectual obstacles as well as physical ones.

What's more, once analysts began looking into the economics of disability, they found that barriers were extremely costly. We cannot review those findings here. They are examined in great detail, however, by Frank Bowe in his book, *Rehabilitating America* (1980). In short, when society ignored the steps that kept people in wheelchairs from entering public buildings, when it refused to stand up to publicly financed institutions that violated section 504, when it turned away from blind people who needed documents transcribed onto tapes, when it failed to ask why there was not a teletypewriter (TTY) in every fire house and police station in this country so that deaf taxpayers would enjoy the same protections as hearing taxpayers, then society had made a choice and it had a moral obligation to recognize the *consequences* of that choice.

More About Barriers: Normalizing Environments

Wolfensberger's study of institutional models, mentioned earlier in this chapter, was written in 1968 for a collection of papers entitled *Changing Patterns in Residential Services for the Mentally Retarded,* published in 1969 by the President's Committee on Mental Retardation. These papers reflected a new way of thinking about services and about disability. They also reflected the 1960s.

President Kennedy came to office with a very personal

concern for the needs of mentally retarded citizens. His administration backed up that concern with legislation. First to be enacted were the Maternal and Child Health and Mental Retardation Planning Amendments. This act, in part, authorized grants for states to plan comprehensive, coordinated services for mentally retarded persons. Congress then passed the Mental Retardation Facilities and Community Health Centers Construction Act of 1963. Again, this act provided that states could receive funds only after they had developed an approved plan of services. Neither act sought to create enough institutions so that every person classified as retarded could have a "space." Rather, these acts encouraged the states to examine the varying needs of a varied population and, whenever feasible, to provide services within the community. In addition, the acts encouraged coordination among the health and social services agencies within each state. That is, the acts did *not* promote segregated services. This philosophy of extracting benefits from agencies which, too often, had ignored certain groups was to become the cornerstone of the Developmental Disabilities Act of 1970.

Although plans differed from state to state, they offered a consistent portrait of a subgroup within the disabled population. Who are the individuals in this group? Where did they live and how did they live? The evidence shows that most of them were not receiving assistance through the state rehabilitation agency and were not considered to have immediate vocational potential. Some were confined to residential institutions, and some were not; those who were in institutions made up a very mixed population. Some were mentally retarded people; some were severely physically disabled people who had been misdiagnosed early in life; and some were multiply disabled people with varying degrees of physical, mental, and medical impairments. Noninstitutionalized persons shared similar characteristics: some had not received appropriate diagnosis or assistance when they were children; many were homebound; many could not dress, wash, or feed themselves; and many did not have access either to disability related services, such as therapy, or to traditional services, such as dental care. It was a sore point among parents that whenever their sons or daughters needed a dentist, they had to find a specialist willing to accept a multi-handicapped patient. Many of the people included in the state planners' profiles had been disabled at birth or early in life. They had missed out on the socialization process that takes place in the classroom and the schoolyard. The architects of the Developmental Disabilities Act of 1970 knew that state reviews delineated a population much larger than the familiar set of persons classified as mentally retarded. They sought legislation that would help advocates plan and coordinate services for those people who, sharing the characteristics we have just described, were most underserved and most at risk.

How severe was a "severe" disability? How does one distinguish between problems stemming from a disability and problems stemming from the scars which accumulate from being treated as "defective"? How much does the stigma of retardation contribute to what is characterized as dependence? These are just some of the issues that emerged in the intense and occasionally emotional debate over what constitutes a developmental disability (Abt, 1977; Neimark, 1978).

Early IL Efforts

The federal-state rehabilitation system was a categorical program, not an entitlement program. The benefits of entitlement programs—such as Social Security or army pension plans—are automatic, contingent merely on fairly straightforward eligibility rules. The benefits of categorical programs, however, will vary with the mood of Congress and with the amount of money the government is willing to spend after military and entitlement items are accounted for. Food stamps, the program which helped elderly people to bring down their energy costs by winterizing their homes, and Head Start are all examples of categorical programs. Categorical programs usually require some kind of matching funds from the states, and give states the right to stay out of the programs altogether. In addition, categorical programs are authorized for a specific length of time. When the time is up, Congress must decide whether to continue the program as is, enlarge it, or allow it to elapse. By the 1960s, when disability advocates came to Washington to call for extension of the vocational rehabilitation program, they were also determined to push for an important new thrust in the legislation: independent living services.

Congressional attempts to authorize independent living (IL) services date back to the late 1950s. In 1959, two bills were introduced to expand the vocational rehabilitation program, enabling it to provide independent living services to severely handicapped persons (The Urban Institute, 1975, pp. 4-10). Neither bill passed. New legislation including provisions for IL services was introduced in 1961. Again, the measure was defeated. The next important juncture for IL legislation was 1972, the year when the Vocational Rehabilitation Act was set to expire. A bill was introduced which would significantly expand the program and the kind of assistance the program could offer. Its major thrust, as Senator Alan Cranston said, was to "eliminate the creaming and shift the focus to harder cases in order to serve individuals with more severe handicaps" (Pflueger, 1977, p. 10). The bill authorized "comprehensive rehabilitation services," including "vocational rehabilitation services and any other goods (including aids or devices) . . . that will make a substantial contribution in helping a handicapped individual to live independently or function normally with his family and community" (Pflueger, 1977, p. 10).

Congress passed the bill over administration objections. President Nixon announced a pocket veto, charging that the new provisions would duplicate existing state services and dilute the program's traditional emphasis on employment. In 1973, Congress passed a similar bill which, although slightly revised, still contained IL provisions. Once again, Nixon vetoed the bill. Those two vetoes have been credited as the impetus that brought together the small community-based disability rights groups that had surfaced across the country (Varela, 1979).

The final version of the legislation, the Rehabilitation Act of 1973, did not make any provision for independent living. It was revolutionary, nonetheless, both for what it contained, and for the way the burgeoning disability rights movement used its mandates. The 1973 act contained several provisions that proved critical to the movement. First, the act required state rehabilitation agencies to establish methods of selection to ensure that severely disabled people were not bypassed. Though the act retained its vocational focus, it served notice that state agencies had a responsibility to severely disabled people. Second, section 130 of the 1973 act authorized the Comprehensive Service Needs (CSN) study to explore methods for serving severely disabled people. Section 130 also authorized six research and demonstration projects as part of the CSN study. At last formal federal support for a significantly broader state rehabilitation program seemed within reach, and not a moment too soon. Rehabilitation providers were beginning to feel the barb of the growing ranks of disabled activists who had begun talking about curb cuts in the fifties and sixties and were now charging that most programs did not meet the needs of their community.

To these activists, the six CSN projects symbolized the beginning of a new wave of community-based services to help people who, previously, had nowhere to turn. In the 1970s, state rehabilitation agencies began using innovation and expansion (I and E) grants to provide seed money for independent living projects and for nonvocational adult services. As we indicated earlier, the I and E program had its roots in the rehabilitation amendments of 1954, which sought to give the system a little elbow room by authorizing some research activities. The I and E provisions, thus, became a sort of safety valve, allowing the system to test new ideas.

The 1973 act also contained various client rights and civil rights provisions, the most important of which was section 504. In the 1970s, "504" would become a rallying cry as important to disabled activists as the phrase "black power" had been to civil rights activists a decade earlier. Section 504 prohibited federally supported programs from discriminating against disabled persons. Thus if a medical clinic relied on federal funds, persons in wheelchairs had to be able to get into the building where that clinic was located so that they could exercise their right to the same services other citizens were receiving. Historically, vocational rehabilitation had been a service program important primarily to disabled people who wanted to find jobs.

Section 504, however, made the 1973 act important not just to those who were looking for jobs but also to those who wanted to use the same clinics as everyone else, who wanted the same choice of apartments, and who wanted to get into the polling places on election day.

Disabled people were stirred by the politics of the 1960s, in particular by the example of other minority groups demanding the right to define their own identities. Disabled people were actively demonstrating in the 1970s. But even before that happened, a few groups had begun their own self-help programs.

IL on and off Campus

Bruce M. Brown, who once served as a senior analyst in the research section of the California State Department of Rehabilitation (CDR), has traced the roots of Berkeley's Center for Independent Living (CIL). Its founders met as college students at the University of California at Berkeley, where they were taking part in an experimental program to see if persons with severe spinal cord injuries could live on campus. The first two students in the program, Edward Roberts, now director of CDR, and John Hessler, entered the university in 1962. They were housed at Cowell Student Health Service Hospital. Both were CDR clients. As the number of students in that program grew, they formed a mutual support group; they brainstormed to figure out ways of paying for attendant care through Medicaid and of getting and getting along in their own apartments off campus. In a sense, through their mutual support, they were developing campus "street skills." In 1970, some members of the group applied for a grant from the Federal Office of Education so that they could provide assistance to other disabled students. Through this grant, they established the Berkeley Physically Disabled Students Program (PDSP) at the university (Brown, 1978).

By late 1971, the PDSP experiment had encouraged activists to set up an off-campus organization to help severely disabled people live in the community, away from hospital settings. The off-campus program, which provided training, and information and referral from a streetwise, self-help perspective, was called the Center for Independent Living.

According to Lex Frieden, a leading spokesman in the IL movement, these were vital years in the struggle to find alternative support systems. As we have observed, since the 1950s people involved with the rehabilitation field had been arguing for new programs that would serve individuals who were in institutions, who were homebound, or who had fallen through the eligibility cracks of the programs then available (Chizmadia, 1978). In Houston, a group of former patients from the Texas Institute for Rehabilitation and Research (TIRR) drafted plans for a cooperative living residential project. Sponsored in part by TIRR, the project opened in Houston in 1972. Project members lived in a barrier-free, dormitory-style building near the downtown area; in addition, they "hired and managed their own attendants, arranged for their own transportation on a shared basis, and generally practiced the skills required in order to live independently" (Frieden, 1978, p. 6). The project evolved into a TIRR-sponsored transitional living training program known as New Options. Efforts in other states followed. In 1974, Dr. Frederick Fay and other Massachusetts activists helped establish the Boston Center for Independent Living (BCIL). Like its predecessors, BCIL was designed as a client-run project.

Self-help, of course, predates the 1970s. Tanbrier House at the University of Illinois was established in the 1950s. Students at Tanbrier House hired staff, managed the budget, and set policies. Still, CIL, the Houston project, and BCIL drew attention to self-help at a time when the field was being challenged to meet the needs of severely disabled people. IL became a frequent topic in rehabilitation journals. Although the IL literature contains a myriad of definitions and models, a number of themes recur, some of which point to consensus and some to division.

First, the literature reveals a consensus on those services most closely identified with IL centers. The early projects described here were started by people who didn't want to live behind hospital walls. The services they needed, and first sought to provide, included attendant care, information on income and benefit rights, and, often, a base of operation from which to organize reviews of accessibility, lobbying campaigns, and discussion groups. Discussion groups and peer counseling were the primary IL center responses to the interpersonal needs of people in the community. IL service programs were often funded through Title XIX (Medicaid) and Title XX (social services) of the Social Security Act. Some also relied on CETA funds (the Comprehensive Employment and Training Act of 1973), Community Development funds (the Housing and Community Development Act of 1974), and assorted research grants. Many peer-controlled centers were begun with seed money from I and E grants, but these could only fund projects for up to three years. Though the legislation to support such services was in place, Congress never appropriated the amount of money that would have been necessary to make them available to all, or even a significant number, of the disabled people who needed them.

In addition, the literature revealed a sharp difference between the way disability rights spokesmen viewed IL and the way spokesmen from other sectors of the rehabilitation field viewed it. As Jean Cole of TIRR observes, many professionals claimed that independent living was merely a new label for goals that their particular discipline or agency had been pursuing all along (1979). Staffers from medical rehabilitation facilities held that the best way to make people independent was to help them reach their optimum physical functioning; placement specialists held that jobs were the key to independence in our society; and counselors who placed high value on behavior modification held that to become independent, disabled people must learn to set realistic, attainable goals.

IL movement leaders did not and do not oppose good physical functioning, jobs, or goals. However, when they write about independence they stress choice, risk, and self-determination. As DeJong has noted, many of the services most closely ociated with the IL movement, such as training people to hire and manage attendants or to get the income benefits they are entitled to if they are out of work, involve giving disabled people the information they need in order to do more of the things they want to do (1979, pp. 42-43).

This distinction, in turn, leads to a third theme: the centrality of the disabled person in IL service delivery. Traditional providers would claim that in order to set up an IL program, one must identify needs, set objectives, and develop plans for meeting them. Movement spokesmen are likely to ask: How many disabled people are involved in identifying the needs and setting the objectives? Do disabled people constitute a majority of the policy-making board for the program? Who administers the program, and how many disabled people are on staff? These questions precede decisions over program content. For IL leaders, they are the marrow of what independence is all about: freedom from the consequences of other people's attitudes toward your disability. As Judy Huemann has said: "To us, independence does not mean doing things physically alone. It means being able to make independent decisions. It is a mind process not contingent upon a 'normal' body" (Stoddard, 1978, p. 2).

Though the debate continued, and though new programs sometimes adopted more of the movement's slogans than its specifications, enough disabled people set up peer support programs and were able to point to enough success stories to prove that client control need not be inimical to effective service delivery. By proving this disabled leaders were in a better position to challenge the authoritarian premises of professional services, and to compete for service funds (Steinman and Traunstein, 1976).

That is what Congress was being told in 1978 as it drafted new rehabilitation legislation. The new law, entitled the Rehabilitation, Comprehensive Services, and Developmental Disabilities Amendments of 1978 (PL95-602) was the single most far-reaching piece of legislation ever offered to the disabled community. Among its provisions was Title VII, extending program assistance to severely disabled people who might not have vocational potential and who might be ineligible for services under other provisions of the amendments. (Title VII *did not* establish an "either/or" two-track system of segregated services, rejecting the assumption that IL clients were, by definition, ineligible for vocational rehabilitation services.) Part A of Title VII authorized state rehabilitation agencies to provide comprehensive services. Part B was a grant program for independent living centers. Part C authorized grants to provide IL services for older blind persons. Only Part B was funded, at levels so far below the amount authorized in the amendments that critics charged the government with not being committed to IL centers. Still, Title VII was remarkable for the degree to which it mirrored the principles of the IL movement.

For example, Part A required state rehabilitation agencies to "provide assurances that not less than 20 percent of the funds received by a State under [Part A] shall be used to make grants to local public agencies and private nonprofit organizations for the conduct of independent living services..." (PL 95-602, sec. 705 (A) (8)). Congress, in other words, gave its backing to the idea of community-based services offered by pri-   , nonprofit organizations.

Throughout the 1970s, Congress heard from Frederick Fay, Lex Frieden, Judy Huemann, Edward Roberts, and a host of other disabled activists who had had hands-on experience in IL center program design. That Congress listened is evident from section 711 of Part B, which listed some of the services IL centers could offer. This section specifically mentioned a number of the ideas most closely identified with the IL movement: peer counseling, attendant care, and information and advocacy on income rights and benefits.

At the same time, Congress finally endorsed the principle of consumer control. In light of the attitudes of the past century, the consumer involvement mandate contained in Part B is noteworthy: "an application by a public or nonprofit agency or organization for [an independent living center] grant shall (1) provide assurances that handicapped individuals will be substantially involved in [the] policy direction and management of such center, and will be employed by such center" (PL95-602, sec. 711 (c)).

Legacies and Lessons for the 1980s

Attitudes and definitions are at times ephemeral, as, indeed, are congressional promises. In the spring of 1981, UCPA again held its annual conference in Washington, D.C., where it returns every four years following presidential elections. During briefing sessions before the quadrennial trek through Congress, the conferees learned that the Reagan administration wanted to abolish a host of categorical programs, including the vocational rehabilitation program and the independent living grants authorized through the 1978 amendments. The money which would have gone into these programs—and a disparate array of other programs such as food stamps and Aid to Families with Dependent Children—was to be cut 25 percent and then sent to the states as a block grant for social services. Each state would have the authority to decide which programs, if any, to support, and at what level. The prospect raised the spectre of teachers pitted against welfare mothers and welfare mothers pitted against disabled activists for a shrinking share of social service funds. Officials within the administration also wanted to rewrite the 504 regulations, under the guise of giving individual states more flexibility.

President Reagan's block grants program did not get through Congress. Scaled down versions of the program, which the administration referred to as the New Federalism, were circulated among the nation's governors and mayors, but attracted weak support and no consensus. The battle over revising the 504 regulations continued, but disability rights advocates mounted so much pressure that the administration gained new respect for their determination.

Though the disability rights movement could legitimately claim victories, the battles left advocates in a somber and reflective mood. What issues would IL activists, service providers, and researchers be struggling with in the 1980s? Two questions, in particular, seemed to stand out as the unfinished legacy of the IL movement.

Who Will Meet the Needs of Severely Disabled People? As the 1980s opened, concern over tight money and social services cutbacks again drew attention to the issue of creaming, which had haunted the federal-state rehabilitation services system practically since its inception. Creaming, as we noted, was the tendency to concentrate services on individuals who were only mildly disabled and stood a good chance of finding work.

Through the 1960s and 1970s advocates had pushed for more services for severely disabled people. State rehabilitation officials joined in that crusade. By 1981, however, disability rights advocates were beginning to wonder how long it would be before state rehabilitation agencies went back to creaming as a way of demonstrating the cost-effectiveness of the program.

What Are IL Needs? One cannot read about the IL movement without being struck by its vitality; indeed, by its audacity. Disabled leaders dared to draw comparisons between themselves and the civil rights activists of the 1960s. Disabled leaders dared to use words like oppression and self-determination. Disabled leaders dared to say that they could run their own service programs, and then to go out and prove it.

As I argued earlier in this chapter, a central and seminal concept for this movement was that of access, with its roots in barrier removal campaigns of the 1950s. By 1981, the controversy between the activists and the professionals, which Jean Cole wrote about, was going strong. In general, professionals put the emphasis on providing services, while IL leaders focused on the need to eliminate barriers.

Throughout our history disability legislation has reflected how society has dealt with both the issue of who should be helped and of what kind of help should be authorized. Yet, the laws described in this chapter are merely political indicators of a larger struggle: a fight to be free. There has always been someone, somewhere, fighting against laws, attitudes, and practices that restrict personal autonomy. That fight goes on.

3

Developing New Self-Images and Interdependence

Irving Kenneth Zola

The Independent Living Movement represents a direct challenge to current notions of rehabilitation (see Gerben DeJong's discussion in Chapter One). It offers a unique challenge, spearheaded not by new technical advances but by a new social awareness, and formulated not from within, by medical personnel, but from without, by lay groups. In another sense, however, it is but the latest incarnation of an old theme in American life—the idea of self-help. The history of self-help, as traced in this chapter, illuminates the problems and prospects of the Independent Living Movement.

Mutual aid societies in the United States reach back to

Note: This chapter is a revised and expanded version of an article that appeared in the October 1979 issue of *Archives of Physical Medicine and Rehabilitation.* The article benefited from the editorial and substantive suggestions of Edith Lennenberg, Mara Sanadi, and Beatrice Wright. This version owes a considerable debt to the contributions of Marsha Saxton.

frontier days. As early as the first part of the nineteenth century, Alexis de Tocqueville (1961) noted the American pen-
chant for joining groups; by 1900 there existed a directory list-
ing over 250 independent, national, voluntary lay organizations.
The goals of most such organizations, though central to their
avowed reasons for existence, were generally rather distant from
the members themselves. The early societies sought either to
help the community at large or to ameliorate some specific condition or disease.

The transition from voluntary associations organized to
help others to mutual aid societies organized to help their own
members was not an easy one. Although some historians have
found examples of such associations in early agricultural cooperatives (Katz and Bender, 1976), the mass waves of immigration in the late nineteenth and early twentieth century most
clearly stimulated their proliferation (Handlin, 1959). Thrust
into a nation which offered few formal services to aid their survival, the new arrivals responded by creating mutual aid societies. Membership in these societies was based primarily on some
shared social characteristic, such as race, religion, or country of
origin, and, initially, the aid given was of the most material sort.
Interestingly, the cost of a funeral proved by far the most popular of benefits. Money-lending ran a far distant second. It would
take a giant effort to move from this tangible kind of service to
aid of a more psychological nature.

How diffucult a step this was is best illustrated in the
example of polio victims and that best known of illness-oriented
voluntary organizations, the March of Dimes. Most polio patients were young children, and the rehabilitation problems
they faced were enormous; yet there was no "coming together"
of the afflicted. When it is remembered that polio patients were
never isolated from one another, and even had clinics, wards,
and whole hospitals devoted to their treatment, the fact that no
support organization, however informal, ever arose is even more
surprising. In retrospect, it appears there must have been an implicit assumption that such activity was inappropriate, that
everything that could be done already was being done—*for* the
patients. Disabled people were expected to suffer quietly and

keep their problems to themselves. As a result, they remained locked into a system that prevented them from doing much about their situation and isolated from others who might share their concerns.

Three Barriers to Self-Help

From such data, we can infer that there must have been a number of barriers impeding the development of health-related self-help organizations. The three that seem most basic were the nature of the problems which such groups addressed, the nature of the help offered, and the nature of the personnel best suited to give that help.

In the first place, the problems with which mutual aid societies dealt were long considered socially offensive. The societies dealt with loss and deficiency—umbrella categories that included everything from loss of function to the inability to control certain behaviors. The taboos placed on disability were hierarchical; losses of hearing, seeing, or mobility were far less stigmatized than facial disfigurement or having a colostomy, which in turn were far less stigmatized than drug abuse, alcoholism, and overeating. Toleration for persons who are less than perfect is a very recent phenomenon. Many of the older generation are still bothered by even the most accepted of handicaps: they scream at those with no hearing, avoid mentioning the beauty of scenes to the blind, and reprimand their children for being curious about someone with a limp. All of this is complicated by the American belief that there is *no* problem that cannot ultimately be solved. Given this belief, unsolved problems or diseases represent failure, and the disabled become constant reminders of national inadequacy. Historically, the general response has been to put them, as much as possible, out of sight and out of mind (Zola, 1981).

In the second place, the nature of the help that disability entails seemed threatening. Even today, being in need of help is not an accepted condition in the Western world, and particularly not in the United States. This attitude may be summed up in the aphorism, the Lord helps those who help themselves.

Until recently, independence was the byword and achievement against all odds the measure of success. Horatio Alger, for many years the embodiment of the American ideal, was someone who overcame great limitations in his background to attain success. So, too, the folk heroes of disability and chronic disease have been not the millions who came to terms with their problems but those few who were so successful that they *passed*: the polio victim who broke track records, the one-legged pitcher who played major league baseball, the great composer who was deaf, the famous singer who had a colostomy. They were all so successful that no one knew of their disability, and therein lay their glory.

The emphasis on such successes has done more harm than good for the majority of people with disabilities, because it masks the real kinds of help that those with chronic conditions need. Management in daily living does not involve dramatic tasks, but mundane ones. Examples of persons who overcame their disability once and for all mask the time element required for such achievements. Most aid can neither be given nor utilized in a short series of encounters. Moreover, the problem for the majority of the disabled is not a temporary one but one that will last a *lifetime*. How uncomfortable this makes people feel is seen in the frequently negative response to those mutual aid organizations such as Alcoholics Anonymous, the early Synanon, Re-Evaluation Counseling, and the current Independent Living Movement that explicitly state this lifetime commitment.

In the third place, widespread acceptance of mutual aid has been slowed by our worship of the technical expert, especially the physician. Modern medical care has been, and to a large extent still is, the exclusive province of doctors. It has been hard enough for the physician to give up tasks, and therefore responsibility, to a growing army of paramedics. But paramedics have remained at least nominally under his authority. Self-help organizations, on the other hand, are essentially lay groups and, as such, largely outside medical control. As a result, any good that they might do was at first scarcely noticed. Even when positive results of mutual aid were reported in, for example, group therapy and encounter groups, they received little professional recognition and were dismissed as second-choice alternatives. At best, they might be viewed as something for patients to do to keep themselves occupied and out of trouble. Such forms of help represented self-treatment which, next to chiropracty, was regarded by most medical professionals as perhaps worse than no help at all.

Because people with severe disabilities tend to have chronic medical problems, they have been thought to need rather close medical supervision. As a result, many of their needs have been overmedicalized. When it was shown that many tasks —even catheterization—could be self-taught with minimal difficulty, such examples were dismissed as the exceptions. Again, when it was shown that untrained people, even some with relatively low IQs, could become excellent personal care attendants, the professionals argued that attendants also required medical supervision and, moreover, that without it, such services would not be reimbursed by third-party payers (see Chapter Nine for further details).

Agents of Change

With such formidable forces ranged against the severely disabled, how did self-help ever get off the ground? There is no single answer; rather, a number of events combined to pry open the door. For example, World War II had an enormous impact upon Americans' ability to ignore the more unpleasant aspects of life. The war ended American insulation once and for all. Ordinary Americans, particularly those in the armed services, came in contact with different cultures, and thus with different ways of defining and handling problems. One could argue that the civil rights movement truly got underway then, as whites and nonwhites were forced to come to new definitions of themselves and each other. One might have expected this to have taken place much earlier, with the waves of immigration that inundated America in the nineteenth century. However, Glazer and Moynihan (1963) argue that the impact of those migrations was blunted both by the vastness of America, which permitted most citizens to remain isolated from the newly arrived, and by the philosophy of Americanization, which, accepted by immigrants and encouraged by residents, consciously attempted to extinguish all traces of the heritage immigrants brought with them.

Equally as important was a change in the concept of disability, occasioned by changing patterns of disability. As a host of infectious diseases came gradually under control, more and more people were surviving to middle age and beyond. As a result, many latent or previously numerically insignificant disorders suddenly loomed large: arthritis, diabetes, mental illness, heart disease, multiple sclerosis, spinal cord injury, stroke, cancer. Moreover, these were disorders which were more often disabling than immediately fatal, and for which no magic bullet either in prevention or in care was forthcoming. The majority of persons so disabled could require medical management for extended periods of time, even for life.

There was something more to these disorders: they fundamentally altered the doctor-patient relationship. They forced a shift from cure to care. No longer did treatment involve the doctor doing and the patient receiving. For treatment to succeed at all, as in psychotherapy, the patient had to be an active participant. It would take some time for this fact to be fully accepted by both the former patients and their former caretakers.

Psychiatry's coming of age had a special impact. Because it made abundantly clear the importance of behavior in all aspects of disease, from how one gets sick to whether or not one recovers, it reemphasized the oneness of a person's mind and body. This phenomenon is perhaps most evident in the ever expanding number of disorders identified as psychosomatic. In the context of medical care, *support* was no longer just something to consider if one had the time. In fact, it stood at the very core of helping. Yet the supporting role was not one for which many health personnel felt trained or inclined. Even had they been willing to actively undertake such a role, it's not clear that, numerically, they could ever have filled the need. Moreover, as long as America's current commitment to specialization in medicine continues, the shortage of physicians is unlikely to disappear. As a result, many medical tasks—from taking history and counseling, to prescribing drugs, giving injections, and performing certain forms of surgery—have come to be done by people who are not doctors.

The biggest leap forward, however, has come not with the delegation of responsibility to less-trained personnel but with the assumption of many therapeutic tasks by people who *had been there*. In short, it began to be recognized that patients could have the expertise to help both themselves and others.

It has been a struggle to attain this recognition. The world in general and the medical world in particular still too often feel that only they are in a position to know what is in the best interests of the disabled. Often, they contend that their years of experience and lack of personal involvement permit them to understand disabled people's needs more clearly than they do themselves. A personal experience shows how occasionally ludicrous this claim can be. One day, I entered the workshop of a prosthetist who had been in the business for over fifty years. Noting that I had had polio and use a cane to walk, he motioned me to come near.

He:	"I wonder if you'd try this cane."
IKZ:	"I did."
He:	"Well, what do you think?"
IKZ:	"It seems solid enough."
He:	"Now watch this."

He then took the cane from me, pushed a little button about three inches from the handle, and out popped a twelve-inch blade. Before I could say another word, he went on: "This one is even handier. Look!" Taking another cane, he again pressed a button and now brandished what might be called a ten-inch iron blackjack. "You know," he said, "in times like these, with so much crime in the streets, this self-defense cane should come in pretty handy."

"Yes," I replied in my best tongue-in-cheek fashion, "particularly if the thief lets me lean on him for support while I dismantle my cane."

In one sense, I feel that no matter how sophisticated, tolerant, or even understanding the unafflicted become, those with a disability ultimately have to see to their own needs by banding together and pushing. This is not merely because the general public does not care but because, in a very real sense, they do not know. It is not accidental that major changes in the architecture of public buildings have been pushed by paraplegics; that drug maintenance costs have been reduced through the efforts of *mended hearts*; that extensions of medical insurance coverage have been accomplished by ostomates and new speech therapies by laryngectomates; or that a new profession, enterostomal therapy, was created and originally staffed by former patients. As Michael Harrington points out in *The Other America* (1962), public interest is not stirred solely by large populations of "problem-bearers." There have always been millions of poor, millions of blacks, millions of consumers. It takes something more than numbers to stir society to action.

The passage of section 504 of the 1978 Amendments to the Rehabilitation Act represents a major shift in national disability policy away from benevolent paternalism and toward the legal protection of civil rights. The enactment of section 504 was brought about largely by the activism of disabled people themselves. A number of sit-ins took place before the appropriate regulations were finally issued. The militance of these sit-ins, inspired by the successes of the civil rights movement, demonstrated that the plight of the disabled is due not just to physical limitation but to systematic and pervasive discrimination. It vividly contradicted the stereotype of the disabled person as powerless.

The Continuing Struggle

While there is strength in numbers, the very act of categorizing and tabulating disabilities creates a dilemma. In trying to find strict measures of disability, or focusing on "severe," that is, visible, handicaps, we make distinct categories of what is, in fact, a continuum of disabilities. By agreeing that there are 20 million disabled or 36 million, or even 100 million, we delude ourselves into thinking there is some finite number of disabled people. In this way we try to distance ourselves from the reality of disease, disability, and death. But our safety is illusory.

Any person reading the words on this page is at best momentarily able-bodied. That person will, at some point, suffer from one or more chronic diseases and may be disabled, temporarily or permanently, for a significant portion of his or her life.

That we persist in this denial means that the necessary steps to reverse it are difficult to acknowledge as well as to undertake. But several steps do suggest themselves. First of all, we who have chronic diseases and disabilities must see to our own interests. We must free ourselves from the physicality of our conditions and the domination of medical professionals (Illich, 1976). In particular, I refer to the number of times we think of ourselves, and are thought of by others, in terms of our specific conditions. We are polios, cancers, paras, deaf, blind, lame, amputees, and strokes. Whatever else this does, it distracts our attention from our common social disenfranchisement. Our forms of loss may be different, but the resulting invalidity is the same (Zola, 1982a).

While organizing around specific diseases may occasion great success in raising research monies, it has divided our strength and caused one disease group to vie against another. This has led not only to overspecialization of services but also to underdevelopment of our consciousness. It has made us so dependent on others—the medical world for treatment and the general public for money—and so personally accountable that we often feel we have no rights. We, patients all, perhaps the last and potentially the largest of America's disenfranchised, must organize on our own behalf. Cutting across specific diseases, we must create mutual advocacy, consciousness-raising, counseling, and resource groups (Bowe and others, 1978). And wherever and whenever possible, staff and members alike must have some disability, whether a chronic disease or a physical handicap. I do not claim that no one else can help or understand us; rather, I would argue that, as with women and blacks, we have reached that point in history where having been there is essential in determining where to go.

Providers must rethink their traditional notions of help and independence. One-way giving keeps the recipient powerless. Care-givers must act as advocates, assisting their clients to act for themselves. The notion of independence must be expanded to include considerations of the quality of life. It is not always necessary that persons do everything for themselves, or do always what they are capable of doing, such as walking long distances, if that effort proves healthy but exhausting. The energy lost in physical exertion cannot be used elsewhere. A powered wheelchair might well diminish the amount of exercise an individual gets, but at the same time it enormously increases his or her social capabilities and networks. The Independent Living Movement argues that it is more important for us to have full control over our lives than over our bodies. We will give up doing some things for ourselves if we can determine when and how they are to be done.

The self-help movement is but one part of the struggle. While a prerequisite for change, it is neither the sole nor the sufficient avenue. We have to take into account social arrangements as much as self-conceptions; the one, in fact, reinforces the other. The problems of those with a chronic disability should be stated not in terms of the incapacities affecting physical functioning, but in terms of the obstacles placed in the way of daily social functioning. What should be asked is not how much it will cost to achieve a society completely accessible to all with physical difficulties, but rather why a society which excludes so many of its members was created, and why it is perpetuated.

There is a growing awareness that this exclusion is not an accidental byproduct of postindustrial societies. Just as religion and law were beginning to lose their power as absolute arbiters of important social values, Darwin unwittingly ushered in the age of biological determinism. One critic of the times, who realized the social import of Darwin's work, exclaimed, "Sir, you are preaching scientific Calvinism with biological determinism replacing religious predestination." The fixity of the universe and the hierarchical relations once attributed to God were suddenly being justified by science. The ensuing hundred years have seen an expansion of the influence of science in general, medical science in particular, such that science has in some ways replaced religion and law. Where once a social rhetoric referred to good and evil, it now prefers healthy and sick.

We have experienced a gradual increase in the use of medicine as an agent of social control. While some have argued that this is the humane way to deal with social problems, the concepts of health and sickness still locate the source of trouble in individual capacities, instead of in social arrangements, where it properly belongs (Zola, 1977).

It is politically and economically expedient to have a portion of the population declared physically unfit. Health occupations figure among the fastest-growing and best-paid, and health-related industries among the most profitable (Health Policy Advisory Committee, 1971). Until the day when no one benefits economically, socially, or psychologically from those who are dependent on them, there will always be categories of exclusion.

Regardless of whether we join activist groups, support those who do, or seek in other ways to change the social, political, and economic structure of America, we must at least examine ourselves. If morality or justice do not provide sufficient motivating force, perhaps personal survival will. All of us must contend with our vulnerability. Increased life-expectancies may yet make independent living services necessary for everyone. Not to recognize this can only leave us unprepared for the exigencies of life. As medicine enables us to survive, sick or disabled, for ever longer periods of time, we will experience a triple sense of powerlessness. First, we will be more physically and socially dependent; second, through our previous denial, we will have deprived ourselves of the knowledge and resources to cope; and third, in the realization of what we have done to those who have aged before us, we will feel that we have lost our right to protest.

In this light, it is especially important to remember what Erik Erikson said about society's continual denigration and isolation of the aged: "Any span of the [life] cycle lived without vigorous meaning at the beginning, in the middle, or at the end, endangers the sense of life, and the meaning of death in all whose life stages are intertwined" (1964, p. 133). So it is that what we do to the physically handicapped and chronically ill, we do only to ourselves.

Part Two

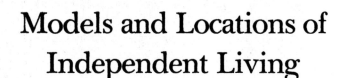

Models and Locations of
Independent Living

The IL movement began as an idea—as a new way of perceiving people with disabilities. From that idea came the tangible programs and support services that have made autonomous living possible. Authors of chapters in this section look at some of the program structures that have emerged, at responses to needs in various geographic areas, and at the influence of environmental factors on IL options and programs.

    The first three chapters provide an overview of IL program types in the United States and in other countries. They explore the reasons for differences and evaluate the strengths and limitions of various approaches. For example, some IL programs provide housing, either on a transitional or on a long-term basis. Others provide no housing at all but focus on counseling and other services. Location as well as philosophy affects the structure of a program. In urban areas clients can come to the centers, while in rural territories the opposite is true. One of the chapters in this section describes effective services in rural areas and explores ways of improving delivery to a widely scattered constituency.

The last two chapters were written by architects and deal with the effect of physical space on IL concerns. Distance, one author points out, is a barrier, too, and much more attention should be paid to the way buildings that will be extensively used by disabled people are located. An inaccessible or restricted environment drastically curtails the activities available to a person and consequently reduces the richness of his or her life, while an environment that facilitates activity has the opposite effect. The last chapter in this section shows how the constructed environment—including homes, public buildings, sidewalks, and parks—can be made to function as a support system.

4

Understanding
Alternative Program Models

Lex Frieden

An *independent living program* can be defined as a community-based program with substantial consumer involvement that provides directly or coordinates indirectly, through referral, services severely disabled individuals need to increase their self-determination and to minimize dependence on others. Those services most usually provided include housing, attendant care, reading and/or interpreting, and information about other necessary goods and services. They may also include transportation, peer counseling, advocacy or political action, training in independent living skills, equipment maintenance and repair, and social or recreational services (Frieden and others, 1979).

More specifically, independent living programs are designed to serve the needs of a population in one particular community, as opposed to a region, state, or nation. The programs

Note: This chapter is an updated and revised version of an article that first appeared in *Rehabilitation Literature,* 1980, *41.*

depend on the people and resources in the community for direction and subsistence. They depend on the people who receive their services to provide leadership and assistance by serving on boards of directors or advisory committees, and by working as paid or volunteer staff. Consumer involvement insures both that programs do not lose touch with client needs and that they will maintain their down-to-earth character. The programs provide whatever services are necessary to enable severely disabled people to live comparatively independent lives in their own communities. In many instances, these services answer basic needs like housing, transportation, and attendant care. In a few cases, these services are primarily oriented toward career goals like education and work.

In an extensive 1978 survey, the Independent Living Research Utilization (ILRU) project identified three major types of program: centers, residential programs, and transitional programs. A federally funded technical assistance project located at The Institute for Rehabilitation and Research (TIRR) in Houston, Texas, ILRU conducts research, offers training and consultation, and sponsors the production of written and audiovisual materials by severely disabled people. After polling more than 450 programs which claimed to provide services for independent living, ILRU identified only 35 programs which actually fit our definition of an independent living program.

Of the 35 IL programs identified, only 12 met the definition of an *independent living center* as originally characterized by the Center for Independent Living in Berkeley, California, described as follows by Cole (1979, p. 458): "The Center for Independent Living (CIL) in Berkeley, California, is the prototype of the community-based program. It was probably the first organization operated by disabled consumers to be established in the United States. CIL is not a residential program, but a multifaceted program of referral services, support services, and research and advocacy projects directed toward removing architectural and attitudinal barriers. The goal of the organization is total integration of people with severe disabilities into community life by providing various kinds of counseling, independent living skills training, and other supportive services. Whenever possible, existing community resources are used, so CIL also refers many people to agencies that provide such assistance as vocational counseling, training and financial support." In this strict sense, as it is generally understood by leaders of the Independent Living Movement around the country, and as codified in California law, the independent living center is a nonresidential, nonprofit consumer-controlled independent living program.

As originally conceived, an independent living center must provide a minimum set of services, including housing assistance, attendant care, readers and/or interpreters, peer counseling, financial and legal advocacy, and community awareness and barrier-removal programs. Because this somewhat restrictive definition excludes programs of a residential or transitional nature, the term *independent living program* has evolved to include independent living centers, residential programs, and transitional programs. As used here, the term *independent living program* is analogous to the term *independent living center* as described in Title VII of PL95-602 (the 1978 Amendments to the Rehabilitation Act). *Independent living program* was chosen for use here because it is a generic term that subsumes the several different types of programs. It is understood that this broader definition was intended by the initiators of PL95-602 when they refer to *independent living centers,* even though in other contexts, *independent living center* has a quite restricted meaning.

An *independent living residential program* is a live-in program that provides or coordinates attendant services and transportation, and may also provide related services. An *independent living transitional program* is one which helps severely disabled people move from comparatively dependent to more independent living situations. The primary service provided by these programs is skill training in such areas as attendant management, financial management, consumer affairs, mobility, educational/vocational opportunities, medical needs, living arrangements, social skills, time management, functional skills, sexuality, and so forth. Transitional programs are usually goal oriented and/or time linked. It is important to keep in mind that both types of program must fit our initial definition of an independent living program. Cole (1979, p. 459) describes two programs that exemplify these models:

The Boston Center for Independent Living (BCIL) is a well-established example of a residential program. BCIL was founded in 1974 as a consumer-run self-help community where severely disabled individuals could develop independent living skills. Since then it has evolved into a nonprofit corporation that coordinates 3 different forms of independent living in the Boston area. Since its inception BCIL has made transitional living facilities available to interested severely disabled individuals. The program includes skills training to prepare participants for independent living in the community. For participants with more developed independent living skills who desire a more private lifestyle, BCIL has located an apartment building that makes cluster housing available in modified apartments with a pool of personal care assistants. BCIL has also been working to locate facilities and funding for individuals who wish to share an accessible apartment with a personal care assistant and live independently.

New Options in Houston is an example of a transitional training program that provides information and first-hand experiences to prepare participants for independent living in a short period of time. The residential program includes a 6-week cycle of instructional modules emphasizing the skills needed to live and work with a minimum of assistance.

Participants can enhance their personal, physical and functional skills through the New Options Program. They learn to work with personal care assistants, are introduced to educational and vocational opportunities and alternative living arrangements, and experience the community through fieldtrips. New Options also has an extensive independent living research project which is used to trace the influence of the program on former participants.

The three types of independent living program are similar to the extent that they are community-based, have consumer involvement, and provide services designed to facilitate independent living by severely disabled people. They differ according to whether they provide ongoing or transitional services, whether they are residential or nonresidential, and whether they are controlled by consumers or merely provide opportunities for substantial consumer involvement. These differences may seem subtle and unimportant to the uninitiated observer. In fact, these differences are extremely significant, often prompting heated debate among supporters of independent living.

It is not difficult to explain why. Some people argue that independent living programs must be controlled by consumers in order to be viable. Others argue that consumer involvement on a lesser scale is sufficient. Some people hold that residential programs are institutional, segregated, and do not promote optimal normalization in the community. Others argue that they provide suitable alternatives to institutionalization for severely disabled people, that they represent one step on a continuum of independence, and that they need not necessarily be segregated. Some people argue that transitional programs are simply residential programs in disguise, that they are too much like traditional rehabilitation programs, and that they do little to insure the long-term support of severely disabled people in their communities. Others hold that transitional programs differ significantly from residential programs in that they force participants to move into the community after a specified period of time, or after the participants have met certain goals. They argue that transitional programs are much more cost-effective than other sorts of independent living programs and that they enable severely disabled people to live independently in their communities without the need for ongoing services other than those provided to the general population.

These differences of opinion should not discourage the adoption of any one type of program, but should lead to questions which may help determine which types of program are most appropriate to meet the needs of severely disabled people in particular communities. Instead of competing with one another for preeminence, these three types of program should complement each other. It has been the case in some instances that all three types of programs are needed in a given community.

In addition to the basic features, programs can be described in terms of a number of variable features. These features are useful in classifying programs and in determining how those programs fit into any given community. The principal features surveyed by ILRU in 1978 and discussed by Pflueger in her monograph *Independent Living* (1977) are service setting, service delivery method, helping style, vocational emphasis, goal orientation, and disability type served. Other features which may be important include program sponsor, management structure, geographical setting, and primary funding source.

The term *service setting* pertains to whether a program is residential or nonresidential. *Service delivery method* pertains to whether services are provided directly, by the program, or indirectly, through referral to other agencies. *Helping style* pertains to the extent to which consumers are involved in the operation of the program. *Vocational emphasis* pertains whether or not vocational goals are prerequisites for participation in the program. *Goal orientation* pertains to whether the program is transitional or ongoing. *Disability type served* pertains to whether the program focuses on people with a particular type of severe disability or whether the program provides services for people of many different disability types. *Program sponsor* pertains to whether the program is sponsored by a health service, social service, or rehabilitation service agency in the community, or whether it is an independent entity. *Management structure* pertains to the amount of control retained by an organization's board of directors, as compared to the executive director, or to the power of the director as compared to that of the staff. *Geographical type* pertains to whether the program serves an urban area with dense population, or a rural area with scattered population. *Primary funding source* pertains to whether the program is supported primarily by fees, or by grants and donations. It is important to recognize that these features are not exclusive, and that they simply constitute dimensions across which programs may vary.

Existing Program Models

Although the Center for Independent Living in Berkeley, California, has most often been cited as the epitome of an independent living program, many others are worthy of attention. Two in particular are the Ann Arbor Center for Independent Living (Ann Arbor CIL) in Michigan, and the Community Service Center for the Disabled (CSCD) in San Diego, California.

Both the Ann Arbor CIL and CSCD are located in highly

populated urban areas. They each serve over 500 clients per year, drawn from all major disability types. Both report that they serve male and female clients in equal numbers and that nonwhite persons represent at least 25 percent of their clientele. In addition, disabled persons make up more than 50 percent of the staff at both centers. Their primary services include advocacy, community consultation, and community education. Both provide referral to housing, attendants, and transportation. With annual budgets in excess of $100,000, both programs rely on multiple funding sources including federal, state, and foundation grants, as well as individual and group donations. State agencies represent primary source of income for both. In spite of substantial support, both programs list inadequate funding among their major problem areas.

Data on other centers are not lacking. The ILRU project is presently updating its 1978 survey of independent living programs. Data obtained thus far seem to indicate that the number of independent living programs in the United States has nearly quadrupled during the three years since the original survey was done. There are now more than twenty programs in California alone. There are at least five programs each in Massachusetts and Texas, and at least three programs each in New York, Kansas, Michigan and Washington. The great majority are located in urban areas. In fact, only three truly rural programs have been identified. In the past, many programs were located adjacent to university campuses. However, newer programs tend to locate away from campuses, in order to better serve the community at large. Residential and nonresidential programs seem to be equally represented among existing programs; indeed, several programs provide comprehensive services in both residential and nonresidential settings.

It is clear that nonresidential programs serve more persons on an annual basis than residential programs do. On average, nonresidential programs serve more than 500 persons per year, while residential programs serve fewer than 50. More than two thirds of the existing programs serve persons with different types of disabilities. Of those which focus on a single disability, spinal cord injury is the type most often served. There are twice as many ongoing independent living programs as there are transitional programs. In fact, very few of the recently established programs are transitional. With respect to vocational emphasis, the programs are evenly divided. About half have a strong vocational focus, and half an only incidental focus on vocational issues.

About half of the existing programs are staffed primarily by handicapped individuals, and the other half primarily by nonhandicapped persons. Those programs which are not staffed primarily by handicapped people generally are directed or managed by handicapped individuals. Most programs provide both direct services and referrals to other agencies. While a few of the older programs provide only direct services with no referrals, the majority of recently organized programs place tremendous emphasis on information and referral services. This appears to reflect a trend toward better utilization of existing community services. It also reflects the growing emphasis on advocacy which has led to the expansion of existing health and social service programs to include severely disabled persons among their clientele.

The most frequently cited service provided by independent living programs is residential service in housing owned and operated by the center itself. The next most frequently cited are peer counseling and training in independent living skills. Other services frequently cited include attendant care, advocacy, financial aid counseling, transportation, social and recreational activities, and mobility training. Most programs are recently organized, private, nonprofit entities governed by a corporate board of directors who in turn employ an executive director to manage day-to-day program activities. A few programs are affiliated with comprehensive rehabilitation centers, voluntary agencies like Goodwill and the National Easter Seal Society, or state vocational rehabilitation agencies. These programs are generally managed by a project director who is employed by the sponsoring agency and who reports to an advisory committee which includes strong consumer representation.

Almost half of the existing programs rely on four or more sources of income to support their programs. The older programs rely more heavily on income from fees for services rendered (paid by consumers, vocational rehabilitation agencies and the like, or insurance carriers), while the newer programs rely more on grants from federal, state and local governments. Donations by individuals and corporations form a secondary source of funding for most programs, while foundation grants are still of incidental importance. Almost two thirds of existing programs depend on state rehabilitation agencies as their primary source of funds. While nearly as many list federal grants as one source of income, very few depend on them as a primary source. About one quarter of all programs have only one source of funding. On the other hand, another quarter rely on at least five sources of income, and, with one exception, each of these programs serves more than 500 persons annually.

Not surprisingly, the older programs, established in or .ore 1976, tend to be the biggest. In particular, those programs which serve the most people tend to have the largest budgets, and to serve the largest communities. In many respects, the older programs are characterized by the prefix "multi": they are usually multiservice, multidisability, multifunded, and multifocused.

Information gathered about the successes and failures of existing programs can be useful in planning new programs. If one were to ask what kind of independent living program was best, most experts answer that that depends on the needs of disabled people in any given community, on the availability of existing community resources, on the physical and social make-up of the community, and on the goals of the program itself. Nonetheless, a few rules hold true for all programs.

Successful programs tend to be those that incorporate the major tenets of the Independent Living Movement. In particular, provision must be made for the substantial involvement of consumers in program planning, management, operation, and monitoring. Programs should be community-based, and the services they provide should be directly related to community needs. Programs should provide a set of core services not available to disabled people elsewhere in the community, and they should coordinate and provide referral to existing services in the community. They should also provide a combination of ongoing and transitional services.

Programs should establish straightforward management policies modeled after other successful community-based social service programs. They should maintain sound fiscal management and adopt effective accounting procedures. They should obtain consultation and assistance from existing programs and other sources of technical assistance, and they should establish program evaluation methods. They should develop multiple sources of funding, and they should be accountable both to funding sources and to their own clientele. They should develop strong relationships with local and state rehabilitation agencies, as well as with the private sector in their own communities. They should struggle to avoid compromising principles in the face of pragmatic concerns. Finally, they should strive to be inventive.

Future Trends

It appears that new programs will continue to be established at the present rate for the next two to five years until each state has on the order of five to thirty independent living programs. This means that by 1985 there may be as many as 300 to 500 programs in the United States. Based on the fact that there are now about 135 active programs in the United States with budgets averaging $150,000 per year each, we can assume that about $20 million is being spent on independent living programs today. Some $15 million of this represents federal appropriations under Title VII. Furthermore, given an additional $3 million appropriated in fiscal year 1982 under Title VII, primarily to establish new programs, it is not impossible that enough funding will be available in 1985 to support the anticipated 300 to 500 programs.

Again, judging by recent trends and the prevailing opinion of experts, one can predict that future programs will emphasize consumer control, will be community-based, and will avoid providing residential services. Given additional funding, one could also predict the establishment of more than one program in a single metropolitan area. These programs would be of several different types—some transitional, and some ongoing. Also, they would be likely to focus on different disability types. For example, one program might provide services primarily for mentally retarded adults, another for mobility impaired individuals, and yet a third for persons with visual or communication disorders.

With the growing movement toward independent living for severely disabled people, there will come a greater demand for integrated, barrier-free accommodations. Public attention and political clout will focus more closely on elimination of work disincentives, provision of barrier-free public transportation, and establishment of community-wide referral programs for attendant care, readers, and interpreters.

However, with the rapid proliferation and expansion of independent living programs, a number of programs will fail due to overexpansion and mismanagement. This could lead to an effort by the federal government to impose strict controls on funding, and to require program standardization or perhaps even licensing. Rapid program development could also lead to the evolution of the independent living specialist. If all these changes came to pass, institutionalization would be inevitable, and the Independent Living Movement would likely wind up a part of the nursing home establishment, the mental health/mental retardation establishment, or some similar bureaucracy.

In conclusion, let us look once more at the present state of development of independent living programs. Right now, in the United States, nearly thirty thousand severely disabled people are living more independently than they were three years ago. These thirty thousand are people who have been and are being served by independent living programs. By 1985, at the present rate of growth, as many as half a million severely disabled people may be living comparatively independent lives, integrated throughout our communities as a result of services provided by independent living programs.

5

Developing Programs
in Rural Areas

Lois O. Schwab

Rural Americans are a self-reliant group who make up 27.7 percent of the country's population (Beale, 1981). Nearly sixty-three million individuals have chosen to live and work on the farms and in the small towns found across the length and breadth of the country. Of all people, they are the most dependent on the land-based economics of agriculture, forestry, and mining. They bring the uniqueness of their situation to their individual lives, to their communication, to their associations, and to their outlook on the future. Swaczy points out that "economics factors, local history, social traditions, geography and proximity to urban centers mold the characters of different rural areas. A tenant farmer in the Southeast and a rancher in Montana have different outlooks. A miner in the Appalachian coal fields lives in a small town far different from the trailer town of a Wyoming coal miner" (1979, p. 3).

Rural areas are defined as those "where the majority of the people in a political subdivision (county, state, or section of

73

a state) live in an open country setting or in small towns"
(Swaczy, 1979, p. 3). Thus, aligned with a farm population of
six million are another fifty-seven million persons who have
chosen to live in nonmetropolitan rural and small town communities. The term *nonmetropolitan* refers to all counties lying
outside of metropolitan areas, which are defined as areas containing urban centers of 50,000 people or more. Counties adjacent to urban centers are considered metropolitan if they meet
certain criteria, such as the number of community workers and
the degree of urbanization. According to preliminary 1980 cen-
sus figures, nonmetropolitan areas have increased in population
by eight million during the last decade. Furthermore, all parts
of the United States experienced population growth in rural and
small town communities. Regionally, this growth exceeded 31
percent in the western states, with an average increase of 15.4
percent for the nation. Furthermore, except in the South, rural
areas and small towns are growing faster than the nation's
metropolitan areas for the first time since 1820 (Beale, 1981).

Disability found in rural areas of America differs in both
kind and rate of incidence from that found elsewhere. A 1978
Social Security Administration publication entitled *Work Disability in the United States* analyzes disability in the 18–65 age
group for all parts of the country. In the southern states, 17
percent of the population have some degree of disability; this
figure encompasses the 9 percent who are "totally disabled"
and the 8 percent who are "partially disabled." In the north
central and western states, the total is 14 percent; 6 percent
"totally disabled" and 8 percent "partially disabled." In the
New England states, 7 percent are "totally disabled" and 6 percent are "partially disabled," for a total of 13 percent (U.S. Department of Health, Education and Welfare, 1978a).

Because programming needs differ across the country,
this discussion will focus on three points: first, a unique pioneer
project which continues to meet the needs of rural persons; second, the outreach into rural areas of the state rehabilitation
services and the newly organized Independent Living Centers;
and third, the grassroots rehabilitation programs devised and
carried out by home economists in the Cooperative Extension
Service.

Development of a Statewide Service Model

In 1966, a mobile, self-contained unit called Homemaking Unlimited was developed as part of a rehabilitation program designed to enable individuals with physical limitations to try out ideas for simplifying activities related to daily living (Nebraska Division of Rehabilitation Services, 1972). A first of its kind, the coach was made possible by a grant from the Nebraska Heart Association to the then School of Home Economics at the University of Nebraska. It initiated a teaching program for homemakers, both men and women, with cardiovascular conditions, amputation, paraplegia, arthritis, visual impairments, and other physical disabilities.

Homemaking Unlimited was modularly planned so that any one idea could be tried independently of the others. Work simplification principles were incorporated throughout. The kitchen centers provided for working while seated—a feature adopted especially for persons using a wheelchair or having limited energy. Devices for persons with the use of only one arm were displayed. Other displayed items included cleaning and laundry equipment that was easy to see, reach, grasp, and handle, and grab bars for the bathtub and toilet that had been designed for use by persons with various kinds of physical limitation.

Illustrated material drew special attention to a balanced diet that helped persons with limited physical activity to control their weight. A continuous slide show depicted a physically limited mother caring for her child. Clothing with easy-to-put-on features and adaptations for specific disabilities was displayed at another demonstration center. Well-illustrated bulletins were prepared for free distribution.

The Homemaking Unlimited program was scheduled through the University of Nebraska Cooperative Extension Service. University staff worked closely with local advisory groups composed of Extension Service staff and representatives from the medical profession, health agencies, and civic groups to develop plans for intensive use of the coach when it came to the community. The program also served as a basis for research projects and field experience for graduate students enrolled in a training program made possible under the first teaching grant in home economics awarded by the Vocational Rehabilitation Administration (now the Rehabilitation Services Administration). The program generally concentrated on rural areas where approximately 20 percent of the population was over sixty-five years of age.

In seven years of existence, the Homemaking Unlimited program covered every part of the state. During that time, thousands of persons with disabilities toured the coach. Each person was given the opportunity for an in-depth trial of all the items that might prove useful. The usual interview lasted an hour. Subsequently, hundreds of persons were referred to the Nebraska Division of Rehabilitation Services and the Nebraska Rehabilitation Services for the Visually Impaired for further assistance in the development of their capabilities.

By 1968, the number of persons requesting additional services had become so great that the Nebraska Division of Rehabilitation Services decided to do something to meet the expressed needs. Through an innovation grant, a second Homemaking Unlimited coach was built and a second homemaker rehabilitation consultant (a graduate of the University of Nebraska master's program) was hired. The home economist, who had had special training in homemaking rehabilitation and rehabilitation counseling, was sent to travel around the state. The first two years were largely spent planning procedures, informing counselors of the new service, and building a caseload. Between January 1, 1970 and January 1, 1972, forty-two cases were closed. Of these, twenty-two were closed "rehabilitated" at a cost ranging from less than $100 to $4,896 for new rehabilitation services. The mean cost per client for services was $271.01. The mean cost per client, including services and administrative costs, was $582.01. These individualized services required any-g from one month to slightly over two and one half years, with an average case time of 9.2 months. Clients ranged in age from twenty to over sixty years. Those in the 40–50 age group received more services than all other age groups combined. The physical disabilities of the clients were diverse, although the greatest number of clients (24 percent) had multiple sclerosis.

In 1974, the Nebraska Division of Rehabilitation Services developed a comprehensive, statewide system, originally called the Residential Services Program, to provide a variety of consultation and training services to clients eligible for Vocational Rehabilitation (VR). Now called the Independent Living Services (ILS), this program was started with an establishment grant from the Rehabilitation Services Administration to the College of Home Economics, University of Nebraska. After the first two years, the project was taken over by the Division; subsequently, two separate innovation and expansion grants assisted the development of three in-state independent living laboratories.

The present statewide ILS program employs a staff of ten full-time and one half-time specialists who are located throughout the division's six geographic regions. They are housed in the local VR offices, where they act as consultants to agency counselors and provide direct services to individuals. Each specialist has received an undergraduate degree in home economics plus additional training in the development of functional skills for independent living.

Hoffman (1979) explained the operation of the program as follows:

> Upon completion of the initial evaluation by the ILS specialists, eligibility is established for the program and a consultation is held with the client and counselor. A treatment plan is developed for the delivery of IL services and is incorporated in the client's Individualized Written Rehabilitation Program (IWRP) as an intermediate objective. Services are provided by the IL specialist at no cost to the individual while case service funds provide necessary equipment and related materials needed by the client to develop as independent a life style as possible.
>
> Services offered through the Independent Living Program are designed to be flexible and adaptable to the needs of each client. All clients are served on an individualized basis, and services are generally provided in the client's home. The ILS Program provides three broad categories of service which include Counseling and Guidance, Barrier Removal, Transportation Consultation, and Activities of Daily Living Training. All service systems interface with "traditional" VR services to provide a comprehensive service program.
>
> Counseling services are structured to help clients explore

their disabilities and psychologically cope with their situations and responsibilities. Major subject areas include problem solving, decision making, family relations, child rearing and goal setting.

Guidance services are organized to help clients live more efficiently. These service areas deal primarily with home management problems which may be aggravated by the advent of disability within the family. Included are money and time management; efficient use of energy; storage adaptation; nutrition, meal planning and preparation; and clothing selection, modification and repair. Other consultation services are made available or developed according to the needs of the client and family.

Helping clients overcome barriers and mobility problems in the home, community and at the job site is the intent of this group of services. ILS program specialists are available for consultation to both private and public agencies on architectural barrier removal. Clients may also receive consultation and assistance in the modification of personal vehicles.

Individual training in feeding, dressing, personal hygiene, grooming, home management, transportation usage and mobility is available for clients, family members, and attendants.

After several years of operation, the ILS Programs staff decided to explore the possibility of developing training and evaluation laboratories where clients could more effectively and efficiently be served. This led to the development of a network of innovative centers known as Independent Living Laboratories.

Established by two separate I & E Grants, these nonresidential laboratories are located in three strategic geographic areas in the state (Scottsbluff, Norfolk and Lincoln) and are operated by ILS Program specialists.

The laboratories provide a wide range of evaluative, diagnostic, and treatment services and serve as a "testing ground" for various assistive devices. In many instances, clients can experiment with several types of equipment prior to purchase, and architectural modifications can be tested prior to making alterations at the client's home or work station. Clients can be served in small groups of four to six in the laboratories—an advantage for some types of skill building and counseling activities [pp. 25-29].

In fiscal year 1980, the Nebraska Independent Living Program served 10 percent of the total Vocational Rehabilitation program, or 1,061 persons, and provided consultation services to 559 other individuals and agencies. Altogether, 298 individuals

Figure 1. Caseflow Within the Independent Living
Services Program.

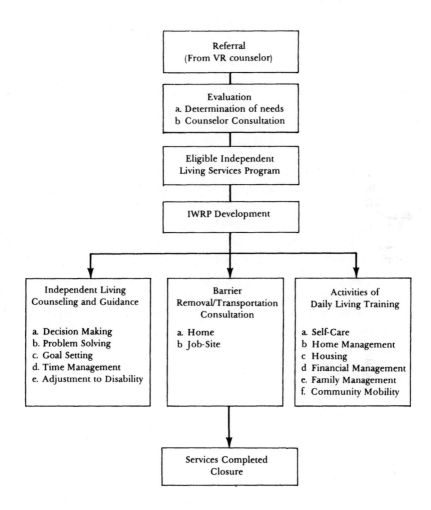

Source: Hoffman, 1979, pp. 25–29. Used by permission.

were brought to successful closure in the area of independent
living. Of the 298, 141 individuals were rehabilitated as homemakers.

Rural Outreach Through Independent Living Programs

The California Department of Rehabilitation has developed a comprehensive, statewide system of independent living services through its more than twenty centers. During the period 1970-1980, this system has shown that California's over one million severely disabled citizens can be reached through community-based programs. In 1979, the state legislature passed legislation to provide $2 million to assist in maintaining core services in these centers.

The impetus to start most of the centers came from groups of disabled individuals. Four centers were started with support of local chapters of the California Association for the Physically Handicapped; others were started by members of the disabled community at large with financial help from various sources. The California Department of Rehabilitation, the United Cerebral Palsy Association, and the Easter Seal Society provided funds for these pioneer efforts.

The need for services was assessed in several ways. Some centers determined community need according to the experience of their own staff and other persons with disabilities; others formally surveyed the disabled community to ascertain where service gaps existed. Still others patterned themselves after the Center for Independent Living in Berkeley.

Thus, no two centers offer an identical array of services because each reflects the needs of local consumers. The number of services ranges from as few as two—usually information or referral and counseling—to as many as fourteen separate services.

Although six independent living centers serve some rural populations, there is still a lack of independent living services for severely disabled individuals in rural areas, where high unemployment and high poverty levels prevail and few community services exist. Under Title VII, Part B, of the Rehabilitation Act, funds have been appropriated to establish a center in a rural area of Kern County, California. The center will concentrate on reaching prospective clients through use of appropriate media, such as English and Spanish language radio announcements, labor union newsletters, and notices on community bulletin boards.

New York State's nine centers are located in urban areas but serve multicounty region encompassing rural areas. Outreach to rural communities is obtained through public service announcements on television and radio. In addition, referrals are made by staff of the state rehabilitation agency, the Visiting Nurses Association, and the New York Department of Social Services. Most centers have a van to transport disabled persons from rural areas into the center.

The Alaska Division of Vocational Rehabilitation utilizes a computer system to help deliver independent living services. The IL center will soon have access to an electronic mail system hooked up to the Vocational Rehabilitation Agency's offices and to fifty-two school districts. This system will provide information and referral on a statewide basis. Advocacy and small service groups will be used for local organizing, while the center will provide technical assistance.

In Pennsylvania, the Erie Independence House Center reaches out to a thirteen-county area that is predominantly rural. This center operates primarily as a referral service. For example, the center holds classes and seminars on independent living topics throughout the area, using television, radio and newspaper announcements to reach disabled persons.

The independent living center established at the University of Wisconsin at Stout by the Wisconsin Department of Health and Social Services serves primarily rural populations in nine counties. This program started by identifying those persons in need of independent living services. Individuals who need generic services receive an appropriate referral. The center focuses on unmet needs in the areas of housing, transportation and development of daily living capabilities.

In Missouri, The Whole Person, Inc. not only serves metropolitan Kansas City but also reaches out to rural areas of six counties to assist persons with physical disabilities. Among other services, the center acts as a common channel of communication within the disabled community; as a spokesperson in the news media, and before legislative bodies; as an advocate on questions of housing, employment, transportation, accessibility, recreation, and education; and as a source of referrals to available services.

In Viburnam, Missouri, the Disabled Citizens Alliance for Independence was the first independent living program in the nation to be located in an exclusively rural area. Serving four counties, the staff trains disabled people to live on their own. The alliance operates within a fifty to sixty mile radius of its headquarters. Outreach aides tour the rural area calling on persons with disabilities, to determine the nature of their handicap and needs.

In neighboring Kansas, another rural model called Operation Link serves nine counties. Offices in Stockton, Hays, and Smith Center provide special services to persons with physical, mental or emotional impairments. Services provided (or coordinated through referral) include: attendant care, counseling, generic services, housing, training in independent living skills, job development and placement, peer counseling, advocacy, readers and interpreters, transportation, information about goods and services relevant to independent living, equipment maintenance and repair, socialization, and recreation.

A unique feature of this project is its method of case management. The project employs four case managers, each of whom has completed nineteen hours of training in individual program planning. The case manager acts as an advocate for the client, serves as a counselor, and helps to coordinate a variety of services. Clients range in age from nineteen to fifty-four, and their disabilities include mental retardation, emotional disturbance, multiple sclerosis, and hearing impairment. The project is supported with federal funds from the Developmental Disabilities Office and the Rehabilitation Services Administration and with state funds from the Kansas Planning Council on Developmental Disabilities and the Kansas State Department of Social and Rehabilitation Services.

Maine's independent living center, headquartered in Augusta, reaches out to rural areas through self-help meetings in twenty rural towns. At these meetings, persons with disabilities are brought together to work on self-advocacy and program development within the community. A traveling van is being equipped with personnel and tools to repair wheelchairs, TTYs, and prosthetic devices.

In New Hampshire, the Granite State Independent Living Program works out of Goffstown to serve the residents of an essentially rural state. Outreach begins with contacts to local hospitals, to find persons with new injuries and those who are homebound or mobility-impaired. Initiated with a statewide needs assessment, the program is now run by the Spinal Cord Injury Foundation.

In South Carolina, the Vocational Rehabilitation Department located the independent living program at the Dill Beckman Comprehensive Center in West Columbia. While operating primarily in a large metropolitan area, the program utilizes the services of the Clemson University Home Extension Service for homemaker instruction, training in independent skills, and similar activities.

The Vermont Center for Independent Living, operating out of Montpelier, provides comprehensive, statewide services. These include a peer-counseling program to provide assistance in solving problems; training in independent living skills and self-advocacy for persons with severe physical disabilities; information referral; newsletters and other information; and accessible housing, transportation and attendant services. Individuals with disabilities are now being prepared to serve as interns and advocates in the program.

In Kentucky, the course of independent living has been influenced by the special needs of blind persons across the state. In a newly initiated program, most of the state's blind persons (estimated to number over 6,000) are to be given specialized training in adjustment, orientation, mobility, and other activities of daily living. Previously, only individuals judged to have rehabilitation potential for employment were afforded this opportunity.

The Cooperative Extension Service

The Cooperative Extension Service, operating under the United States Department of Agriculture, has programs in all fifty states, the District of Columbia, Guam, Puerto Rico, and the Virgin Islands. Each local program determines its own structure. The Extension's nearly 4,000 local home economists are all professionally trained and experienced educators. A newsletter issued three times a year, and distributed nationally, keeps persons interested in working with disabled persons informed of new resources and services. The Cooperative Extension Service also runs 4-H programs for mentally retarded, physically disabled, emotionally disturbed, blind, and deaf youth between the ages of nine and nineteen.

The National Extension Homemakers Council, which has 600,000 members in forty-two States, is conducting an educational awareness campaign on accessibility in the home. Builders, contractors, and others are being informed of the means by which homes can be made accessible to persons using wheelchairs, canes, crutches, and other aids.

Independent living services in Minnesota can be traced back to 1958, when an Extension program, Homemakers Limited, began to offer interdisciplinary educational services. More recently, another Extension program, Ability—Not Disability, has developed brochures and audiovisual materials for disabled homemakers. These documents are widely used by cooperative extension programs in other states, including Alabama, Arkansas, Ohio and West Virginia.

Clothing for persons with disabilities is a subject of great interest to many home economics programs of the Cooperative Extension Service. Arizona Extension personnel have conducted research on the clothing and other daily needs of handicapped persons. The fruits of this research include an annotated bibliography and resource list as well as slide presentations exploring clothing solutions for particular disabilities.

In Nebraska, special clothing for children with disabilities has been developed, and consultations are held with most disabled children who pass through the University of Nebraska ical Center. Health fairs conducted by the Extension program feature devices and clothing for persons with physical disabilities. Cornell University has developed leaflets containing clothing suggestions for persons with disabilities. New articles of clothing for persons with special needs are constantly being developed through these programs.

In addition, unique projects have been undertaken in many states. For instance, in Alabama, Extension personnel have issued numerous press releases for local newspapers, indicating various ways in which homemaking can be carried on despite disabilities. In Maine, Extension has run a summer camp stressing independence for children with disabilities. In North Dakota, groups have been formed to teach persons who are mentally retarded to cook using a workbook, *Cooking From Pictures*. In Ohio and Missouri, Extension specialists keep blind persons up-to-date on best buys, recipes, new products, and other homemaking needs, through radio reading programs for the blind. Additionally, Ohio Extension sends program assistants hired under CETA directly to the homes of disabled persons to help them develop their independent living skills. At Clemson University in South Carolina, an Extension housing specialist helps plan adaptive kitchens for persons using wheelchairs. In Wisconsin, house parents and developmentally disabled adults are offered lessons on nutrition, food preparation, and sanitation in the home. Adapted step-by-step cookbooks are used.

Cooperative Extension programs are available to *all* persons across the United States. In contrast with most rehabilitation services, which rely on individual consultations, Extension home economists structure most of their programs as group activities. This includes demonstrations, field trips, and the development of peer support.

Independent living rehabilitation services for persons in nonmetropolitan areas are being provided at best only in a random manner. The Independent Living Center program as funded by the Rehabilitation Services Administration has established several projects for rural areas but these touch the lives of only several thousand persons. The need remains to reach the rest of the 8 million persons with physical and/or mental disabilities who through chance or choice live in the rural areas of America. Such an effort can be made; there are systems and networks, some of which are described in the following sections, that reach into and function throughout rural America, and that might well be used to extend IL services.

Cooperative Extension Service. The Cooperative Exten-

sion Service (described earlier) is a national network, established
to raise the quality of life for rural America through educational
and demonstration programs. Presently, there is sporadic interest in educational programs which have precise information for
persons with disabilities. The various lessons and inclusion of
persons with disabilities are shared through a national newsletter. But these are only to be taken up as the members "vote
for" the lesson. Nebraska's exemplary program should be taken
up by the entire system as a model for public education. It resulted in referrals and information being made available to
thousands of persons.

Educational Service Units. The consolidated service units
for schools in rural areas that provide special education programs could extend their assistance to disseminating information and referrals. Many state rehabilitation services are under
the auspices of education, just as rehabilitation services at the
federal level are within the federal Education and Rehabilitation
Administration. It would be a natural extension of this existing
service to give assistance in the independent living field.

Traditional Vocational Rehabilitation Services. The fed-
eral/state program for vocational rehabilitation has made considerable progress over the years in most states. Section A of
Title VII of the 1978 Amendments to the 1973 federal Rehabilitation Act provides for the extension of services through already established channels. Again, the Nebraska model whereby
an independent living specialist is available for all clients requiring independent living services should be activated. Under Section A funding, these independent living services could be extended to persons of all ages regardless of vocational capability.
The expertise of the professional rehabilitationist would be
utilized to bring individuals to maximum level of function in
care of self and environment.

Integrated Health Services. Small hospitals and doctors
offices exist throughout the rural areas. Rehabilitation generally
has been referred to as the third phase of medicine—but the
practitioners of medicine have not recognized their referral obligations to disabled people. Independent living specialists should
be located in private hospitals, just as other special units are

allocated for accessibility. Intensive education of present and future practitioners in both the medical and therapeutic field is called for to establish such a system on a national basis.

Other human service systems, such as Social Security and various welfare programs, have the potential for extending independent living services to all persons in the rural areas. It is imperative that such services be made available so that all persons, regardless of age, location, sex, or financial means, may have the opportunity to live as freely, creatively and responsibly as possible.

6

Learning from Methods
Used in Other Countries

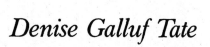

Denise Galluf Tate
Thomas A. Lee

Attempts to assure the disabled person's integration in all aspects of life depend on many factors, such as national resources, social structure, the attitude of society, and other influences. Besides the United States, several other countries, notably Sweden, Denmark, the Netherlands, and Great Britain, are searching within their own economic, political, and social contexts for reasonable solutions that address the needs of severely disabled individuals in the areas of housing and environmental adaptation, education, transportation, and personal care. Canada and Australia are prominent among the non-European nations that have been active in this endeavor as well. This article reviews the

Note: This chapter is an extensively revised and expanded version of an article by D. Tate, R. Jarvis, and G. Juhr that appeared in the October 1979 issue of *Archives of Physical Medicine and Rehabilitation.*

most current information presently available in the United States regarding independent living efforts in the above-mentioned countries.

Sweden

Sweden has been recognized as one of the most advanced countries in providing services for the severely disabled. As noted by Purtilo (1981), the United States and Sweden are two of the most affluent postindustrial nations in the world, with comparable levels of economic growth as reflected in their standards of living and gross national products. Furthermore, each country spends approximately 8 percent of its gross national income on health care, which places them among the most health-costly in the world.

Documents published by the Swedish Institute for the Handicapped (1979, 1980) and the Ministry of Local Government (1978) indicate that Sweden has both a strong central government and extensive local government. Public bodies at all levels—central government, county council, local authority—are responsible for most services provided to disabled persons, such as housing, employment, education, medical care, and social welfare.

In order to increase the opportunities for contact between government authorities and organizations of the handicapped, special coordinating bodies—councils for the handicapped—have been set up at the different governmental levels to participate in political decision making. As reported by Gardeström (1978), there are about twenty-five organizations for the handicapped in Sweden. In addition to their coordinating function, these organizations have been active in setting up local social and recreational activities and group travel programs. Some associations for the most severely handicapped have set up their own hospitals, convalescent homes, and rehabilitation centers.

In comparison to other countries, Sweden has no general law aimed at securing the rights of handicapped persons. Instead, special paragraphs concerning handicapped rights have been inserted in certain laws, for example, the Building Act and the

Child Care Act. In the case of other laws, such as the Education Act and the Work Environment Act, it is either considered self-evident or it is stated in the legislative history that handicapped persons are also covered by the law. The exception to this rule is the Act on Provisions for Mentally Retarded Persons of 1968, which gives the county councils full responsibility for the mentally retarded. This law is intended to respond to those requirements of the mentally retarded not met by social resources at the disposal of all citizens.

With respect to education, the Swedish Education Act makes the municipalities responsible for almost all compulsory educational services below university level. Efforts to integrate disabled children and youngsters in normal schools are promoted continuously by state grants.

In 1970, a National Board of Attendant Service was established. The board has two principal aims: first, to make personal service (attendant care) available to severely physically disabled persons who are studying at universities, colleges, and high schools; and second, to provide housing, personal assistance, and medical care to physically disabled and other severely handicapped persons enrolled in secondary schools.

Environmental planning and housing for severely disabled persons are emphasized in Sweden. As described by the Swedish Institute for the Handicapped (1979), the Building Act has special provisions that ensure adequate housing accommodations and accessibility for "persons whose mobility or orientational ability is reduced as a result of old age, handicap or illness" (pp. 10-11).

There is a special government housing allowance to enable a dwelling to be designed to meet the handicapped person's individual requirements. It may be granted for all types of handicap, for example, reduced mobility, defective vision, allergy, epilepsy, psoriasis, colostomy, extremely small stature, or mental retardation. This allowance is intended for such measures as are necessary to provide for the primary housing functions of sleeping, resting, attending to personal hygiene, preparing food, eating, and moving around in the dwelling.

Opportunities for independent, integrated housing for severely disabled persons do not only depend on the dwelling's technical design. In many cases, access is needed to personal assistance in the form of a home help service as well as to technical aids. Twenty-four-hour attendant care is provided for those living in special service flats. Government subsidies cover 35 percent of the cost of this service.

An experiment in individual integration has been carried out in Sweden by the Fokus Society and more recently in the Netherlands. The Swedish Fokus Society provides well-adapted flats—currently, 280 distributed among thirteen towns—and access to personal assistance for severely disabled persons. Flats are available for single persons or families and are located in one apartment building in order to make the day and night service easier. There are also flats for nondisabled people in the same building. Disabled people lease flats on the same terms as other tenants. It is up to disabled people to demand the help they need from assistants. They take responsibility for their own meals, medical attendance, and so on.

It must be pointed out that many of the severely disabled encounter difficulties in living during their first six to twelve months in the new environment. Exchanging a sheltered existence for an independent life with full responsibility is sometimes very difficult. However, of the approximately 300 young disabled persons currently living in the thirteen towns, none wish to return to their earlier situation. A survey of what Fokus has accomplished in two years shows that approximately 80 percent of the tenants now have jobs or are pursuing a purposeful course of study. Before moving in, 90 percent had been receiving an invalid's pension.

Integrated homes of the kind that the Fokus Society provides have also proved to be an economical solution for society. The total cost of rent and attendant care service is considerably lower than the corresponding cost of living in an institution and only half that of a long-term clinic. In addition to accessible housing, the Swedish government makes provisions for adequate transportation for the disabled. However, there are still many difficulties for persons with severe handicaps in using streets and public transport. All handicapped persons who cannot use the public transport system are entitled to use a special service. It is open to people with varied disabilities including those with blindness, orthopedic impairments, cardiac diseases, and mental retardation.

Most communities provide a specialized transit service, "färdtjänst," for disabled and elderly citizens. These systems utilize subsidized taxis and special vans to transport people who cannot use public transportation from one point to another in the community. Handicapped persons who are working or studying and are unable to use public transport can, through the National Labour Market Board, receive a state grant of up to SKr 33,000 to buy a car. Any extra equipment they need to be able to drive the car is granted to them.

A new transportation service for the most severely handicapped is currently underway in Sweden. The "riksfärdtjänst" requires that disabled passengers pay only for a second class railway ticket, whatever transport is used. This nationwide system allows disabled people to travel in trains across country borders (for journeys of sixty miles or more) and is to be used for recreation and other private purposes. In explaining this system, Kallman (1981) points out that severely disabled persons in need of assistants can have the government cover the fare for the assistant.

With respect to efforts to integrate mass transit, Frieden and Frieden (1981) state that many subway stations have been equipped with elevators. One interesting aspect of the subway adaptations is that these elevators use the escalator tunnels for shafts. Elevators move diagonally at the same angle as the escalators. By using existing tunnels, the expense of installing the elevators was apparently minimized.

The definition of independence in its broader sense includes not only the fulfillment of basic needs such as housing and transportation but also the option of being employed. Ettarp (1980) discusses the employment situation for the disabled in Sweden in an article entitled *Vocational Rehabilitation During a Recession.* He explains that in attempting to leapfrog the economic recession resulting from the oil crisis of 1974–1975, Sweden combined antiinflation measures with a traditional labor market policy aimed at sustaining full employment. One of the premises adopted was that job opportunities for the handicapped must be viewed as an integral part of the labor market policies undertaken in order to maintain employment in Sweden. The measures to protect employment for the disabled were organized along two main lines: (1) to avoid lay-offs and dismissals occasioned by short-term cyclical factors, and (2) to adopt policy measures that could create new employment options for the most disadvantaged outside the regular labor force.

To implement these two policy lines, the 1974 Security of Employment Act stipulated that an employer must have substantial grounds for giving notice. Reduced work capacity due to handicap or infirmity does not normally constitute acceptable grounds for dismissal. Another measure gave state subsidies to firms that had announced impending lay-offs or dismissals. These subsidies are used to provide laid-off workers with in-plant training during working hours.

State grants for semi-sheltered employment may be given to organizations hiring severely disabled persons who are unable to obtain work in the regular labor market. At present, these grants amount to 75 percent of total wage costs for the first year of employment, 50 percent for the second year, and 25 percent for the third and fourth years. Furthermore, as indicated by the National Labour Market Board (1978), more substantial grants may be awarded to employers who hire severely disabled youngsters. Concurrently, the Swedish Government Commission on Long-Term Employment Policy (1978) reports that the definition of disabled in Sweden is being expanded to include a large proportion of young persons who have social, medical, or occupational handicaps, often combined with mental disturbances and drug abuse. State grants may also be awarded to the employer if the disabled employee is in need of someone to assist with certain work tasks.

It is particularly noteworthy that the recession and the deepening problems of the labor market never led to a lowering of the standards of labor market policy. On the contrary, several government bills reaffirmed the principle of universal entitlement to employment. It was stated quite unequivocally that the right to work must also apply to persons with severe disabilities. No minimum work capacity should be stipulated in order for a handicapped person to be entitled to work. Unfortunately, these political ideals were not matched by a similar economic effort to increase the number of sheltered job opportunities.

In order to make the future organization of sheltered workshops more uniform and effective, all 370 of the country's sheltered workshops were brought together in 1977 in a new conglomerate called Public Enterprises. Public Enterprises is the seventh largest industrial group in Sweden, with a turnover exceeding $750 million. The group employs about 22,000 disabled persons. Its establishment has been hailed as a major step forward in hiring the severely disabled.

Generally speaking, these policies have kept unemployment in Sweden at a lower level than in other western European countries, except Austria and Norway. However, we cannot disregard the fact that many elderly and severely disabled persons have disappeared from the labor market statistics because they have retired on disability pensions, not always because of employment difficulties. People who would formerly have been obliged for economic reasons to accept very adverse working conditions in order to gain a livelihood are now able, on reasonable economic terms, to choose not to work.

The Netherlands

In the field of rehabilitation, as in all other fields of welfare, the Netherlands has a two-tiered system. Blommestijn (1978) states that while the government and the provincial or local authorities have a coordinating, stimulating, advising, and financing function, the provision of services for the handicapped is mainly the concern of private nonprofit organizations having a religious, ethical, humanitarian, ideological, or non-denominational basis. The Netherlands Central Society for the Care of Disabled has acted as the central organizing body for rehabilitation activities since its founding in 1899. At present, the Netherlands is witnessing a movement toward coalition between organizations of professionals in the field of rehabilitation—

mainly represented by the National Rehabilitation Association-and associations representing disabled consumers. According to Laurie (1977), these groups are now working together to influence politicians, policymakers, administrators, and the general public on issues important to disabled people.

Historically, the Netherlands has placed strong emphasis on traditional institutional programs and less emphasis on generic service programs and legislation. The current Dutch philosophy is that a range of facilities should be offered from which handicapped persons can choose for themselves. Three types of housing development are presently in evidence: congregate living centers such as the Huize Barendsz Centre at Velp, clustered living centers such as Het Dorp, and integrated housing units such as the units at Zwijndrecht. Greenstein and Leonard (1976) note that single dwelling units for handicapped persons outnumber collective living units in the Netherlands.

Huize Barendsz is typical of housing built by the Dutch in the last twenty years for physically disabled persons who require such services as meal preparation, bathing and physical therapy. The emphasis is on the provision of common living facilities: double dormitory-type rooms built around a common living room, dining room, and bathing facility. As this arrangement is not conducive to individual privacy, single rooms are provided in recent extensions.

Brattgard (1973) argues that "the most comprehensive social experiment of group integration is the community of disabled named Het Dorp in Holland. When society did not open its door to receive the disabled, a community of their own was built for them" (p. 5). Known throughout the world, Het Dorp (the Village) is a community of 400 dwelling units built in 1964 on forty-four acres of wooded and hilly land near Arnhem in eastern Holland (Greenstein and Leonard, 1976). The concept behind the project, as Tate, Jarvis and Juhr (1979) mention, was to demonstrate that when inappropriate institutionalization is replaced by accessible facilities that promote self-care, the physically disabled can grow in independence, productivity, and self-esteem. The project consists of a mixture of two-, three-, and four-story units carefully situated so as to be accessible from the outdoors. A system of elevators facilitates internal mobility. Floors of the buildings are organized in groups of ten individual units. Nine residents and one staff attendant comprise a living group, and social contact is promoted by the group's having its own large living-dining room equipped with kitchenette.

At the onset of the project, interviews were conducted with disabled persons to determine their specific needs in construction and design of the buildings. As a result, a sophisticated approach making use of such conveniences as radio-controlled door-openers, electric wheelchairs, specially designed kitchens, and accessible bathrooms has been implemented. Commercial and service facilities, including a supermarket, restaurant, gas station, and travel agency, are centrally located and accessible by the residents, thus encouraging interaction with outsiders, primarily the citizens of the nearby residential districts. These facilities are also used by members of the outside community who, however, rarely venture into the central area or become involved with the daily activities of the residents. The villagers are able to travel to Arnhem either in their electric wheelchairs (which frequently break down) or in small buses supported by the project. However, as the cost of the bus service is prohibitive for those who have not previously contributed to social insurance plans (and are thus not adequately covered), the amount of integration achieved has been less than initially intended.

Although Het Dorp provides an opportunity for the severely handicapped to live independently and to have free access to the outdoors, it is unlikely that the Dutch government would support the building of a similar center for a number of reasons. First, the location, design, and size do not facilitate interaction between the handicapped residents and the surrounding community. Second, the costs of operating the village are much higher than originally projected. Third, as the residents become older they need more and more care. Furthermore, most of the businesses in the village are managed and operated by nondisabled people and most of the residents of Het Dorp are unemployed (Frieden and Frieden, 1981).

Integrated housing at Zwijndrecht consists of several hundred new units, about 10 percent of which are for the handicapped. The buildings, according to Greenstein and Leonard (1976), are two-story townhouse units clustered in groups of six to eight. Units for the handicapped are distributed throughout the development, typically occurring at the end of a string of townhouses. The two houses at the end of a selected string of units are designed so that the two lower levels are combined into a single two- or three-bedroom unit for a family with a handicapped member.

At present, a government agency is sponsoring experimental clustered living projects at Enschede, Delft, and Groningen. The Fokus Society (funded by the Netherlands Ministry of Health and Social Affairs) is developing similar projects at Almere and Woongarm. The most important difference between the two independent living projects appears to be the method of financing attendant care services. The Fokus Society pays subsidies directly to the disabled residents who may then purchase services from private vendors, whereas the government furnishes the care services, eliminating the opportunity for the disabled person to choose, pay, and, when necessary, fire the attendant.

The Netherlands has a national program to provide technical aids to disabled people. Although a comprehensive system of aid centers does not exist, there is a mechanism for recommending, prescribing, purchasing, replacing, and paying for the repair of many different kinds of aids and devices. A government agency, the G.M.D. or Joint Medical Service, is responsible for reviewing applications for aids and equipment, including automobiles. In order to encourage independent living among disabled people, administrative provisions exist to ensure that disabled people will have as much responsibility as possible in purchasing equipment and services. The G.M.D., by means of follow-up visits, ascertains if the equipment has been purchased and is being properly used.

As Frieden and Frieden (1981) report, there is a significant service gap for disabled people in the Netherlands in the area of transportation. The Dutch National Railway system is almost totally accessible. There are portable ramps for boarding trains at nearly every station. Every train has at least one car adapted for use by people in wheelchairs, and personal assistance is generally available upon request. However, there is virtually no accessible intracity public transportation. The limited amount of local transportation that exists for the handicapped is provided by voluntary organizations such as the Red Cross, by police and fire departments, and by private agencies transporting clients to and from sheltered workshops, activity centers, and training programs.

Denmark

Normalization, or integration, which has been the target of services in Denmark for decades, means that disabled persons should be given conditions of life as close as possible to the normal and that services should be provided in accordance with individual needs. In reviewing Danish legislation, Bank-Mikkelsen (1980) explains that in 1976 the Rehabilitation Act of 1960 was repealed by the enactment of the Social Assistance Act. The Rehabilitation Act of 1960 had aimed to limit the consequences of invalidity or disease through the provision of technical aids and special medical treatment as well as through tuition, retraining, vocational training, and other occupational training for disabled persons.

The new Danish legislative and administrative reform, which came into effect in January 1980, had several unique features. First, all special legislation concerning specific handicaps was abolished. Second, general legislation concerning social services, education and health now included all citizens. Third, all categorizing of handicapped persons was abolished, both as to the traditional groupings, such as the blind, deaf, epileptic, speech defective, physically and mentally handicapped, and also as to groupings within these categories. Fourth, persons with special needs now receive services according to the needs of each individual. This approach should ensure equalization and individualized service. Fifth, the responsibility for services for handicapped persons was transferred to regional and local government (consisting of 14 counties and 275 municipalities), so that services for handicapped persons now come under the same authorities as are responsible for services for the rest of the population. Sixth, a consumer council with representatives from organizations of the handicapped will be established in every region. According to Bank-Mikkelsen (1977) these councils will follow developments within each area and can make proposals to the local authorities.

Integration in education has been established over a number of years. Jorgensen (1979) points out that of the 125,000 children receiving special educational treatment, 100,000 students are placed in integrated classes receiving supplementary education, 15,000 students are placed in special classes at ordinary schools, and 10,000 students attend special schools. Furthermore, writing about the role of special education, Dyssegaard (1981) explains that the new Danish law on special education secures the right to special education, as needed, for all handicapped persons both before and after the age of compulsory education.

In Denmark, current government policy aims to help disabled and elderly persons remain where they have been living if they so desire (Jorgensen, 1981). Government financial support is available to cover rent payments. As of February 1978, Denmark legislated accessibility requirements that affected all housing except single-family houses built for owner-occupiers. Public loans are made available to adapt apartments or houses as necessary.

In Denmark, integrated living for disabled persons is best demonstrated by the founding over the past fifteen years of a series of collective houses by the National Association of the Disabled. In 1971, this agency, through the Cripples' Building Society in Copenhagen, established nine collective houses throughout the country containing 1,100 flats. Eight additional buildings with 900 flats were planned at the same time, and negotiations were in progress for five more buildings with 700 flats. Goldsmith (1976) indicates that the Danish strategy is to concentrate in collective houses those persons with severe physical disabilities who need clinical support and who are not managing in family housing. As with the Fokus Society in Sweden, one of the primary objectives of the collective houses is physical and social integration with nonhandicapped peers.

The thirteen-story collective house at Hans Knudens Plads in Copenhagen, constructed in 1959, was the first of its kind in the world and serves as an example of the collective house concept with 170 apartments adapted for the disabled. Integrated living with nondisabled peers is attained by virtue of the fact that one third of the flats are reserved for the disabled, while the remainder houses orthopedic hospital nursing staff and the general public. In addition to a special nursing home for persons disabled by polio who require respiratory equipment, this collective house also contains a hostel for younger disabled singles, workshops, and a communal restaurant. Essential differences between the collective house and the Het Dorp concept have been observed. Both propose that normal society has failed to cope with severely disabled people on their own and that efficient clinical service is best achieved by concentrating the disabled population. But where the collective house attempts integration with nondisabled persons, Het Dorp opts for more segregation. One might question, however, whether complete integration is possible in a housing project that was originally built to accommodate a predetermined number of severely disabled persons and medical staff.

Describing the Danish housing system for the disabled, Laurie (1981) states that nursing homes are planned for people who need constant nursing care. Day nursing homes function similarly. Day centers provide no nursing care but offer activity and social contact. Sheltered housing, which is often built adjacent to nursing homes, may consist of a small number of apartments for disabled people who seek limited independence by using the personal care, housekeeping, and other services of the nursing home. Hostels with domestic help are provided for young severely handicapped persons who are not able to live in ordinary hostels, to assist them in the transition from home and school to adult life.

A home help service for the physically disabled is run by the local government's social security program. The helpers provide personal care, cooking, and cleaning services. They are given a six-month comprehensive training course that includes psychology and understanding the disabled. The disabled recipients pay a little from their pensions but never more than two hours of service. The remaining salary is paid by the municipality. Depending on the needs of the disabled, individual home help assistance is available 8-12 A.M., 2-4 P.M., and 6:30-8:30 P.M. Most significantly, family members are paid to take care of a disabled person in their family. The pay is approximately the equivalent of the pension of a retired person. One example would be a family with two boys disabled by muscular dystrophy. Both parents would be paid to stay at home and take care of their sons. A special car and special equipment would be supplied by the local authority. The home help system is effective for disabled individuals who have families or who need a minimum amount of assistance, but inadequate for the severely disabled who require the services of live-in attendants.

Under the Social Assistance Act of 1976, counties can establish centers to supply the communities and handicapped consumers with information concerning technical aids. In comparing Denmark with Britain, Laurie (1981) explains that both countries extensively use equipment to facilitate independence as a supplement to, or replacement for, attendant care. The use of ceiling hoists and clos-o-mat toilets that substitute warm water and air for wiping is common.

The Ministry of Public Works recognizes that an essential contribution to independence for the severely physically handicapped is access to public transportation. Commencing in 1981, the Danish State Railways will provide accessible cars and facilities on long distance trains. Discussions with the State Air Transport Authorities and the Scandinavian Airlines System concerning access to airports and planes are underway. All municipalities provide special buses and taxis adapted to the handicapped. The fare for this service is the same as for public transport. It is offered for transport to and from work and to some degree for shopping, visits, and leisure time activities. Substantial subsidies are available for disabled people to purchase and adapt motor vehicles.

According to Bank-Mikkelsen (1980) another expression

of the growing awareness of the needs of the handicapped lies in the establishment of the Handicap Council, which will include as representatives persons currently responsible for service delivery as well as persons with expertise in housing, regional planning, traffic, work environment, health and social welfare, and training and employment conditions.

Great Britain

Recent findings (Smith, 1980; Laurie, 1977) suggest that in the 1970s, Great Britain significantly improved its efforts to help its severely disabled population. These efforts include: the development of mobility and wheelchair housing within general housing; assistance with adaptations in the home; the growth of housing association movement that is able to respond flexibly to special needs groups and to pioneer unusual independent living arrangements; and the recognition of the need to relieve stress on the families of handicapped people who continue to live at home.

Substantial impetus was given to the independent living movement when a publicity-wise handicapped consumer organization, the Disablement Income Group, mounted a very effective campaign culminating in the passage of the national Chronically Sick and Disabled Persons Act of 1970. This act made it mandatory for local authorities to determine the number of disabled people in their community and assess their individual and collective needs; to provide an effective information service; and to extend the range of their services for the disabled. Further acts of Parliament (the Housing Acts of 1974 and 1980) afford wide discretion for local authorities to assist in the private sector by way of housing improvement grants that are available to disabled people on a wider basis than to nondisabled.

New housing developments for the disabled in Great Britain reflect the desire among disabled people to have the opportunity to choose their own homes. According to survey results reported in a design guide of the British Centre on Environment for the Handicapped, few disabled people felt they would enjoy a special village like Het Dorp, while many regarded as ideal the principle of Sweden's Fokus Society housing.

Official government policy since 1974 has encouraged local authorities and housing associations to build mobility and wheelchair housing. Wheelchair housing was specifically designed for chairbound people and those who need to use a chair in the kitchen and bathroom. Mobility housing was developed starting from the idea that most physically handicapped people can live satisfactory lives in standard housing provided that certain rooms are on the same level and minor details are modified. In her comments about the use of low-cost adaptations in housing, Laurie (1981) explains that the English Department of the Environment, which developed the concept of "mobility housing," estimates that 98 percent of the three million British persons categorized as physically impaired could use mobility housing, while only 2 percent of this population would need special housing.

Although statutory attendant care services recognize the need for support to home care givers, attendants are not usually available at the times when they are most needed, that is, late at night or early in the morning. The report of a seminar sponsored by King Edward's Hospital Fund for England (1980) describes the Crossroads Care Attendant Scheme as a flexible system of locally recruited care attendants available at times that meet the needs of the home care giver. Attendants are found through advertisements in local newspapers.

In Great Britain, the benefits, services, and allowances necessary for a disabled person to live at home are extremely complex. These benefits and services are coordinated by local and national health and welfare authorities. Local authorities provide aids, home adaptations, home helpers, rent allowances, meals on wheels, and residential accommodations, either free or for charges that vary from one locale to another. Health authorities are responsible for home nursing care. Visiting district nurses and other health services are available at the request of the family doctor. National welfare benefits include invalidity pensions and a supplementary mobility allowance or attendance allowance.

As custodial residential care is replaced by adapted housing within ordinary housing projects or by adaptations to existing houses, organizations traditionally involved in residential care have begun to pursue more innovative developments. The Cheshire Foundation for the Sick, a pioneer in providing residential care for the disabled, has recently established so-called bread winner bungalows for couples on the grounds of residential facilities, ground floor apartments for disabled students at Oxford who require personal service, homes for psychiatric after-care, homes for mentally retarded children, and counseling services. The Spastics Society has, since 1957, provided sensitive, enlightened services to cerebral palsied individuals. Gradually shifting its focus towards independent living, it now sponsors such resources as a traveling exhibit of aids demonstrated by an occupational therapist, toy libraries, weekend conferences for disabled persons and staff members, accommodations for severely disabled married couples, and a training college for professional and voluntary staff. The Spastics Society has also sponsored the Holinteg housing project, which provides integrated housing for elderly and disabled individuals in North London. Although the proportion of disabled residents is limited to 25 percent, all units are accessible.

Since the 1974 Housing Act, housing association activity has flourished in Great Britain. Under the act, a housing association grant is available for hostel projects and for projects to meet special needs, including the needs of the elderly and handicapped.

Reagan (1980) describes an interesting pilot project in independent living accommodation. The Grove Road housing scheme at Sutton-in-Ashfield, built in 1973 in association with the Raglan Housing Association, is attracting considerable attention. In this scheme, independent living is facilitated through a combination of housing design, aids, equipment, and a built-in support system. Three ground floor flats for disabled people are connected to three flats for supporting families above by a speech intercom system, enabling the helping families to be called in when needed as agreed in a cooperation clause of the tenancy contract.

Another project, Sheltered Housing for the Disabled (SHAD), has been established to give severely disabled people the opportunity to live in their own houses, enabling them to lead independent and full lives as members of their own community. SHAD's director's house is a prototype for further housing schemes being planned in conjunction with the Threshold Housing Association. Living in the house with the director are four community service volunteers who provide round-the-clock care and support. Volunteers are recruited by Community Services Volunteers, the national volunteer organization, through its one-to-one scheme. According to Laurie (1981), the major housing adaptations include a roll-on–roll-off stairlift and bathroom aids (an autohoist to the bath).

A number of British consumer organizations advocate the rights of the disabled. These include the Spastics Society, the Royal National Institute for the Deaf, the Royal National Institute for the Blind, the Disability Alliance, the Disabled Living Foundation, the Disablement Income Group, the Association of Disabled Professionals, and the National League for the Blind and Disabled (Carnes, 1981). The Royal Association for Disability and Rehabilitation (RADAR) promotes coordination of disablement groups, provides technical information, fosters and funds research, finances diverse projects, and consults with the government on topics important to the disabled.

Canada

In Canada, vocational rehabilitation and independent living services are mandated under the Vocational Rehabilitation of Disabled Persons Act of 1961 and the Canada Assistance Plan. Under the provisions of the Vocational Rehabilitation of Disabled Persons Act, the federal government contributes 50 percent of the costs incurred by a province in providing a comprehensive program for the vocational rehabilitation of physically and mentally disabled persons. A comprehensive program includes such services as medical, social and vocational assessment; counseling; restoration services; and the provision of prostheses, training, maintenance allowances, tools, books, and other equipment. These services are provided directly by the provincial government or purchased from voluntary agencies. Under the Canada Assistance Plan, the federal government reimburses the provinces for 50 percent of the cost of assistance to persons in need and for 50 percent of certain costs of improving or extending welfare services that prevent dependency and help recipients achieve self-support.

In 1977, the federal government adapted and legislated a Human Rights Act protecting handicapped people from discrimination in federal employment. However, as Jones (1979) points out, the act does not provide protection for the handicapped from discrimination in the areas of services, facilities, housing, commercial occupancy and public accommodation. In 1981, the Special Committee on the Disabled and the Handicapped recommended that "physical handicap be a proscribed ground of discrimination for all discriminatory practices listed in the Canadian Human Rights Act" (Smith, 1981, p. 19). Provincial governments, notably those of New Brunswick and Manitoba, have enacted more comprehensive human rights legislation in the areas of public accommodations, services and facilities, property rental and occupancy, publications, and signs.

Falta (1975) describes efforts that have been undertaken throughout the country to make the concepts of normalization and integrated living an integral part of service provision to the handicapped. Canada Mortgage and Housing Corporation was established as a Crown Corporation in 1964 and given the responsibility of administering the National Housing Act of 1944. In a publication entitled *Disabled Persons in Canada* by the Ministry of National Health and Welfare (1980), Canada Mortgage and Housing Corporation is presented as active in promoting barrier-free design and modification of programs to allow construction of a wide variety of accessible dwellings. Furthermore, Smith (1981) explains that it has been recommended that the National Housing Act be amended "to enable groups to develop more nonprofit cooperative and group homes for physically and mentally disabled persons, including clusters of group units in apartment buildings" (p. 73).

A significant development in integrated living in the 1970s is represented by Project Normalization, which was established by a team attached to the Canadian Paraplegic Association (Quebec Division). This project demonstrated that young quadriplegic adults can live happily in independent living units that are barrier-free and require a minimum of design modifications and expense. Instead of specifying special features to be built into apartments, this project has emphasized the use of occupational therapists and industrial designers to teach specific maneuvers and develop simple adaptations that, coupled with good equipment, increase individual functioning. Public agencies responsible for housing, welfare, home care, education, manpower, and transportation provided significant help in designing the overall goals of the project.

Since 1975, the Montreal Municipal Housing Bureau has regularly provided accessible and functional dwelling units in its high-rise projects. The National Building Code of Canada does not prescribe requirements for accessibility for handicapped persons; however, during the 1970s, government departments and provinces increased their commitments to dealing with the problem of access. All ten provinces have amended in varying degrees legislation bearing on accessibility for the disabled. The redesign of social service and health delivery in Quebec has included proposals for decentralized consultation and home services for disabled individuals living in the community. The Department of Education has adjusted student scholarships for the handicapped so that funds for living expenses are available to quadriplegic students residing off-campus.

Numerous transitional homes and apartments for disabled persons discharged from long-term institutional settings have been established over the past ten years and are assisted by the Canada Mortgage and Housing Corporation. Examples include the Paraplegic Lodge in Vancouver, British Columbia; Participation House, in Markham, Ontario; 1010 Sinclair, in Winnipeg, Manitoba; the Wheelchair Housing Centre in Winnipeg, Manitoba; and the Point Pleasant Lodge in Halifax, Nova Scotia. The Cheshire Home Foundation, originally founded in England and chartered in Canada in 1971, operates numerous long-term group homes in Ontario and Saskatchewan to provide a normalized home environment for physically disabled adults. The way of life is as close to normal living as possible, with residents being free to come and go as they choose. Work opportunities are arranged where possible and social activities are organized by the residents (Laurie, 1977).

Falta (1980) describes the integrated housing options in Canada in terms of four principal models.

1. Group homes, which can be of two types: a half-way house accommodating eight to twelve residents and fully staffed on a twenty-four-hour basis, or a smaller home of from three to a maximum of six disabled persons, for whom physical aid is provided by means of a paid live-in helper.
2. A grouping of approximately six to ten handicap-adapted apartment units, dispersed as much as possible within an apartment building. Personal physical help is provided on an on-call basis by a small in-house staff.
3. Adapted apartment units in accessible buildings, located anywhere within the community, where a disabled person can live in a fully integrated manner. Personal attendant services are available once a day on a fee basis.
4. Renovations to render a home or an apartment accessible, utilizing government subsidies.

Because of the different levels of local initiative and government commitment within the ten provinces, wide discrepancies in the actual quantity and quality of housing exist.

As a result of a complaint concerning a disabled person denied access to a passenger train, the Canadian Transport Commission ruled in 1981 that VIA (a Crown Corporation responsible to the Canadian government for providing passenger rail services within Canada) must provide manual lifting service at stations across Canada. It further ruled that self-reliant handicapped persons in wheelchairs should be permitted to travel unaccompanied by an attendant. Attendants with non-self-reliant disabled persons should be allowed to travel free of charge. In a 1980 article, VIA is described as preparing to make new and rebuilt cars, as well as stations, more accessible.

In the past few years, numerous agencies throughout Canada have been involved in the development of integrated living projects that provide disabled persons with comprehensive rehabilitation services. For example, the Canadian Paraplegic Association, with a division in each of the provinces, operates one of the world's largest comprehensive rehabilitation systems for the spinal cord injured. The association supplies and maintains equipment, and provides counseling, employment guidance, vocational training, educational supervision, and assistance with housing and home care services. The Ontario Crippled Children's Centre in Toronto is involved in all phases of the production and delivery of prosthetic devices and houses an internationally known rehabilitation engineering service. The Canadian Rehabilitation Council for the Disabled has recently established a non-profit organization entitled Technical Aids and Systems for the Disabled with the objectives of stocking aids in a central warehouse and coordinating community or provincial delivery systems.

Australia

In Australia, a stronger emphasis has been placed on physical rehabilitation per se than on the broader goals of independent living. Australia, unlike the United States, has no laws mandating specific services for the severely disabled. According to Parmenter (1980), however, both consumers and professionals have been significantly influenced by the development of the Independent Living Movement in the United States.

At present, comprehensive rehabilitation services are primarily developed and delivered by the Commonwealth Rehabilitation Service with support from other government and non-government agencies in the areas of sheltered employment, activity therapy and training, and home care services.

A network of independent living centers is being established across Australia to display and provide information about orthoses, prosthetic equipment, and aids to daily living. The first center was opened in 1977 by a voluntary agency, the Yooralla Society of Victoria. Currently, these centers emphasize display of information relating to the physical aspects of disability. Services for severely disabled individuals are limited, although some counseling is given in the areas of mobility, communication, self-care, home adaptations, and recreation. Because of the country's geographical size and its relatively small population, consumer activity tends to be fragmented and isolated. Thus the projected independent living centers seem an excellent vehicle for enhancing consumer involvement.

Several programs have been established throughout the country to assist severely disabled persons to develop more independent lifestyles. The Yooralla Society of Victoria, in addition to operating an independent living center, also provides a wide range of services and facilities to assist the rehabilitation of physically disabled children and adults. These services include parent and family counseling, short-term care, vocational training, employment in workshops, activity therapy programs, recreation, and accommodation programs.

The House With No Steps in New South Wales, established in 1962 as a sports and social club for the handicapped, has evolved into a network of residences, workshops, and training centers. In 1966, a vocational training center opened to provide an array of vocational and independent living services. Then, in 1969, the project established twenty independent living units for individuals able to live without assistance.

The Phoenix Society in South Australia provides employment under sheltered workshop conditions and, if opportunity exists, in the regular job market. It also offers professional assessment and training in personal care, interpersonal competence, community survival, and work skills. Recreational, social, and cultural activities are also offered by this program.

The Regency Park Center for Physically Handicapped Children in South Australia exemplifies an integrated independent living model that includes intensive training in those skills required to enter either open or sheltered employment. The emphasis of the program is on frequent evaluation of progress, and on integration of work and interpersonal skills training.

International Perspectives

In order to compare development of independent living services in different countries, it is first necessary to understand differences between concepts of independent living. Problems of definition bear both on cross-cultural differences among countries and on differences within a specific country.

As stated in Chapter One, historically there have been two different concepts of independent living in the United States: the professional concept and the consumer concept. Both are reflected in Title VII of the 1978 Amendments to the Rehabilitation Act.

Independent living is defined by most rehabilitation professionals as an alternative to vocational goals. Independent living rehabilitation, as distinct from vocational rehabilitation, includes medical and social services that enable a disabled person to live in the community short of being gainfully employed. According to the consumer concept, however, independent living and vocational rehabilitation are not viewed as competing policy goals. Rather, vocational rehabilitation is seen as subsidiary to the independent living goal: gainful employment is one of several ways a person can become independent. This concept emphasizes a person's ability to become productive not only through employment but also through other contributions to family and community life.

The professional concept of independent living is endorsed by countries such as Sweden, Denmark, and the Netherlands where the government, assuming an almost paternalistic role, provides substantial benefits to disabled persons and spreads the cost of disability throughout the society. The emphasis is placed less on open market employment opportunities than on sheltered workshops, self-care within the home, activities of daily living, and care within the community.

Severely disabled persons in these countries are provided with attractive options to avoid participation in the competitive labor market. They are given opportunities for extended paid education, and educational leave from work is viewed as a right. In addition, semi-sheltered employment is made available in regular places of employment. The Netherlands has the most extensive sheltered workshop system. The system, however, has been criticized for reducing the motivation of disabled persons to seek regular employment.

On the other hand, the professional concept of independent living in Scandinavia differs somewhat from that in the United States. Vocational potential, as defined in the United States, was never an issue in Scandinavian countries. Services for the severely disabled with no vocational potential were not provided in the United States until the passage of the 1978 Amendments to the Rehabilitation Act. However, in most Scandinavian countries these services have been provided since 1960 regardless of the issue of vocational potential. This line of thought represents a strong endorsement of the consumer concept. Consumer groups are highly organized, sophisticated, and financially well-supported in most countries reviewed in this article.

Two features of IL programs in other countries may have implications for the United States because of their importance in minimizing the cost of services. The first is the emphasis on family support services. In Denmark, families are paid to take care of disabled family members. Home care is shown in most cases to be more cost-effective than nursing or hospital care. The second is the preference for simple, low-cost technology over sophisticated environmental adaptations. Two examples cited in this chapter are the Swedish subway station elevators that use escalator tunnels for shafts, and the English concept of mobility housing.

Independent living in the international context is probably best represented by the expression *integrated living*. The extent to which various alternatives to institutionalization satisfy the needs and preferences of disabled persons has yet to be comprehensively evaluated. Likewise, the trade-off between degree of integration and adequate proximity to medical care cannot be expressed in a generally valid equation, but can only be weighed for each individual. Regardless of individual need and preference, however, the available evidence indicates that community placements, even those requiring a full range of modifications and services, invariably prove to be less costly to the community than institutional placements. For this reason, both handicapped consumers and the communities in which they live will benefit from continued examination of international activity in rehabilitation through independent living.

7

Overcoming Distance as a Barrier

John Malcolm Phillips

The goal of this chapter is to show how to ensure that future housing for disabled people and specialized facilities (where they are still necessary) are rationally located with respect both to one another and to all the places that disabled people want to visit. In this chapter I will outline the principles of determining appropriate distance as well as some of the problems involved in implementing such an approach.

Many people do not fully appreciate the emphasis that should be placed on distance in determining the location of housing and other facilities for disabled people. Part of the problem is that most decision makers are mobile. Over short distances, they are able to walk quickly and to carry goods in both hands. Over longer distances, they can use their cars, and can travel on routes of their choice at the times of their choice.

Most disabled people, however, are not so mobile. Many of them must rely on public transportation, for reasons of economy. The options of owning a car or using taxis are generally available only at a considerable sacrifice. Even special buses can be costly to use often. Also, such buses are not available for impulse trips; generally they have to be booked hours or even days in advance. Furthermore, special systems segregate their users from the general public.

Housing and Distance

Before we consider housing options that require little or no transportation, let us define what we mean by housing and distance in this context. Housing for the disabled can be classified in four main types, according to the degree of accessibility each offers the disabled person. *Inaccessible housing* is that which anyone using crutches, a walker, a cane, or a wheelchair would have trouble entering. *Accessible housing* allows any person to enter through the front door and move around in at least some of the rooms. *Mobility housing* is that which anyone using crutches, a walker, or a cane can enter and move around in with ease. A person in a wheelchair can enter each room, although possibly with some difficulty. The main difference between accessible housing and mobility housing is the door widths. *Wheelchair housing* is fully accessible to all disabled people. Design features include wide doorways, extra space for wheelchair maneuvering, and convenient placement of switches, controls, and window handles. Optional features might include height-variable shelving and counters.

Four types of distances should concern us when we consider the location of any facility.

Distances Within a Facility and Within its Grounds. It is to be hoped that in the future there will be fewer buildings for disabled people that will be large in themselves. However, there may be large complexes, covering several acres, with mobility suites and wheelchair suites dispersed among several buildings. In this case, we would be concerned with the total distance from the suites' front doors to the primary contacts.

Distances to Primary Contacts. Frequency and necessity of trips to primary contacts make these distances important. Examples of primary contacts include accessible transit stops or stations, activity centers, bars, places of worship, dentists' or doctors' offices, drugstores, grocery stores, health centers, libraries, banks, meeting halls, and restaurants.

Distances to Secondary Contacts. Distances to secondary contacts are not as important as the *means* of reaching the contacts. If we assume that in the future, some buses on some routes will be accessible, then a convenient bus stop (a primary contact), with reliable, frequent, and direct service is most important. Secondary contacts are often downtown or in a district center. Since many residents may not choose to live downtown, then they must travel to reach secondary contacts. Examples of secondary contacts include department stores; hospitals and clinics; lawyers' offices; the main library; parks and zoos; movies, music, and hobby shows; special events; special stores and offices; theaters; and treatment centers.

Distances to Special Facilities. Distances to any buildings designed to be used by disabled people for recreation, therapy, counseling, or work must be reasonable from the point of view of users who live in the neighborhoods of their choice and must travel to these buildings. This goal can sometimes be achieved by building two or three small facilities in various parts of town rather than enlarging an existing facility or rather than building a large facility to start with. The optimal size of any one facility will depend in part on the population and geographic areas to be served overall.

Establishing Guidelines

Much work has been done in establishing such standards as the minimum width of doors, the maximum slope of ramps, and the ideal height of toilet seats (Goldsmith, 1976). However, there is very little, if any, information on distance as a barrier to people with mobility problems. In part, this is because people with disabilities vary so widely in their abilities and motivation. Moreover, writers and policy makers may be unaware that a more precise standard of distances would be valuable. Instead of precise figures, in the literature references to accessible facilities employ such terms as *close to* and *near*. This allows for great latitude in interpretation.

Several recommendations can be offered to people who

are trying to advise and to legislate on this complex problem. First, the distance problems of different groups should be treated separately. At the very least, the requirements of the mentally handicapped should be considered apart from those of the mobility-impaired. Where a person is disabled in both respects, then the more stringent distance criteria (those that apply to mobility) should be used. Second, maximum distance criteria should be stated as explicitly as possible, even in the absence of research data. Third, maximum distance guidelines need to be developed and incorporated into legislation.

What should the maximum distance be from the door of the mobility suite to a primary contact? At present, physiotherapists and occupational therapists are studying whether such a standard can be set. Until definitive data appears, this writer considers that 800 feet, door to door, is a reasonable maximum in terms of locating mobility and wheelchair units. This limit would apply to the location of buildings frequented by disabled persons who do not own their own cars.

One way to determine reasonable limits is to measure the time required to travel to primary contact points. A person with limited ability to withstand unpleasant or even hazardous conditions, such as low temperatures, should have to spend no more than ten minutes in going to the convenience store (one way). This translates into a distance of 1,000 feet for an active person in a wheelchair, including two street-crossings within that distance, or 500 feet for a person requiring some rest stops or using a walker or canes.

Assessing Variables that Affect Mobility

Several secondary factors need to be considered when determining maximum distances for travel. Obviously, individual ability is the most important factor. A graduate of a rehabilitation center might be capable of performing two-wheel tricks with his wheelchair and capable also of traveling a half mile (2,640 feet) roundtrip to a store and back. However, to a frail elderly lady, incapacitated by arthritis, a travel distance of 400 feet would pose a problem. However, motivation may be an important, although somewhat unpredictable, factor; overall attitude—the degree to which one sees oneself as healthy or sick, happy or depressed—may be involved. The specific occasion will also affect the distance that a person will travel; some trips are simply more interesting or important than others.

Environmental conditions need to be carefully assessed in determining maximum distances. The successful use of canes, walkers, crutches, hand-propelled wheelchairs and powered wheelchairs is, to a large degree, determined by the environment. In every case, distance is a barrier. In addition, anyone using an aid or having problems with balance or limb control experiences the environment in terms of all the surfaces that he or she moves over, sees, and touches: their configuration, their size, their attitude or slope, their width, their breadth. The condition (and even the existence) of sidewalks and streets, the existence of curb cuts or ramps, and the safe operation of properly located traffic lights are all critical factors. One group home that we surveyed looks well-located on the map. But in order to reach the closest grocery store, one must travel along 500 feet of gravel sidewalk to a main road, and then along another 20 feet of sidewalk to a curb ramp leading to a crosswalk at a blind corner. All other stores are over half a mile away. In effect, all the residents of this home are prisoners because they cannot move off their property without help. This is not what is meant by independent living.

Weather can influence mobility from the point of nuisance (wheelchair users' hands become muddy during and after a rain) to the extent of impasse (a snowfall can prevent movement not only while it is still snowing but also until snowbanks or even relatively thin drifts are removed). Extremely hot or cold weather also presents a danger, especially to persons who move slowly.

Yet another difficulty is posed by slopes, which vary from the nearly level to the prohibitively steep. The prohibition point varies with the strength of the person, the length of traverse, and the opportunities to stop and rest at points along the way (American Public Works Association, 1977).

The problem of traffic must be considered both as it is

today and as it is likely to be in the future. In one instance, mobility suites and a group home were provided on a quiet street within easy wheeling distance of a comprehensive shopping center. This journey required crossing at the center of the block, and the practice could be condoned because of the quiet character of the street at the time. Subsequently, street patterns in the neighborhood were changed, and the quiet street became a dangerous one-way thoroughfare with a speed limit of forty miles per hour. To be safe, the journey then required traveling along the street, which has a slope, to an intersection with a traffic light. The one-way distance became 3,000 feet, putting the shopping center out of independent reach by the majority of the residents. Planners should be careful, therefore, to measure *safe* distance, which is not necessarily the direct distance, and ⌄ to try to ensure that the system will not change in the future.

Failures of Planning

The cities we have surveyed demonstrate a relatively low incidence of success in locating housing, despite the availability of advice and despite restrictions set by funding agencies. Although there is, as yet, no evidence to suggest that other geographic areas have had any better success, we urge that evaluations similar to ours be made in other cities.

In a nearly completed study of a Canadian prairie province (Phillips, 1981), this author has found that 76.5 percent of facilities built for people with mobility problems are located more than 1,000 feet from the closest grocery store. In most cases, distances to the post office, the bank, and the drugstore are even greater. Distances were measured from 102 housing complexes the majority of which include several living units. Eighty-eight of these complexes include a significant proportion of wheelchair and mobility units, while 14 consist entirely of specially built units.

Table 1 gives distances from housing locations to convenience stores and grocery stores in two Canadian prairie cities, each with a population of about 500,000. Each location contains from two to five mobility or wheelchair suites, within a larger complex. Table 2 compares distances to various community contact points in four Canadian cities.

Table 1. Distances from Mobility Units to Closest Convenience Store
or Grocery and to Closest Major Grocery.

Distance to Closest Convenience Store or Grocery	Distance to Closest Major Grocery
Of 47 locations measured in City 1:	
38 (80 percent) exceeded 800 feet	40 (85 percent) exceeded 800 feet.
32 (68 percent) exceeded 1,000 feet	34 (72 percent) exceeded 1,000 feet.
14 (30 percent) exceeded 2,000 feet	18 (38 percent) exceeded 2,000 feet.
10 (21 percent) exceeded 3,000 feet	11 (23 percent) exceeded 3,000 feet.
Of 32 locations measured in City 2:	
24 (75 percent) exceeded 800 feet	27 (84 percent) exceeded 800 feet.
20 (63 percent) exceeded 1,000 feet	25 (78 percent) exceeded 1,000 feet.
10 (31 percent) exceeded 2,000 feet	17 (53 percent) exceeded 2,000 feet.
5 (16 percent) exceeded 3,000 feet	7 (22 percent) exceeded 3,000 feet.

Note: Data for both kinds of stores is displayed because convenience stores lack variety, do not necessarily carry all necessities for daily living, and in most cases charge more than major groceries. Thus, some researchers might choose to consider only major groceries.

For several years, guidelines on location have been given in books on planning and in advisory bulletins that are distributed to organizations requesting funding (Canada Mortgage and Housing Corporation, 1977; Goldsmith, 1976; U.S. Department of Housing and Urban Development, 1979). Why, then, has the success rate been so poor?

Clearly, there must be factors that consistently lead organizations away from good planning. The most obvious are the cost of land and the availability of land. Bluntly stated, the importance of distance has been outweighed by considerations of mortgaging and financing.

Part of the problem springs from organizations having been encouraged to use cheap, available land. For example, the Michigan State Housing Development Authority has urged organizations developing group homes to "find sites in the com-

Table 2. Numbers of Locations Exceeding 1,000 Feet
to Community Contacts.

Exceeding 1,000 feet to the closest convenience store *or* grocery:

City 1	32/47	68 percent
City 2	20/32	63 percent
City 3	4/ 6	67 percent
City 4	3/ 3	100 percent

Exceeding 1,000 feet to the closest major grocery:

City 1	34/47	72 percent
City 2	25/32	78 percent
City 3	4/ 6	67 percent
City 4	3/ 3	100 percent

Exceeding 1,000 feet to the closest drugstore:

City 1	37/47	79 percent
City 2	26/32	81 percent
City 3	4/ 6	67 percent
City 4	3/ 3	100 percent

Exceeding 1,000 feet to the closest post office:

City 1	39/47	83 percent
City 2	27/32	84 percent
City 3	4/ 6	67 percent
City 4	3/ 3	100 percent

Exceeding 1,000 feet to the closest bank:

City 1	32/47	68 percent
City 2	23/32	72 percent
City 3	4/ 6	67 percent
City 4	3/ 3	100 percent

munity that can be acquired for very little cost or no cost at all. School boards, city and State agencies, churches, industry and occasionally individuals who are philosophically committed to development of this kind will sometimes provide land at either a minimal cost or donate it" (Michigan State Housing Development Authority, 1978, p. 27).

Some state agencies consider land either as equity or as a statement of serious intent to build on the part of a society. In many instances, a society, frustrated by being unable to find suitable land, will clutch at any possibility, especially if cost is a factor. However justified the motives behind such actions, we feel that they must be reexamined in light of the low success rate in locating the mobility housing units.

Similarly, integration has tended to defeat policies regarding distance. North Carolina's Special Office for the Handicapped states that "residential units accessible to the physically handicapped must not be segregated from other units. For example, in large apartment complexes all the units for the disabled may not be placed in one building but must be dispersed throughout the complex" (Special Office for the Handicapped, 1980, p. 9). However, this means that if a grocery store is 200 feet from one corner of the site, and if the complex is 1,000 feet across, then some living units would necessarily be beyond our recommended travel maximum. Even if the disabled people who inhabited the distant units were able to drive, they would be discouraged from making impulse trips in their wheelchairs.

State and local agencies and private societies should be encouraged to survey a fair sample of their most recent and representative housing for disabled people. By measuring distances to contact points, they would be able to evaluate their success rate for themselves.

Recommendations

What suggestions can we make to improve decisions about site selection in the future? First, each community needs to evaluate its existing mobility and wheelchair accommodations. The study should include a tabulation of distances to the closest community contact points, an evaluation of the actual success of design, and a survey of the occupancy rate of mobility and wheelchair units.

Given present knowledge, however, we cannot predict how many facilities of various kinds each city should build. Perhaps in the next three to five years we will be able to project how many mobility suites, how many wheelchair suites, how many places in group homes and/or cluster apartments, and how many houses modified or built for families should be provided in a city of a given size. Within these guidelines, specific decisions will naturally take into account the needs of the local disabled community.

Caution will have to be used in comparing city with city.

The size of a city will be a factor; larger cities and cities with universities will be likely to have active rehabilitation centers. Rehabilitation program graduates often stay near the centers, partly because of the barriers they encounter in outlying areas. Cities with rehabilitation centers could expect, then, a larger number of disabled people, as could those cities with other attractions, such as a superior climate or a superior network of social services. Other important factors include the age distribution of the population and the nature of industry in the city.

In planning for the future, it would be unrealistic to suppose that any type of housing for disabled people will be fully occupied on opening day. People move for many reasons: they become old enough to leave home, they require a higher level of support services or can manage a lower level, they are evicted, or asked to leave, their economic condition changes, they finish an educational course, they move from another city, or they are discharged from a rehabilitation center or hospital. Clearly, none of these events are controlled by the opening of new housing space.

The prospective tenant wanting to move will have general preferences regarding neighborhood, type of housing, and type of complex in which the housing is situated. He or she may also have specific requirements, such as the need to keep a pet or the need to keep away from animals. Other considerations may include financial limitations, the desire to be on a certain floor, or feelings about residing in a complex inhabited by elderly people. Because of this, any prospective tenant will have a low probability of encounter with any particular housing complex.

Another reason that some disabled people fail to apply for new accessible housing is that they are afraid of the unknown. They prefer to put up with the inconveniences that they know rather than risk a move for conveniences that they fear might cost them more or that might have hidden disadvantages. Therefore, they avoid arranging to move or they cancel at the last minute.

Vacancies occurring at the start-up of a facility must not be criticized. In several cases, nonprofit societies have opened a facility, only to find that it takes a year, or even two years, to fill it to capacity. One can imagine the concern of such a society's board members in the face of criticism from opponents questioning the need for construction of such a facility.

So far, data on the occupancy of wheelchair suites by disabled people are available from only one Canadian prairie city. They show a very low proportion of appropriately occupied suites in that city (see Table 3). It is certain that many wheelchair suites in other Canadian cities are occupied by nondisabled people. In all probability, this situation is prevalent wherever a mechanism for appropriate placement does not exist.

Table 3. Occupancy in One City of Wheelchair Suites
by Disabled Persons.

Agency Providing Suites	Number of Disabled/ Number of Wheel- chair Suites	Percent Occupied by Disabled Persons
Agency A	33/93	35.5 percent
Agency B	5/44	11.4 percent
Agency C	25/63	39.7 percent
Total	63/200	31.5 percent

Note: These suites are all included in larger complexes housing the elderly, low-income persons, and other populations. Seven of these complexes have built-in administrative capabilities that may ensure more appropriate occupancy of wheelchair and mobility suites. If these seven complexes, representing fifty-seven suites, were removed from Table 3, the occupancy rates for Agencies A, B, and C would drop to 24 percent, 0 percent, and 10 percent, respectively.

In order to protect the newly-built or vacant accommodation for use by disabled people funding that will allow empty units must be provided or else a policy that will allow short-term use of the accommodation by nondisabled people must be established. However, no agency is likely to promote the concept of an empty suite very actively, in part because of the importance of satisfying lenders and insurers. The most attractive system would be to lease the space on a short-term basis to a less appropriate tenant. This person must be made to understand that he or she will be asked to leave when a mobility-impaired person applies for tenancy.

A Mobility Accommodation Registry

Developing a mobility accommodation registry would be an important step in matching, appropriately and effectively, prospective tenants with accommodation as it is built or becomes vacant. In cities where such a registry does not exist, newly built, accessible units are likely to be filled by nondisabled people. (I do not suggest a reduction in the number of mobility or wheelchair suites to be built. Having more units than disabled tenants will allow for the predicted future increase in the number of disabled people, and also allow for a diversity in choice of location and type of unit.) The registry should have its office at an accessible location, preferably on several bus routes, and in a barrier-free building. In cities with a population of less than 300,000, the registry could be an adjunct of a larger registry, or of an organization serving disabled people.

In addition to its housing function, such a registry would promote both efficiency and effectiveness. In several cities without registries, it has been found that the majority of mobility and wheelchair units (with the exception of those in specially built projects) are not being used by disabled people. As we have seen (Table 3), one city, in assessing mobility accommodation built integrally with regular housing, found that the number of mobility suites occupied by disabled persons was a very low 63 out of 200, or 31.5 percent. Furthermore, the survey included several large complexes that have organizations that are active in securing disabled tenants; thus, the success rate for those without such organizations was even lower.

Other roles that a mobility accommodation registry can play include:

  Being a resource center for equipment, furniture, and related information
- Providing educational material
- Ensuring that the neighborhood is accessible
- Establishing and administering a system for holding accommodations open for appropriate disabled tenants
- Making recommendations to funding agencies and to legisla-

tors on ways to increase the housing stock most appropriately, based in part on the kinds of research mentioned earlier
in this chapter
- Monitoring adherence to the requirements of the funding
  and/or approving agency
- Monitoring the adequacy of design solutions
- Conducting research; that is, registering preferred accommodations, and surveying perceived needs and problems and
  seeking solutions
- Surveying existing accommodations for effectiveness

The following are crucial features of a registry:

1. Accommodation information. A registry should maintain a master list of accommodations, broken down by type. The
list would be used as an index, and the only information needed
would be a reference number, name (if any), and street address.
A dossier of individual accommodation units would also be necessary. It would include reference number; name of building, if
any; address of building; number and kind of barriers or partial
barriers; distances to community contact points; any restrictions, such as those regarding children and pets; specific suite
number; names of adjacent streets; description of accommodation; floor where accommodation is located; available services, if
any; amount of rent; information on subsidy, if any; name, address, and phone number of contact person; name of owner;
name of funding or sponsoring agency; exterior and interior
photographs; and distances to accessible transit stations or stops.

2. Composite map of the city. A composite map would
consist, in part, of an opaque base map of the city (generally
available from the city's engineering or transportation department), on which would be marked points of interest such as the
downtown area, entertainment centers, hospitals, zoo, and well-
known landmarks. It is useful to show branch post offices, as
their locations indicate business and shopping areas.

Over this base map would be placed one or more trans-
parent overlays, on which the locations of accommodations can
be shown by symbol or colored dot, together with the same reference number that has been used in the master list and dossier.

The precise number of overlays needed would depend on how crowded (and therefore confusing) the inventory of accommodation was.

3. Prospective tenant information. A systematic record would need to be kept of some or all of the following information on prospective tenants: name, address, date of application, type of present accommodation, present rent, disabled person's name (if different from tenant's), age, comparable data on relatives if multiple accommodation is required, special needs (for example, attendant service), preference for furnished or unfurnished accommodation, source(s) of income, maximum rent, moving date(s), name of person who provided referral, preferred area of city, final disposition of case, and date of final disposition.

A Planning Method

Although a registry is the best means of providing disabled tenants with the right housing, it does not necessarily follow that it is the appropriate agency for planning and development. In the first place, planning involves a wide range of facilities, and in the second place, registry staff may be inexperienced in planning.

Any planning method will have to rely in part on data available regionally or locally. In this regard, disabled people, town planners, and health planners represent important human resources. Physically disabled people can provide information regarding where they live, where they would like to live, how they would like to live, and where they want to go. Town planners can provide population data, predict population shifts, predict future changes of traffic routes, advise on the suitability of sites, the existence of barriers, and similar matters, and provide maps, showing streets, bus routes, centers of commerce, recreation areas, neighborhoods, barriers, flat districts, and existing buildings that house or are used by disabled people. Health planners can provide specific population data, other research data, and reproducible models.

Let us now look more closely at some techniques for rational, coordinated planning. Planning facilities for disabled persons involves a number of basic assumptions:

- that there are advantages in having disabled people remain in their own neighborhoods, or live in neighborhoods of their choice.
- that people who have mobility impairments can travel a limited distance.
- that for any population served, the size of the facility is positively correlated with the size of the area from which clients or residents are drawn.
- that there will be accessible buses on some normal city bus routes, that these buses will be of use to some disabled people, and that because of higher capital costs, the buses, and thus the routes, will remain limited.
- that any list of barriers that includes steps, slopes and unsuitable surfaces must also include distances.
- that a range of housing options is advantageous.

With these assumptions in mind, it is possible to begin actual planning procedures. The first step should be to establish criteria for locating any facilities that will be built primarily for physically disabled people. The next step is to agree on the optimal size for each of the facilities that could be provided. Some may not have optimal sizes, but most will. Then, it is important to determine the numbers of disabled people who would make use of each of the different types of facilities. By dividing the number of disabled people in the region needing each type of facility by the size of the facilities, the number of required facilities can be determined. For example, if one hundred persons in a region could benefit by living in group homes, then twenty-five group homes of four persons each, or eight boarding homes of twelve persons each, or any combination of these numbers, would best serve their needs. Projected population figures can be used to give building targets five and ten years into the future.

The next step is to develop a master map for the region. Like a registry map, the map should show streets and block patterns, bus routes and other transit routes, accessible bus routes and stops, and accessible transit stations, post offices, and all existing buildings or parts of buildings used by physically disabled people. From this map, one can determine the best neighborhoods for later location of sites. Conversely, one can eliminate those neighborhoods with known barriers. While it is important to establish priorities for development, it is equally important not to let priorities override opportunities. Once the map is developed, it will be possible to use it to determine the best location for any new building or complex. In both immediate and long-range terms, the result will be a network of facilities that reflects the rational approach taken in the region, incorporating information and ideas from the most knowledgeable people, including some of the users themselves.

Once the registry and planning method are in place, selection of suitable areas on accessible transit routes can begin. Gaps in accommodation can be filled. Barriers around existing housing can be removed. Accommodation can be evaluated, and, where necessary, improved. Selective rehabilitation of older, partially accessible units can take place. Guidelines for designers and developers can be drawn up. They should include such items as instructions to measure distances from the door of the suite rather than the edge of the property. They should also prescribe current technology such as flexible counter heights and appropriate plumbing fixtures to enable the unit to be used by people of varying disabilities or of differing stature, whether disabled or not.

The social and financial benefits of implementing these suggestions are several:

- Disabled persons who can use accessible public transportation will be able to do so most advantageously. This will mean more independence and greater freedom of choice in traveling.
- Those able to use accessible public transportation, and others, can live in the neighborhoods of their choice.
- Sites for buildings and complexes will be chosen with a strong emphasis on the accessibility of the surrounding area.
- All buildings and complexes will be built with a close relationship to other elements of living.

- Governments will have to spend less on special transportation and taxi allowances and will be better able to utilize accessible buses, which are expensive.
- Because of reduced transportation expenses, disabled persons will have more to spend on other items.
- The registry will help ensure appropriate matching of people and accommodations, and minimize the use of wheelchair suites for nondisabled people.

Summary

In this chapter, I have investigated the possibilities of using town planning methods to establish a network of accessible housing and facilities for persons with disabilities. Certainly, many people will choose to live and work outside of the network. But, in the same way that school planners take into consideration the safety and mobility limits of children in locating elementary schools, I advocate city planning techniques that take into consideration the needs of adults with mobility problems. In particular, I advocate a distance limit of 800 feet and the setting up of a registry in each city.

Greater public awareness of the problems of disabled persons is also needed. In two major cities which this writer surveyed, less than 5 percent of the intersections adjacent to wheelchair housing units had curb ramps. While one branch of government had spurred the development of hundreds of mobility and wheelchair suites, another had failed to follow through by linking these suites successfully with the local community. This is but one example among many, but it underlines the need for the kinds of changes suggested here. Buildings are capable of standing for a hundred years or more. The importance of locating them in the right places, from the beginning, cannot be overestimated.

8

Designing Supportive Physical Environments

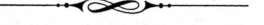

Raymond Lifchez

Until recently, accessibility of the physical environment to handicapped persons has been a peripheral matter in the practice and teaching of architecture. Environments have been designed primarily with able-bodied persons in mind and the consequences of this narrow point of view confront us today; the environment is largely inaccessible and few, if any, design methods recognize the needs of the handicapped user. Recently, however, federal legislation and active campaigning by handicapped persons have resulted in a growing awareness of these needs among architects and architectural educators.

Generally, in their efforts to solve the problems of acces-

Note: This chapter is adapted from *Design for Independent Living: Environment and Physically Disabled People* by Raymond Lifchez and Barbara Winslow (The Whitney Library of Design and the Architectural Press, 1979; University of California Press, 1982). It appeared in its present form in the October 1979 issue of *Archives of Physical Medicine and Rehabilitation.*

sibility, architects and educators have placed undue emphasis on dimensions and abstract performance criteria. But such emphasis only transforms handicapped persons into objects, for example, into wheelchairs with measurable requirements. These are important criteria, but only as adjuncts to the broader issue of life as a handicapped person in a world constructed for the able-bodied. Understanding this issue requires knowledge and empathy on the part of designers, as well as a willingness to learn about the range of disabilities and their environmental consequences.

For several years the author and his colleagues have been working to understand the needs of disabled individuals with regard to the environment. Rather than focusing on activities that are unique to people with severe disabilities, we have studied the wide range of everyday activities common to all people. Through extended interviews and visits with 150 disabled individuals living in Berkeley, we have sought to learn how they experience the physical environment and how they modify it in order to live in noninstitutional settings in the society at large.

From among the many disabled individuals interviewed, seven were designated as key informants, and they are quoted by name in this chapter. They are a diverse group in terms of personality and lifestyle. Disabled people, after all, are not a homogeneous minority; rather, they represent a true cross section of the population. The key informants are alike in one major respect, however: they are all actively pursuing personal goals.

Our study examined the environment at three levels: the intimate, the dwelling, and the community level. This framework allowed us to draw some distinctions between the types of support disabled people require at each level and to better understand the kinds of interactions that occur there. The intimate environment might include the disabled person and his bed or wheelchair or the disabled person in some of his interactions with his attendants. The dwelling environment might include the actual place of residence or places within the community that serve residential functions—places of work, of education, or of social, political, or recreational activities. The community environment includes both the physical environment of the community and the services and supports it provides to the disabled population. This third scale is especially notable as the environment in which the disabled person is least likely to effect permanent changes suitable to personal needs.

Commonly, people who are disabled, ill, or poor exist in a restricted environment at all levels. The scope of their community may be limited due to lack of transportation and inaccessible buildings. Personal and intimate environments are likely to be affected as well, and such people often lack the money and power necessary to achieve desired changes.

Since behavior exists in an environmental context, the fullest kind of human existence is impossible in a severely restricted environment. Mayer Spivak (1973, p. 46) has given us an important and useful concept for evaluating the environment in psychosocial terms. His concept of an *archetypal place* links together the human experience with the environment of that experience.

When . . . people live in environments restricted to a severely limited range of settings in which to carry out all the behavior that constitutes the human repertoire, their ability to function as individuals and family groups, and the integrity and quality of their society may be impaired. People fail to maintain deep lasting interpersonal relationships, they may suffer in their ability to work, provide or eat food, to sleep in deep renewing comfort, play, raise children, explore and protect territory, to meet with their peers, and make decisions which control the shape and quality of life. Each of the foregoing functions, and others, are associated with thirteen characteristic settings in the physical environment, with the rooms and furniture which focus and support behavior patterns in specific and appropriate ways. Such settings, taken together in their smallest irreducible   p, are archetypal places.

In our study, we found Spivak's view useful in assuring that there would be an appropriate breadth to our inquiry. Therefore we chose the concept of archetypal places as an organizing schema.

Spivak's system (figure 1) permits a great number of environmental needs to be organized under a relatively small num-

Figure 1. Generally Related Life Cycle Stages and Tasks.

Life Cycle Stages

A. *Infancy*   Reflex control; orientation; communicate with siblings and parents

B. *Childhood*   Gain motor, social, verbal, intellectual, emotional competence

C. *Adolescence*   Forge identity; establish peer group relations; social/sexual exploration

D. *Courting-Mating*   Group with peers; pair-bond; obtain sexual privacy

E. *Reproduction, Child Care*   Nesting/nurturing; symbiosis; socialization

F. *Middle Life*   Care of aging parents, reemphasis on worldly affairs, redefine identity

G. *Aging Maturity*   Maintain identity, contact, health; accept care by others, mortality

Tasks

1. *Shelter*   Elemental protection; protection for nesting activities; retreat from stimulation, aggression, threat, social contact; emotional recuperation

2. *Sleep*   Neurophysiological processes; recuperation, rest; reduced stimulation; labor and birth, postnatal care of mother and child; death

3. *Mate*   Courting rituals; pair-bonding; copulation; affectionate behavior; communication

4. *Groom*   Washing; mutual grooming

5. *Feed*   Eating, slaking thirst; communication; social gathering; feeding others

6. *Excrete*   Excreting; territorial marking

7. *Store*   Hiding of food and other property; storage; hoarding

8. *Territory*   Spying; contemplation; meditating; planning; waiting; territorial sentry; defending; observing

9. *Play*   Motor satisfactions; role testing; rule breaking; fantasy; exercise; creation; discovery; dominance testing; synthesis

10. *Route*   Perimeter checking; territorial confirmation; motor satisfactions; social and community control

11. *Meet*   Communication; dominance testing; governing; education, worship socialization; meditation; cosmic awe; moral concerns

(continued on next page)

Figure 1. Generally Related Life Cycle Stages and Tasks, Cont'd.

12. *Compete*   Agonistic ritual; dominance testing; ecological competition, inter-species defense; intra-species defense and aggression; mating; chauvinistic conflict

13. *Work*   Hunting; gathering; earning; building; making

Life Cycle Stages and Tasks Related

A. 1. Protection from elemental extremes; explore dwelling. 2. Recognize bed; learn daily rhythms. 3.— 4. Lose fear of wet face, sudden temperature change; regular grooming as primary contact ritual. 5. Regulate feeding satisfactions. 6. Discover excretion as separate from self; associate with setting and time. 7. Acquire confidence in food abundance. 8. Identify bed as primary secure place. 9. Explore close environment; develop manipulative, cognitive skills. 10. Route connects parts of shelter structures, provides orientation and change; motor satisfaction. 11.— 12. Master frustration in competition with siblings for attention and toys. 13. (See 9).

B. 1. Differentiate subsettings; retreat from overstimulation, threat; emotional recuperation. 2. Associate bed with fatigue; learn volitional control of sleep; illness and recuperation. 3.— 4. Learn to bathe, dress oneself. 5. Coordinate feeding tools; communication; differentiate food from symbiotic source in mother. 6. Autonomously control excretion. 7. Learn to prepare food. 8. Establish play "turfs"; orient to neighborhood; play protect territory from lookout; plan, wait. 9. Role modeling; interact with peers; fantasy, exercise, exorcism, creation, discovery, dominance testing. 10. Enlarge route maps; differentiate settings, provide social encounters; learn safe wandering limits. 11. Regular play/ meeting rituals and places; elaborate functions; dominance testing. 12. Games; fight; agonistic ritual; dominance testing. 13. Acquire intellectual, motor skills.

C. 1. Find alternate private shelter; auto, attic, stairwell. 2.— 3. Meet with opposite sex in private, public settings; obtain sexual privacy anywhere: autos, barns, etc. 4. Groom for mating encounters. 5. Communicate with peers over food and drink. 6. Privacy in excretion. 7.— 8. Expand territory into intellectual domains, job. 9. Learn autonomous hobbies. 10. Provide social contact with opposite sex. 11. Meet with peers, both sexes; establish new rituals. 12. Sexual display: cars, sports, clothes (see 3). 13. Refine work skills.

D. 1. Find new shelter. 2. Share bed with mate. 3. Select mate; achieve couple privacy. 4.— 5. Share food with mate; increase food abundance. 6.— 7. Enlarge larder for family. 8. Expand territory to include mate. 9. (See 12.) 10. Maintain community of contacts. 11. Meet with couples. 12. Personal display, ecological, mating competition. 13. Apply skills toward life support.

E. Expand shelter for offspring (see 5). 2. Maintain sexual privacy against invasion by new young family. 3.— 4.— 5. Increase abundance; feed

Figure 1. Generally Related Life Cycle Stages and Tasks, Cont'd.

family; gather, communicate w/ family. 6.— 7. Increase capacity and variety of food. 8. Expand territory to include young and check frequently. 9.— 10.— 11. Expand functions, contacts; governing, educating, mystical awe. 12. Display in common values; conspicuous consumption. 13. Improve capacities, performance.

F. 1. Shelter contracts as young leave. 2. through 7— 8. Territorial needs contract as young leave shelter. 9 through 13 XX

G. 1. Maintain location or adjust to imposed change; adapt surroundings to needs. 2. More time in bed, sleep less; possible confinement, compression of world to bedside. 3. Adjust sexually to changing libido; possible illness or loss of mate (see 2). 4. Possible inability to care for self. 5. Arrange special diet; reduction of taste, smell spectra. 6. Possibly require aid and equipment; lowered mobility may reduce functional dependability. 7. Possibly require assistance gathering and preparing food. 8. Passive observation of archetypal activities performed by others. 9. New leisure activities to fit changing capacities. 10. Reduction in home range scale; fear of exposure to attack. 11. Need for contact with and support from peers. 12. Probable withdrawal from competition/defeat by young; defensive, evasive postures. 13. Less active roles within former context; fend off retirement.

Source: Spivak, 1973, p. 46. Used by permission.

ber of basic human requirements, so that the former can be seen as nuances of the latter. Thus, for example, the need for security, in its many forms, can be discussed under the more general rubric of *shelter*; in this way the breadth of requirements the residential environment must meet in order to adequately satisfy this basic need can be indicated.

Of Spivak's thirteen archetypal tasks *shelter* and *mate* present two very different sets of issues. Shelter is so commonplace a need that it is here we normally focus our attention in achieving an accessible environment and it is here that some of the most interesting innovations are made in tuning personal space to personal needs. Mate, on the other hand, is a difficult concept because able-bodied people do not usually think of physically disabled people as sexual beings. This stereotyping has had negative repercussions on the way physically disabled persons see themselves. Therefore, it is important to present here the whole-bodied perspective of those who have physical disabilities.

Shelter

Shelter can be broadly viewed as a place of retreat: a place to escape from aggression, stimulation, threat, social contact, and the elements, and a place for nesting activities. The behavioral needs that are met by shelter are physical comfort and security. These needs exist in a continuum from the intimate to the community level and must be satisfied at each level.

An important aspect of growing up and developing a full set of environmental expectations is the evolution of a concept of personal shelter. From infancy, children begin to seek a shelter, first by crawling into and under things, hiding in small places, and selecting a small corner rather than a whole room as the setting for their play. As they grow older, this need is expressed by building forts and treehouses, digging caves, and fiercely protecting *their* property. Adolescents express their developing independence by seeking an alternative shelter; the car or van, the attic or basement room, the distant city to which one runs away in fantasy or reality are substitutes for the rejected shelter offered by and tied to the family. Ultimately, leaving the family home to live alone or with a mate is a cultural signal of independence; it is a sign of being grown up and assuming the rights and responsibilities of adulthood.

Each of these maturational experiences is laden with symbolism. Both in the mind of the maturing child and in the eyes of the world, the gradual development of independence is tied to the expression of a separate shelter. Confidence in the ability to do things for oneself is built by gradual successes in the effort to make a place of one's own; personal as well as geographic boundaries are developed by the possession of a space whose access can be controlled by the individual.

Those who are disabled from early childhood often miss or only partially experience these activities. They may be so sheltered by concerned parents that there is no need or opportunity for them to develop a concept of shelters on their own. Playing outdoors without attendance is almost impossible in a wheelchair. Those classic child-made environments, forts, are generally inaccessible, and treehouses are hopelessly out of reach. The severely disabled child, under the best of circumstances, may be excluded from play with others that involves creating shelters. Alone, the effort required, the difficulty of handling materials, and the need for assistance are enough to overwhelm most efforts.

Shelter is often viewed by the disabled child as the protection and comfort that is provided by others. He is likely to view himself as having little influence on his surroundings: adaptations and changes are made by others. Because the spaces he occupies are rarely his own, the disabled child often lacks privacy. There are no places in which to hide, no retreats from other people. Mary Ann recalls her childhood as a time of always being protected and sheltered, looked in on, and cared for. Confined to a wheelchair that she could not move herself, Mary Ann could never retreat. The expressions of distress so common to the escaping child—slamming the door, hiding behind the furniture, locking oneself in one's room—were not available to Mary Ann.

Adolescence is usually a time of testing. Many small separations are undertaken in preparation for the larger separation to come. Among able-bodied people, resolution of the endless and inevitable conflicts of this age is often reached by separation. The adolescent finds alternative places with an identity that belongs to him and perhaps to his peers. The room is only one alternative among many. Teenagers frequently choose to be absent from the home to find alternative environments. For some disabled teenagers, their room may begin to serve this function. One young disabled woman describes her room as her "home base." She spends all her time there surrounded by her own things, maintaining her privacy by escaping into continuous schoolwork, an escape acceptable to both herself and her parents. However, there are inevitable difficulties in changing the image of a room that has functioned as a symbol of unity with the family into one that symbolizes independence. These problems are heightened if the room must also serve as the scene for family assistance in moving about, bathing, and so on.

As adults, most people have the experience of selecting, acquiring, modifying, and occupying a home or shelter of some form. This home is important not only for all its practical functions as a shelter but also as a symbol of self or, in Clare Cooper's terms, an image of its occupant that is constant in his own eyes and in those of the community (1974, p. 144). For the disabled individual, there has been little opportunity, historically, to create this symbol. Houses or institutions were selected, built, and adapted to meet the needs of caretakers. With increasing numbers of independent disabled people, however, the situation is changing.

Numerous severely disabled Berkeley residents own or occupy homes alone or with others and find it rewarding. John takes an active role in planning and controlling his personal environment and associates this with good health, building self-confidence, and discovering himself.

Conflicts sometimes arise from the necessity for environmental appendages, which ensure access to a home but also declare the disability of the occupant to the world. Carmen's house has two large and essential ramps to permit wheelchairs to travel from the house to the garden and from the garden to the street; both ramps are disguised as part of the garden itself, invisible from the street. The reasons are both practical and psychological. The police recommend locating ramps where they will not call attention to the increased vulnerability of the occupants. At the same time, Carmen wants the house to look as normal as other houses in the neighborhood. Ramps do not fit the image of normalcy.

The problem of selecting, adapting, and occupying a house of one's own is further complicated for the individual who has been disabled from birth or early childhood. Lack of experience in controlling the surroundings, either directly or by directing assistants, presents major difficulties for newly independent home seekers who are armed only with a brief experience at a rehabilitation center or with no experience outside of the family home or convalescent hospital. They must deal with an unfamiliar and complex set of realities in their search for shelter. Housing must be found that is accessible. Too often, a lack of understanding of all aspects of accessibility, such as room and door sizes, counter heights, or turning radiuses, prevents even essential needs from being met.

Finding and adapting acceptable housing that integrates with the network of community association and services and that provides security and elemental protection can offer psychologically rewarding experiences on both the personal and interpersonal levels.

The Intimate Environment. The most intimate forms of shelter are associated with personal space. Clothing and protective devices, such as umbrellas or sunglasses, offer both elemental protection and some shelter from psychological invasion. For disabled people, these devices are supplemented by prosthetic devices and equipment. The wheelchair is so closely related to its occupant that it extends both the physical and psychological space occupied by the individual. While it provides a protective metal shell in the material sense, it also makes the occupant more visibly distinct and psychologically accessible to those who do not see disabled persons as people with the same rights to privacy as others.

On the personal scale, basic needs are related to physical and emotional security. The immediate surroundings of most disabled individuals include a variety of devices—manual, mechanical, and electrical—that enable them to meet their basic needs. Varying in nature from catheters and legbags through wheelchairs and mechanical beds to electric door openers and voice-responsive phones, these devices extend a person's existing abilities and furnish the assistance he requires to make possible an independent life. If these devices fail, many disabled people are literally helpless. Late-night wheelchair breakdowns have left many stranded on the street, immobile and vulnerable.

Electrical failures can both immobilize electric wheelchairs and deactivate voice-responsive telephones. The most minor accident, such as dropping the slideboard used for transferring, can isolate a disabled person in a situation that he may be unable either to change or to leave. Physical security at the personal level implies the need for backup systems for any crucial electric or mechanical device, because any such device can fail. This need is frequently met by the presence of other people who can assist in emergencies, particularly able-bodied individuals. Being dependent on attendants or machinery and being helpless for those hours of the night when there is no one around to help decreases feelings of security. As Mary Ann, who has a disabled roommate, notes, "You think about being alone at night, thinking that if something happens at night, you can't get yourself out of bed, like in a fire or something."

Physical security for the disabled person can mean more dependence on elemental control than it does for the able-bodied person. Spinal cord injury frequently affects the metabolism; the body is less able to adjust to temperature change and may be unable to sweat. The usual responses of exercising to warm up and of sweating to cool down are not available, so comfort is possible only at temperatures within a restricted range. Tom's room is always kept between 70° and 80°; his windows are not open on even the hottest days, in part because of the great difficulty of opening windows without assistance. Lennis can frequently be found sitting in the full sun, often wearing a sweater and often slightly sunburned. One of his major requirements in choosing a place to live is that the windows face south or west so that he can sit in the sunshine. For individuals with metabolic dysfunction, it is essential to provide a heating system that permits each individual to control the temperature and ventilation of the space he occupies.

Other disorders, such as multiple sclerosis, tend to reduce tolerance for heat; comfort may be possible only in spaces that are cool and breezy. Two male informants, both afflicted with multiple sclerosis, have chosen apartments with large windows that can be fully opened. They prefer natural air currents to the chill of air conditioning.

For individuals with temperature sensitivity, a major requirement is flexibility and the opportunity to control comfort personally. Responses to this need vary from being prepared with extra sweaters and jackets (kept within easy reach and carried on all excursions), to keeping the body constantly supplied with liquids (a water bottle or glass and straw are permanently affixed to many wheelchairs), to restricting the selection of spaces in which to live and work to those with accessible and flexible temperature-control systems.

Dealing with the elements is often complicated by various factors related to disability. Asked about how she deals with the elements, Mary Ann responded, "I hate them all. Rain makes your wheels and brakes slip, and it's hard for cars to see you. Cold makes your circulation poor." In Berkeley, the weather is usually mild, it almost never snows, temperatures are moderate, and rains are confined to a few months of the year. Passivity tends to be the common approach to elemental protection there. When the weather is inclement, activities that necessitate going outdoors are simply postponed.

Lennis, who describes himself as a "flexible survivalist," says, "I deal with the problem by contingency planning. For instance, if I need to miss a class, I make sure I have all the books and there is someone there who will take notes for me. I just have to switch gears, not let the situation bring me to a grinding halt."

Other souls can be seen in the midst of rainstorms in a wide assortment of protective coverings. Hoods, capes that cover the back of the chair and keep the seat as well as the driver dry, and umbrellas that are fitted into special slots on the back of the chair are common. Two of our informants described the devices they would most like to see invented for use in rainy seasons. One was a hood similar to that on a baby carriage, which would fold away but always be there when needed, and the other was a "golf cart type cover, a canopy which would keep the whole chair dry."

John finds the elements a pleasing aspect of the environment. "Berkeley is an accepting place. It has places of power. The bay is like open arms to fog, ocean, the elements. I see more people enjoying the rain here than in other places."

Security from the threat of physical harm by others is a constant concern for many wheelchair occupants. They feel that the chair itself is an advertisement of their vulnerability and inability to resist attack, and many regard themselves as moving targets for purse snatchers and muggers. A less obvious threat is posed by the unconscious fears and hostilities many people feel toward disabled people. While typical street violence may be avoided by careful selection of times and routes, the danger of unpredictable violent assault by an individual who feels threatened by disabled people can inhibit potentially rewarding contacts.

Peter stresses that while security is an important consideration, and one that he is constantly aware of, "danger is just a part of it all; part of being disabled is accepting that a lot of things are going to be harder, more time consuming, less safe. Most of us are very accustomed to being in some form of danger. We are susceptible to infections, injury, and so on; but you can't let that get in the way of leading your life. So, you just accept the danger, and if you want to do something, you do it."

One can never be certain about security from attack. Most disabled people are extremely careful in their planning to avoid areas that have a dangerous reputation, time periods during which streets are likely to be deserted, situations in which they are likely to be isolated with an unknown individual. The desire avoid difficult situations, however, may result in spending more time at home than is actually desired.

The Dwelling Environment. The dwelling provides the primary shelter; it offers a retreat from all hostile forces and provides comfort. For most disabled individuals, the dwelling is the only environment in which a real sense of both physical and emotional security is possible. The importance of direct control of the surroundings is a critical element in this feeling. The home of the disabled person is generally more specifically adapted to the needs of the individual than that of an able-bodied person.

The dwelling must serve as a sure escape from threatening situations. This implies ramps that are easily maneuvered, no barriers like curbs at streetside, and door hardware that is workable. Handles with lever action, keys on extenders, adequate space for wheelchair manipulation to open and close doors, good lighting, and accessible doorbells are some common adaptations. Special devices such as intercom locking devices controlled from the bed are also in use.

Once indoors, the disabled person must feel secure from invasion. Locks must be effective and easily operated. Many of the best locks in terms of security are dependent upon small-muscle control for their operation; large-scale versions which are more manageable or differently designed are preferable. One informant noted:

> When I go out, I lock everything—every window. When I come back it's really hot, but it's better than being ripped off. I'm not as worried about being ripped off in this place, 'cause while this place is accessible, I really go to great pains to see that it doesn't happen; and after I've done all I can, if it happens, it happens, and well, I am insured and I do have my stuff marked with my name. I will keep my doors locked if I'm not expecting anybody. And the whole thing behind that is that I have taken a self-defense course, and I would give somebody a pretty good battle. I'm most vulnerable when I am lying down, it's sort of like someone pulled the plug on me. But it's not one of those things that I can just sit around and worry about all the time.

Windows that permit the occupant to see the visitor before admitting him are important. They must be low enough to be used from a wheelchair and located so that the chair can be moved into an effective viewing position. For those who are restricted to a single room, a voice-activated communications and access system may be desirable.

To find an effective balance between security and social isolation is a problem for those who need to spend long periods of time in bed and who cannot leave the bed without assistance. Admitting visitors personally is impossible. There are various ways to handle this problem. Peter often leaves his door open; visitors and attendants come and go freely, and he counts on the constant flow of a number of people through his home to provide security. His apartment is located in a building in which neighbors can hear any disturbance, which supports this approach, as does his decision to share his apartment with another active disabled man, who also brings a steady stream of visitors into the space.

Carmen handles the problem by sharing the space with a number of able-bodied people who can respond to visitors. Regular callers are given keys and the doors are kept open during active hours. Mary Ann and her roommate solve the problem by giving keys to attendants and other frequent visitors. They schedule all other visits in advance so that they are prepared to greet the guest. Due to the high turnover of attendants and the inherent danger of distributing many keys, this approach requires periodic lock changes.

The security problems posed by the necessity of hiring attendants and providing them with access before their reliability has been proven is a constant worry for disabled people. Attendants are often hired from among street people. Most are conscientious, reliable, concerned, and value working with people. However, others are untrained, irresponsible, or simply out to take advantage of an easy victim. Stories are told about homes robbed after attendants were hired, given keys, and then never seen again. Screening programs and referral systems attempt to control this problem, but the undeniable vulnerability of those who are dependent on assistance is a continuing problem that even the security of the dwelling cannot overcome.

A sense of security is sometimes enhanced by the presence of a telephone, which provides another means of communicating with people. This link with help, however, is not always reliable, particularly when it cannot be easily or quietly employed. Lennis described an uncomfortable situation in which he heard someone in the next room at about three o'clock in the morning. It turned out to be his attendant, but Lennis had some uneasy moments; he hesitated to use his phone line to call for help because when it is activated, anyone in the next room can hear the operator come on the line. When asked if he would feel more secure if there were a lock on the door between the bedroom and living room and on the door between the bedroom and bath, he answered that if he put so much hardware on the doors, he would be in danger of being locked in. He felt that security was, to a large extent, in his own mind.

Too often such concerns as effective security or adequate protection from the elements while entering or leaving a dwelling must be relegated to the status of luxury items. Merely finding a building with an accessible entrance and adequate space in the interior poses monumental problems. Gary has experienced many difficulties simply in finding minimally acceptable housing.

Most apartments, particularly in the newer buildings, are cramped. There's just not enough room to move around. The biggest hassle has been hallways and making turns in hallways. This place that I'm living in now, the hallways are relatively wide in comparison to the other two places that I lived in. I guess that's the first thing; basically, if you can find an apartment that is in an older building, like this, you've got half a chance. If you're going to be moving in with another crip, you'd best get two bedrooms, particularly if there are two electrics; otherwise it's just too cramped. As far as closet space and stuff like that, this is the first apartment where I could even get near the closets. . . .

We'd looked at three or four places, and we said, well, okay, this place is still cramped, but we can do it. For almost a year we did it. And for me, I guess, I'm in a better position to try out things like that, because I'm not, say, a quad or someone who has limited use of their hands. I have good use of my hands and arms, [but still] you develop all kinds of weirdass ways to get in and out of doorways; I mean, I can remember times when I would use my head to help myself get out of a doorway if I had to put some extra push on the chair. I would get myself up against the chair and try to push myself out of the door, and maybe one end would go and the other end would get stuck, so maybe I would have to use another portion of my body to open the door or something like that. When you're in a cramped environment, you learn to use everything you've got, and that can be anything from one extra finger that you didn't think you'd have to use to using your leg to kick something.

Shelter has strong psychological overtones. As well as offering security and access, it must provide the symbols of comfort. Returning to the hearth is more than a literary cliché; the presence of a visible heat source like a fireplace or a sunny, protected patio is an important element in the concept of dwelling. Heating systems that offer even and controlled temperatures are important for the maintenance of physical comfort. Heat sources that offer varying degrees of warmth and the opportunity to adjust to the source are emotionally important. Any heating system to be used in the home of a disabled person should be designed to be easily operated with minimal muscle control. In addition, surfaces that can become hot and cause burns must carry visual warnings as some disabilities destroy those sensations that warn of burns or other injury.

In extreme climates, metabolic problems may tend to confine some people to the home unless temperature-controlled access to transportation is available. Sheltered access to the garage or a heated garage may be a necessity rather than a luxury. A sheltered front entry is important for those who require time to operate locks and opening devices, and nonskid surfaces on outdoor paving may be necessary for those who do go out in rainstorms.

The Community Environment. At the community level, one of the most important aspects of shelter is its environmental message. A town like Berkeley, which has demonstrated its concern for the welfare of the disabled population with visible acts such as curb cuts, timed stoplights, and ramps, sends a message to disabled inhabitants and visitors that clearly says: You are welcome here; this place offers shelter and concern. The physical environment was frequently the first subject mentioned by the informants in discussing Berkeley. It induced an immediate sense of security for many upon their arrival. Said one: "If they care enough to make things physically accessible, which was never true anywhere else, I think that probably they will also be more accepting of me personally."

Berkeley also offers shelter for a wide range of public and semipublic activities. Most restaurants are accessible and have come to function as common gathering places in which one can find shelter from the elements and social companionship. While the private homes of the vast majority of the population cannot be entered, such public facilities play a particularly important role in social interactions among able-bodied and disabled people. They provide both an arena in which to meet and a ground upon which the two populations can participate equally.

Mate

The rituals of mating include courting, pair bonding, expressions of affection, communication, sexual expression, and child care. The formation of intimate relationships and the expression of the feelings generated in these relationships are an important dimension in the lives of disabled people.

Perhaps the most important aspects of mating or courtship are the validation it offers of a person's worth and the meaning it often appears to impart to life. A paraplegic man says, "Being disabled, I feel alienated. I want to be—I like to feel I'm still sexually attractive, seductive. How can I be appealing if I'm still in a chair? I've come to realize life has to offer something more than sex. I'm now searching for that meaning. I want to feel alive."

Children pattern their play and their plans for the future after the behavior of the adults around them. One of the most important aspects of this patterning is the concept of family: of marriage and the possibility of having children as expressions of adulthood. This process is as important in the development of most disabled children as it is in the lives of their able-bodied peers. They grow up as part of a family, and their expectations for the future may include the development of their own family. While this may be accepted within the families of disabled people, who see them as whole persons, it is frequently a difficult idea for outsiders to grasp. Some families raise disabled children under the false expectation that they will remain children, cared for by the same family group through adulthood. A few anticipate institutionalization.

Major problems for many disabled people occur as a result of society's unwillingness to view them as sexual beings and potential mates. Institutions traditionally treat them as children, separating the sexes and regarding expressions of affection as a perversion or inappropriate behavior that must be discouraged. Troubled by this negative image, the disabled person must also deal with cultural images that associate sexuality with physical perfection and beauty. As Tom says: "I see myself as having sexual potential, as having marriage potential, but if you took twelve women off the street and lined them up to look at me, I wonder what they would see?"

One effect of this prejudice can be seen in the continuing efforts of the informants to change attitudes. As Peter says, "If there's a little kid on the street and he asks, 'What's wrong with you?' there is a certain responsibility to educate him in disability. The answer must be calm and direct and honest. You are always sort of a representative, and you can influence his attitudes in later life."

In Berkeley, some changes in attitudes can already be seen. John says, "Before I came to Berkeley, I had career potential and I've realized it. Berkeley told me I had sexual potential as well, which means that in some way the community must recognize it. Career potential is always there, but before coming here I was confronted by an attitude toward me of my being asexual. It goes along with the stereotype. The best sex comes from the best-looking people. Righteous turn-on! Rehabilitation center turn-on! People see a disabled person least of all as an ideal society member. It is only since coming to Berkeley that I can see myself as a person important to society."

Developing reasonable expectations of oneself and finding potential lovers are difficult tasks for all adolescents. The teenager who has been disabled from birth must throw off a lifetime of societal assumptions as well as battle the physical difficulties of making contact. Newly disabled people must reassess their own value system, which had awarded points for beauty and athletic prowess. Peter uses the term *physicalism* to describe the value structure that must be overcome; like racism and sexism, it is often particularly important in relationships between the sexes.

The Intimate Environment. Privacy is essential for the development of close relationships and for sexual expression. The problems of working things out so that it is possible for a relationship to begin, develop, and possibly become intimate are particularly difficult when environmental barriers stand in the way. Tom describes his frustration in pursuing relationships that m to show promise: "I used to live in a first-floor apartment with David. The woman upstairs and I were very close. We spent a lot of time together, but there was no elevator so I never saw her apartment, and I had a roommate so we were never alone. There was just nowhere to go. Maybe it wouldn't have worked out anyway, but it never had a chance."

The adolescent years for disabled people can be particularly difficult in this respect. Most teenagers use pushchairs and are dependent upon the aid of parents or friends to move around. Making acquaintances under these conditions is difficult, pursuing them impossible. The acquisition of an electric wheelchair can radically change the life of a person who has rarely had any real privacy; it offers the opportunity to go somewhere alone, to make one's own choices, to control one's mobility. It can permit a relatively equal status among partners in a relationship, even for the severely disabled. When both partners can move about independently and take care of themselves, there is less need for the more able-bodied partner to assume a caretaker role. One Berkeley woman who is slightly disabled herself recently returned from a vacation with a more severely disabled friend. From her unique perspective as both an able-bodied and a disabled person, she expressed her understanding of the difficulties of sustaining a relationship complicated by disabilities: "If you're the person causing the problem, you feel responsible. It can complicate relationships. In some ways, our vacation was a hassle just keeping from becoming upset or making him feel like a burden; yet I had one of the better times of my life just because of who I was with."

The issue of dependency in a marital or romantic involvement is a serious problem for many disabled people; even in cases where the disabled partner has led a fairly independent life prior to involvement there is a constant danger of falling into patterns that lead to dependency. Tom, divorced after eight years of marriage, is now amazed by the extent to which he had become dependent without understanding the destructive effects it was having on his relationship with his wife. A strong quadriplegic, Tom now does everything for himself; he cleans, cooks, drives, works, bathes, and writes without assistance. When he needs help with tasks requiring special dexterity, he hires someone to perform them. Yet, during his marriage, his ability to take care of himself was so eroded that his wife's most serious concern when she left was that he would be completely incapable of managing the simplest tasks alone.

The major factor in the development of this dependence was Tom's failure to adapt the environment to his needs: "It just didn't seem necessary. She drove the car, and as long as I was a passenger and had some help we managed. She did most of the cooking and so forth. It was easier for her and we couldn't change things easily. If she helped me get dressed and pushed me to the bus stop, we could both sleep longer."

The importance of organizing the environment so that each disabled person can meet his needs without burdening a relationship cannot be stressed enough. Attendants who have become emotionally involved with their employers universally emphasize the importance of terminating the professional relationship if they wish to maintain the emotional one. The intensity of physically caring for someone has a dual character; it leads to the development of attractions and closeness and then destroys the same closeness when the caretaking becomes a necessity, neither a free choice made from love, nor a job which can be completed and left, physically and emotionally.

Carmen says, "You should never make a lover out of an attendant. It's true about the mystery—familiarity does breed contempt. On the other hand, it is good to have as a lover someone who has been an attendant to someone else. They understand." When an attendant does become a lover, however, the role must be redefined.

The Dwelling Environment. The homes of disabled people are often the homes of a family—houses containing children, friends, pets, and mates, in addition to the disabled individual. There has been a prevailing tendency for designers to view disabled people as isolated from social contacts and associations. When disabled people are regarded as members of a family, the tendency has been to treat them as a special case, and provide a specially equipped sick room and a space near the kitchen so the homemaker can also function as a caretaker. The rest of the family lives apart.

While this pattern is not appropriate for anyone who is truly regarded as a family member, it is still a spatial necessity in many homes. Two-story houses make up a large part of the residential stock of this country and the upper half is usually inaccessible to the disabled person. When a family member becomes disabled, and the existing home has no accessible private space, arrangements are often made that are difficult for everyone. In one case, the dining room was the only possible place for a disabled young man. His room functioned, however, as a corridor to the kitchen, denying him any real privacy. Furthermore, it could not be closed off completely from the living room and lacked a full bathroom. He was in the unfortunate position of both feeling guilty for the inconvenience of his presence and resenting the lack of any real comfort. The likelihood of a member of any family suffering a temporary or permanent disability is high and should be considered in planning any home.

For the many disabled individuals who do lead active sex lives, both the environment and the personal support system must be arranged to make lovemaking comfortable and convenient. Often, there are the complications of prosthetic devices and transferring, which require the aid of a skilled attendant. Carmen, describing the problems she finds in lovemaking, says: "Most men don't know how to get past the wheelchair, and I don't know how to get past the iron maiden myself. Making love with me is a real trapeze act—the first time is uncomfortable, a little frightening. A lot has to do with bladder problems and my catheter. And there's the time thing: you can't just jump up, take a shower, and douche, and be done. You need all those other hands. By the time you've taken care of one night, you're into the next."

Mary Ann commented on the added complications when the relationship involves two disabled people in wheelchairs. Like many other facts of life for the disabled, lovemaking cannot be totally spontaneous. "You have your plan when you want to go to bed; it can be worked out. It can be any kind of situation when two people become interested in each other. It might be two disabled people with an attendant." Arranging a bedroom space so that it permits sexual relationships to take place with whatever assistance is required, and with privacy as well, is essential.

The Community Environment. The tendency to view disabled people as leading rather isolated existences, or at least relating primarily to other disabled individuals, is reflected at the community level in seating arrangements for disabled people that ignore the presence of a partner. One young woman, frustrated by attending numerous movies and concerts separated from her date, proposed a folding seat for the side of her wheelchair which would permit her date to sit close at hand. "As it is," she says, "when I go out with someone, we are so separated by the chair that he never even gets to put his arm around me. There is no easy sort of progression."

When a couple who are both in wheelchairs are on the sidewalks, a different spatial problem occurs. Two chairs are frequently too wide to travel side by side and when they follow each other, communication is impossible. The most comfortable position for talking appears to be side by side, but facing in opposite directions—an arrangement that also tends to block sidewalks unless a widened area is provided.

The community also tends to express its reluctance to accept disabled people as sexual individuals in the design and operation of hospitals and care facilities. Rooms are rarely provided that have space for a mate to visit for even temporary stays. Beds tend to be single, and privacy is often limited. "For the patients' protection," bedrooms can rarely be locked from within. Such "hands off" messages sent by the environment are reinforced by policy.

In the last analysis, the individual environment—that is, the dwelling, workplace, communal space, and so on—works well only in the broader context. For the dwelling or workplace to be truly accessible, the town or community must have a critical mass of physically disabled residents, a cohort who recognize and support their connectedness. Out of this connectedness spring the small, discrete acts of sharing and communicating between people who understand one another because they share experiences in life and the goal of independent living. Out of this same connectedness springs an awesome potential for political activism, which can help ensure the rights and privileges of those with physical disabilities.

The existence of such a cohort spurs the development of a network of legal assistance, medical and attendant care referrals, equipment service, transportation, housing, jobs, recreation, and other social services. These services are designed to be highly responsive to the special needs of physically disabled persons living in a particular community. Like pioneers in a new territory, the physically disabled often discover their connectedness and collective vitality in the very process of building these networks, which will provide critical support to each person's efforts to live independently.

Part Three

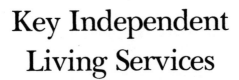

Key Independent
Living Services

Five of the services considered most essential to independent living—attendant care, peer counseling, skills training, transportation, and housing—are featured in this section. A final chapter discusses the contribution of technological innovations. All of these chapters go beyond simply describing needs and services. For example, discussion of attendant care outlines several ways of structuring these programs and demonstrates how the methods chosen by various states reflect their philosophy. The authors also alert the reader to the potential dangers of increased regulation in the form of training requirements for attendants. The chapter on accessible transportation concentrates on urban mass transit, and shows how political and economic factors influence the progress of IL. The discussion of housing is unique in its approach, providing a concrete outline of the steps required for planning and financing special living facilities.

Technology is not in itself an IL service, but it is essential to many aspects of IL programs. One chapter is devoted to technological innovations applied to communication, activities of daily living, education, and employment for people with disabilities. It identifies problems in the development and delivery of today's technology and suggests some specific solutions.

9

Attendant Care

Gerben DeJong
Teg Wenker

Attendant care is one of the services most closely associated with the movement for independent living, especially with regard to severely physically disabled persons, for whom it is most essential. Simple as it is, attendant care is not a well understood service. Confusion arises, in part, because providing attendant care services can involve at least three major sectors of the human services system—health care, income assistance, and social services. Although in itself it is a relatively straightforward service, to understand how attendant care is (or should be) provided sometimes requires a global perspective on human services. Such a viewpoint is rare these days, when categorical

Note: This chapter is revised and updated from an article that appeared in the October 1979 issue of *Archives of Physical Medicine and Rehabilitation.*

grant programs and the like confine most of us to our own niches in the system.

One purpose of this chapter is to cut through the bewildering complexity surrounding the public funding of attendant care services. Although details of service delivery are quite varied from one region to another, all systems can be divided into two general categories: home health services, which are based on the traditional medical model of care, and attendant care services, which are a product of the independent living model. The first chapter in this book compares the medical model of health care with the independent living model. In similar fashion this chapter will contrast the services that flow from those models. Our intent in contrasting attendant care and home health services is to demonstrate how the attendant care model reflects key values and concepts espoused by the Independent Living Movement. However, the attendant care model seldom exists in its purest form. Providing attendant care services through public means makes it necessary to accommodate the requirements of major funding sources, such as Title XIX (Medicaid) and Title XX (Social Services) of the 1980 Social Security Disability Amendments.

This chapter also examines ways that states have used Titles XIX and XX to provide attendant care. We will analyze how the independent living goals of the attendant care model are compromised by employment disincentives that arise from criteria used to determine eligibility for income and medical assistance benefits. Some of the trends that are likely to shape the future of attendant care will also be considered.

Attendant care services are those tasks performed by an attendant when assisting a severely disabled person in bathing, dressing, grooming, toilet care, and other activities of daily living. If necessary, an attendant also helps with meal preparation, food shopping, and household chores. The cost of attendant care varies from minimum wage to about $6 per hour. A handicapped person's need for an attendant varies from about two to six or more hours per day depending on the severity of the disability. An attendant is recruited, hired, trained, supervised, and, if necessary, fired by the disabled consumer. That the consumer, not the provider, directs the provision of care is the distinguishing feature of the attendant care model.

Of all the services and programs associated with the Independent Living Movement, attendant care has acquired unusual significance. It has become the exemplar for independent living advocates because as a model of in-home care, attendant care incorporates many of the values and concepts cherished by the movement. In Chapter One the Independent Living Movement's indebtedness to the contributions of other social movements was noted—the civil rights, consumer, self-help, demedicalization, and the deinstitutionalization movements. The attendant care model incorporates the values and assumptions that characterize each of these movements.

In our society, survival needs such as food, shelter, and health care are often recognized as rights or entitlements. Attendant care must also be viewed as a survival right, a benefit necessary to the physical survival of the individual, since a severely physically disabled person often cannot participate in school, work, recreation, or the political life of the community without it. Because of its indispensable nature, attendant care takes on the character of an inalienable right, with status comparable to a civil right.

Generally, consumer advocates agree that the consumer, not the provider, is best able to judge the adequacy of services and products. Thus, as consumers of attendant care, disabled individuals are best able to evaluate the adequacy and quality of the care they receive. Having the closest possible knowledge of his or her own disability, the disabled individual is highly qualified to establish the level of care he or she requires. The self-help movement goes beyond the consumer movement in assuming that handicapped individuals are not only capable of evaluating service quality, but that they are also able to manage and direct the providers of the services they need. This is the assumption at the core of the attendant care model.

The attendant care concept touches nearly all the themes considered dear to the independent living movement, and the convergence of all these themes and values have helped to elevate attendant care to prominence. Attendant care is viewed in some quarters as a kind of "litmus test" or bellwether service, indicating whether public officials and others truly understand the needs and aspirations of persons with severe physical disabilities. The Social Security Administration, the National Center for Health Statistics, and various university-based research organizations have conducted surveys on the incidence and prevalence of disability. These surveys (Posner, 1972; National Center for Health Statistics, 1972; Nagi, 1973, 1975) indicate that about 1.1 percent of all working-age adults and about 6.5 percent of all elderly need some assistance with personal care. Given the age distribution of the population in 1977, we estimate that this translates to about 2.9 million adult Americans who need such assistance.

These figures include people who need only minimal help (for example, someone to tie their shoelaces) as well as those whose needs are greater. According to a study conducted by Brandeis University (DeJong, 1977a) the number of people whose disabilities are severe enough to require attendant care is only a small fraction of the total reported by the national surveys. We estimate that about 160,000 working-age adults and about 250,000 elderly are functionally dependent enough to require the scope of assistance rendered by a paid attendant.

Home Health and Medical Models for Attendant Care Services

The attendant care model assumes that disabled individuals who are well versed in their own health care needs have the necessary ability and skill to direct and monitor their own personal care. The concept of self-direction, however, is not widely accepted or supported by health professionals. Presently, opportunities are rare within the health services system for severely disabled individuals to manage their own health care. The conventional approach is, in fact, just the opposite, as can be seen in the delivery of home health services.

In the home health system, disabled people do not direct their own care. Instead, care is provided by agency-supervised home health aides. The home health agency functions as the

Attendant Care

specifies the duties to be performed by the home health aide.
Furthermore, the aide's duties are supervised by an agency-em-
ployed registered nurse. The disabled person is a passive recipient of services—in essence, a patient.

Since Medicare is the main source of reimbursement for
home health services, most such agencies shape their operating
policies after those of the Medicare program. Unfortunately, the
disabled individual's ability to direct his or her own care is very
much restricted by Medicare requirements. For example, the
Medicare program requires that home health services be rendered in keeping with a physician plan of treatment, be supervised by a skilled nurse, and be reviewed every sixty days
(DeJong, 1977b).

Professional intervention and supervision are at the core
of the home health model. However, ongoing reassessment by
health care professionals tends to undermine an individual's
confidence and independence. Such professional control can un-
intentionally reinforce dependent behavior. The attendant care
model rejects the submissive, compliant patient role inherent in
the home health model of in-home support services. In the attendant care model, independence is fostered by holding the
disabled individual responsible for managing and reimbursing
his or her attendant.

A comparison between the older home health model and
the more recent attendant care model illustrates significant differences in role expectations:

Home Health/Medical Model	Attendant Care/Independent Living Model
Provider direction	Consumer direction
Physician plan of treatment	No physician plan of treatment
Nurse supervision	No nurse supervision
Aide recruited by agency	Attendant recruited by consumer
Payment to provider	Payment to consumer to provider
Accountability is to physician	Accountability is to consumer

162   Independent Living for Physically Disabled People

Home Health/Medical Model	Attendant Care/Independent Living Model
Patient role	Consumer role
Acute condition	Chronic condition
Restorative/episodic care	Maintenance/continuous care
"Health care" benefit	"Social service" benefit

In the home health model, the disabled person is a patient; in the attendant care model, he or she is a consumer. Yet both models are needed. The home health model is appropriate for providing acute, restorative care during a period of illness or recuperation immediately following hospitalization. The attendant care model is formulated to provide ongoing routine care as an alternative to long term institutionalization. Considering the polarity of their respective goals, these two models of in-home care should also be expected to have equally disparate methods of service delivery.

Services Under Title XIX

The Medicaid program has become one of the main sources of funding for consumer-directed attendant care services. This has been made possible by a relatively obscure federal regulation (42 CFR 440.170(f)) that permits personal care services to be provided in a person's home "by an individual, not a member of the family who is qualified to provide such services, where the services are prescribed by a physician in accordance with a plan of treatment and are supervised by a nurse." This regulation contains many of the trappings characteristic of the medical model in home health services, but because it does not specify the amount of nurse supervision required, it allows great latitude in the amount of consumer participation. A person who is medically stable and has acquired the necessary health maintenance skills would require only minimal nurse supervision under the Medicaid regulations.

The demedicalization debate centers around the concern that there is too much unnecessary medical intervention in problems and life conditions whose etiologies are social and economic rather than medical. In the case of physical disability, the Independent Living Movement asserts that a continuous medical presence is unnecessary once an individual is medically stable. The role expectations of the attendant care model stand in marked contrast to the patient role that comes with medical intervention. In the attendant care model, accountability centers on the consumer, not on the physician. The attendant care model assumes that the consumer does not require the acute/restorative care assumed in the medical model or in home health services. Disabled persons are assumed to be sufficiently experienced to monitor their own physical condition and to seek additional care when needed. Disabled persons are not "sick," do not wish to be exempted from various social and civic responsibilities, and do not wish to be deprived of their personhood.

The features of the medical model that induce dependence are most evident in large-scale institutional programs managed by medical personnel. Attendant care is viewed as an alternative to institutionalization. It allows relatively unskilled individuals to provide, in a community setting, personal care services that would otherwise be provided in an institutional setting. Often a person is institutionalized because no attendant care services are available in the community.

At least fifteen states have used the Medicaid program to finance attendant care services. Among these are Massachusetts and Minnesota, which have had contrasting experience with this program.

Massachusetts. The Massachusetts attendant care program began in 1975 when the state Medicaid program contracted with the Boston Center for Independent Living for the provision of attendant care services. Since then, three other independent living centers have contracted with the Medicaid program: Worcester Area Transitional Housing, Independence Associates, and the Northeast Independent Living Program. The Massachusetts attendant care program is a model program in that it assumes many severely disabled individuals do not need a high degree of medical intervention.

To be eligible for attendant care services in Massachusetts, a person must be eighteen years or older, limited in his upper extremities, psychologically and medically stable, and eligible for Medicaid. Medicaid eligibility is determined by the public welfare department; attendant care needs are determined by the independent living program. A registered nurse and an occupational therapist from the independent living programs complete an on-site assessment of attendant care needs with the prospective consumer. Reassessments are made once each year and sometimes more often, depending on the medical condition of the consumer. The Medicaid program reimburses such assessment services on a fee-for-service basis.

Should an applicant be lacking in any skills needed for the utilization of attendant care services, the independent living program provides training to enhance the applicant's ability to manage his personal affairs. This service is also reimbursed by the Medicaid program.

The responsibility for recruiting attendants falls mainly on the consumer. After the initial assessment, the independent living program acts mainly as an intermediary in the payment process. Time sheets, signed by both the attendant and the consumer, are submitted by the consumer to the independent living program, which in turn sends the bill to Medicaid for payment. The independent living program issues a check to the consumer, who in turn pays the attendant.

The hourly wage for an attendant in Massachusetts, set in 1981 by the state rate-setting commission, is presently fixed at $4.25. The typical consumer needs about four hours of attendant care per day divided between the morning and evening hours. If needed, a night-time attendant is available to turn an individual in bed, to avoid pressure sores. A night-time attendant, who frequently lives with the consumer, receives $6.07 per night. The Massachusetts Medicaid program does not provide enty-four-hour, live-in attendant care services.

About 300 individuals participate in the Massachusetts Medicaid attendant care program. In addition, another 60 individuals participate in an attendant care program supported by the Massachusetts Rehabilitation Commission. The latter program is available to individuals who are employed and therefore not eligible for Medicaid. It is supported entirely with state funds and administered through the various independent living

programs in a manner similar to the attendant care program
funded by Medicaid.

Minnesota. The Minnesota program is centrally administered through the state Medicaid program, not through local independent living programs as in Massachusetts. The program
currently has four hundred eighty participants. As of 1981,
Medicaid pays up to a maximum of $1,000 per month per eligi-
ble participant for live-in or part-time attendants. Many severely
disabled individuals choose to split this sum between several attendants to assure regular care.

The participant is responsible for recruiting an attendant
and a registered nurse to supervise his care. However, for the
most part, the Minnesota program is a provider-based as opposed to a consumer-based system. The attendant and not the
consumer bills the Medicaid program and provides the necessary documentation—for example, the attendant must ensure
that the treatment plan is on record and certified by the physician every ninety days. The physician determines the services to
be provided, the expected duration of service, the frequency of
nurse visits, and the qualifications of the attendant (Minnesota
Department of Public Welfare, 1978).

The Minnesota attendant care program leans to the home
health, or medical, model: the physician rather than the consumer is the principal decision-maker. Moreover, the program
places many responsibilities on the attendant. Because of this,
it largely lacks the self-direction goals of the Massachusetts program.

In Massachusetts, both personal care and housekeeping
services are funded by Medicaid. In Minnesota, most personal
care services are considered to be medical and most housekeeping services nonmedical. The attendant must submit a separate
bill for housekeeping tasks to the state's Title XX social services
program.

Services Under Title XX

A second major source of support for attendant care services is Title XX of the Social Security Act, which allows states
to fund various in-home services without the medical supervi-

sion required under the Medicaid program. California offers an example of use of Title XX to fund attendant care services.

The California attendant care program began in the late 1950s when disabled persons were given a special needs allowance to supplement their public assistance grant under the Aid to the Totally and Permanently Disabled (ATPD) program (California State Benefits and Advisory Board, 1977). When Supplemental Security Income (SSI) displaced ATPD in 1974, the attendant care program was combined with California's new In-Home Support Services program, supported in part with federal funds under Title XX.

Unlike the Massachusetts and Minnesota programs, California's program is administered through county departments of public welfare. The hours of attendant care needed by a disabled person are determined mainly by the county social service worker based on a personal interview. The social service worker may call upon the expertise of an occupational therapist. The consumer may solicit the statement of a physician in documenting his need for attendant care. The number of attendant care hours is to some degree negotiable. The attendant care needs of an individual are reevaluated every six months or more often, depending on the nature of the disability.

Hourly compensation for attendant care is set at or slightly above the minimum wage in California. The total cost of attendant care for any one individual, as of 1981, may not exceed $820 per month. Thus, the maximum number of attendant care hours that an individual can receive is determined in part by this monthly ceiling. Moreover, the disabled individual must take into account outlays for social security payroll taxes and other fringe benefits when computing the cost of attendant care.

The arrangement in California allows consumers to be very much in the driver's seat. They recruit, manage, and pay their own attendants. Neither a physician's plan for treatment nor a nurse's supervision is required. Because of the absence of medical intervention, the California program incorporates the attendant care model in a nearly pure form.

It is difficult to determine how many individuals participate in California's attendant care program. Because administratively the program is part of the state's larger In-Home Support

Services program, it is difficult to distinguish between individuals receiving attendant care and those receiving other forms of in-home care such as chore and homemaker services. Current estimates suggest that at least several thousand disabled individuals receive attendant care services in California.

Work Disincentives

One of the most vexing issues accompanying the provision of attendant care services has been the problem of work disincentives. Until recently, a person would lose several thousand dollars worth of publicly supported attendant care benefits upon becoming gainfully employed. This problem was especially acute for persons in entry level jobs that did not provide sufficient income to cover their attendant care costs. Thus, in accepting employment, an attendant care consumer worked to his economic disadvantage.

The source of this problem was that a person's eligibility for Medicaid and social services was tightly linked to his income. To be eligible for Medicaid or social service benefits such as attendant care, a person also had to meet the categorical requirements of the SSI program. To meet these requirements, a person had to have a medical impairment and be unable to participate in substantial gainful activity (SGA), that is, be unable to work. However, as soon as a disabled person's earnings topped $300 per month, he or she was no longer considered disabled for the purposes of the SSI program. Once working, therefore, disabled persons lost not only their SSI benefits but also their Medicaid and social service benefits, including attendant care—clearly a disincentive to work.

The loss of medical and attendant care benefits could only be delayed if a person participated in a nine-month trial work period (and an additional three-month grace period) or in a time-limited self-support plan. The purpose of the trial work period was to allow a disabled person to test his or her work ability without an immediate loss of benefits. However, after the expiration of the trial work period or self-support plan, the disincentives came back into force.

Under the 1980 social security disability amendments,

many of these work disincentives have been removed or significantly moderated. First, the costs of disability-related expenses such as attendant care can be deducted for the purpose of determining whether a person's earned income exceeds the SGA amount of $300 per month. Second, under a three-year federal demonstration effort, persons who have completed their trial work period and earn in excess of the SGA amount will continue to receive their SSI income benefits and hence remain eligible for attendant care benefits under the Title XIX and Title XX programs. And third, even when their income exceeds the level at which cash benefits under the SSI program are ordinarily phased out, disabled persons can retain their Title XIX and Title XX attendant care benefits under a benefit reduction formula that earlier had been applied only during a person's trial work period.

Not all persons who want to work and need attendant care services will benefit equally from these changes since they apply mainly to those persons receiving SSI-linked benefits. Persons receiving Social Security Disability Insurance (SSDI) benefits, for example, will continue to face certain disincentives since these benefits cannot be retained when earnings exceed the SGA level. However, SSDI beneficiaries will be allowed to have their Medicare coverage extended for up to four years when returning to work. Unfortunately, attendant care services are not available through the Medicare program. (Medicare provides medical coverage to persons receiving "social insurance" benefits, such as SSDI. Medicaid provides medical coverage to persons receiving "public assistance" benefits, such as SSI.)

Some SSDI beneficiaries may benefit from another provision in the 1980 amendments which allows individual states, at their discretion, to provide medical assistance and social services (such as attendant care) as part of a special three-year pilot program. The program is directed to those persons who otherwise would not benefit from the SSI-related changes. Funding for the pilot program is limited to $18 million—$6 million for each of the three years.

In addition, some states have passed their own laws to allow disabled persons to accept gainful employment and still retain attendant care benefits. Financing is borne entirely by the states; there is no federal participation whatsoever. These laws generally predate the 1980 amendments. Both California and Massachusetts have passed such legislation.

The Future of Attendant Care

One important step in solving the problems of attendant care delivery and work disincentives is to divorce eligibility for attendant care from eligibility for income assistance. A persistent feature in the American system of delivering publicly subsidized health and social service benefits is the manner in which these benefits are linked to the receipt of income or income assistance benefits. The receipt of attendant care services should not be related to a person's income or vocational status. Instead, attendant care should be an entitlement service related solely to a person's functional status or capacity.

The new independent living authority under the 1978 Amendments to the Rehabilitation Act (PL95-602) offers a modest opportunity for states to provide attendant care services without regard to income or vocational status. However, funds to implement the new independent living provisions are likely to remain so limited in the foreseeable future that states will have no choice but to continue their attendant care programs under Title XIX and Title XX. It is feared that relatively costly attendant care services would leave few independent living dollars for innovative programs geared to a broader segment of the disabled population.

If anything, pressure to finance more attendant care services under the Medicaid program will continue to grow. Federal appropriations for Medicaid are open-ended while appropriations for Title XX and other programs are fixed. Most states have already exhausted their federal Title XX allotments, which encourages them to refinance services under the Medicaid program whenever possible. Attendant care is one of those services that can be financed under either Medicaid or Title XX.

In the near future, we can also expect attendant care services to be pushed in the direction of the home health or medical model, in part, as a byproduct of Medicaid funding. More importantly, demands for quality assurance are likely to impose new requirements for training and supervision that are more in keeping with the home health model.

This direction is most evident in the HR 3 report prepared by the United States Department of Health, Education and Welfare (1978) in response to congressional concern over the lack of accountability and coordination in such federally subsidized home care services as home health and attendant care. Because the attendant care model conflicts with traditional quality assurance standards that emphasize the training and supervision of care providers, the authors of the HR 3 report recommended that the current Medicaid regulation allowing federal funding for attendant care be rescinded. Instead, the report recommends that attendant care be financed under the Title XX program. However, this recommendation ignores the restrictive income limits imposed by most states to contain Title XX expenditures within federally established state expenditure ceilings.

HR 3 does not adequately reflect the self-determination goals of disabled persons. Rather, it reflects the widespread assumption of agency professionals and policy makers that disabled persons are not self-directed. The campaign of the home health industry to eliminate attendant care services presents a danger that must be faced. Such a campaign is the more difficult to resist when heralded by the politically popular slogan of quality assurance. Given the pressures of provider interests, only consumer vigilance will enable the attendant care model to remain intact.

Personal care is one of the first areas of human activity in which an individual learns to become independent. Yet it is still one of the last areas in which a severely physically disabled individual can become fully independent. To be dependent in the care of one's own body is to renounce much of one's personal autonomy. To manage one's own personal care is to reclaim one's sense of self-worth.

10

Peer Counseling

Marsha Saxton

A young adult, newly spinal-cord injured in an automobile accident, an elderly person recovering from a stroke, a cerebral
palsied person living in an institution. As different as their physical problems are, these individuals will encounter many common experiences in confronting life as a disabled person in our
culture: feelings of despair and isolation, frustration at the inaccessibility of the outside world, a sense of powerlessness, a
fear of being a burden to others. Many attempts will be made to
assist these individuals. Family members, medical professionals,
clergy, social workers, and others will offer varying amounts of
sympathy, reassurance, or guidance. While their attempts will
meet with varying degrees of success, it is likely that one feeling
common to these disabled individuals will remain unchallenged:
"No one really understands what it's like."

I would like to acknowledge the invaluable assistance of Dr. Irving
Kenneth Zola and the peer counselors of the Boston Self Help Center.

171

In a culture that emphasizes youth, rigid standards of beauty, the ideals of physical strength, athletic skill, and rugged self-reliance, it is understandable that most of us are unable to fathom the experience of severe disability. Likewise, the feeling that no one understands is understandably pervasive among the millions of severely disabled people who live in our able-bodied culture.

The statement of one disabled woman regarding her search for a counselor echoes the feelings of hundreds of her fellows (personal communication, Boston Self Help Center counselee, 1979).

When I found myself disabled (with paraplegia), the thing I wanted most was to talk with someone I felt knew the feelings I was experiencing. I wanted to meet a woman who was in a wheelchair and had been there long enough to have put her life back in order. I kept thinking, "All these people are trying to help, but they don't understand." I did not find a peer counselor until almost two years after I became disabled. I can't describe to you how thrilled I was to find her. I was so hungry to know all about her life, her methods for coping with everyday annoyances and difficulties, and especially her ways of coping with feelings. I asked such questions as "How do you get your chair in and out of the car?" I wanted to see if she knew a better way than I had devised. "Do you travel alone or stay in motels by yourself?" At that time, I had not spent a night alone since becoming a paraplegic. I was afraid. "Do you date?" I was real interested in anything she could tell me about dating. You'd think a woman who had been married for eleven years would know how to relate to men. But my experience had been as an able-bodied teenager and then as an adult wife. Now that I was a disabled, divorced woman, I felt totally unprepared to cope with dating. I asked her, "Do you feel less of a woman?" and "How do you feel when people stare?" The most important question I wanted answered was "Are you happy now? Is it okay after five or six years? Does the pain of being different lessen?" All of these questions were ones I desperately needed answered by a relatively well-adjusted disabled woman.

Peer counseling offers someone who understands.

Peer counseling has been used in a limited way by rehabilitation practitioners for years. Former clients have occasionally been asked to report their experiences to new clients regarding such vocational matters as job demands and interviews. Many experienced vocational rehabilitation workers report that they hook clients up with each other without the help of a formal program. Sometimes rehabilitation agencies will hire disabled persons as counselors or placement specialists. This has been particularly true of agencies serving the blind. Client assistance projects in the vocational rehabilitation system are often staffed by former clients or other disabled persons.

While these efforts add up to a promising trend, there has recently emerged a need for a more formalized approach to providing disabled clients with support and input from disabled peers. Such well-known groups as Alcoholics Anonymous and the early Synanon, and newer groups such as Recovery (for ex-mental patients), the National Association for Retarded Citizens, and Parents Without Partners are examples of the five hundred thousand mutual aid or self-help organizations now in operation, involving fifteen million Americans.

Although the American tendency to join groups is not new, the strength of the current trend has no precedent in the country's history. Many factors have spurred the formation of such groups. Among these factors may be counted the increase in the size and complexity of institutions—an increase which, ironically, may tend to render services unavailable or unresponsive to many consumers. As Gartner and Riessman speculate: "People feel unable to control 'big government' and distant bureaucracies and so are drawn to mutual aid groups that enable them to deal with some immediate problems of everyday life" (1980, p. 1). In such groups, individuals are actively encouraged by their peers to take responsibility for their own welfare, thereby increasing their sense of competence and self-respect. Gartner and Riessman argue further that "mutual aid groups are particularly relevant for the major health problems of our society. They provide services inexpensively, but, and most importantly, they address the large numbers of chronic disorders, among them arthritis, diabetes, emphysema, and hypertension, which require only small amounts of medical professional intervention and large doses of caring." (1980, p. 1).

The Independent Living Movement, largely instigated by disabled people themselves, highlighted the need and made known the demand for consumer participation in rehabilitation. In legislation covering independent living programs, this is reflected in the concept of consumer involvement, which mandates that disabled persons be actively involved in policymaking, program planning, and delivery of services.

Peer counseling is a particularly strong example of consumer involvement. The disabled peer counselor, in the role of specialist, can be seen as uniquely qualified for his or her role. An analogous example might be the bilingual speaker who, by virtue of life experience, is singularly qualified to become an interpreter. Similarly, the disabled person possessing the necessary personal qualifications can, with training, offer unique assistance to disabled clients.

Forms of Peer Counseling

Peer counseling is a primary component of independent living services (Griffin and Martin, 1979). The Independent Living Research Utilization project of the Institute for Rehabilitation and Research (TIRR) in Houston, Texas conducted a survey in which it was found that 100 percent of existing centers for independent living claimed to provide peer counseling services while 92 percent reported that peer counseling was a primary service (Board, Frieden, and Cole, 1982). The Urban Institute reported similar results on a questionnaire sent out to all state vocational rehabilitation directors (LaRocca, 1981). Eighty-nine percent of the respondents stated that peer counseling was of major importance in independent living centers, provided that the peer counselors had formal training.

Peer counseling programs vary widely. The Institute for Rehabilitation and Research conducted a survey to determine the characteristics of the many peer counseling programs now in operation (Frieden and Sharp, 1982). From the survey data, TIRR extracted six major program types: the conventional, the field, the rehabilitational, the instructional, the information and referral, and the community. The following descriptions demonstrate the range of approaches to peer counseling as well as the degree of overlap among them.

The conventional approach is the one most generally taken in metropolitan areas and is also the most common across the country. Examples include the Houston Center for Independent Living, the Lawrence Center for Independent Living in Kansas, and the Metrolina Center for Independent Living in Charlotte, North Carolina. Under this approach, peer counseling takes place at the center, closely supervised by a professional, and covers a wide range of topics related to disability. Peer counselors who may be full-time or part-time staff, and may or may not have an academic degree, meet with clients at weekly or biweekly intervals.

The field approach involves peer counselors visiting clients in their homes, nursing homes, congregate housing, or rehabilitation facilities. The amount of supervision and formal training varies widely and most peer counselors are volunteers and provide their own transportation. Much of the counseling may occur on the phone. This approach depends on flexibility and is most appropriate for rural areas where the distance between client and facility may be great. Examples of this approach include Stavros in Massachusetts and the South Carolina Center for Independent Living.

The rehabilitation approach is generally taken by state-run vocational rehabilitation agencies such as those of California and Illinois. These agencies hire peer counselors from their pool of former clients, generally on an as-needed basis. These programs generally have a strong vocational focus and are often highly supervised.

The instructional approach is often taken in transitional living programs such as the Boston Center for Independent Living, the Craig Rehabilitation Center in Denver, and the Warm Springs Center in Georgia. This approach regards peer counselors as educators who train clients in attendant management, use of resources, sexuality, and other independent living skills. The instructional approach is appropriate for metropolitan areas and generally appeals to medical rehabilitation facilities. It is also employed in various educational settings, such as the University of Missouri at Columbia and Widener College in Pennsylvania.

The emphasis in the information and referral approach is on providing information on community resources such as transportation, attendant care, and architectural accessibility; often, the only link with clients is phone contact. This approach is often a component of other program types. Examples include the Berkeley Center for Independent Living in California and Project Independence in Little Rock, Arkansas.

The community approach is a larger version of the support network provided by family and friends. With little supervision or structure to the program, training and education are rarely required of the volunteer peer counselors, who meet with clients through natural helping networks such as church, recreation, and social activities. Programs employing this approach include the Independent Living Program in Shreveport, Louisiana and Hail in Denver.

Role of Peer Counseling

The field of peer counseling is split with unresolved arguments concerning definition and function. A number of terms have simultaneously gained currency: peer counselor, peer helper, peer tutor, peer assistant, peer educator, peer consultant, and peer trainer. All of these terms are valid descriptions of different functions. The term peer counselor is used here because it is the one most widely used in legislation and in the literature of the field. However, the function of the peer counselor necessarily varies with the particular program. A useful general definition is offered by Schatzlein: "Peer counseling is a necessary adjunct to the rehabilitation process in which a severely disabled person who has made a successful transition from institutional to independent community living provides resource information, support, understanding, and direction to another disabled person who desires to make a similar transition" (1978, p. 4).

Specific examples of areas in which a peer counselor can provide help include:

- Management of personal care attendant services, such as interviewing and hiring.
- Activities of daily living, such as dressing, bathing, and bowel and bladder care.
- Equipment purchase, modification, and repair.
- Exploration of available community resources in such areas as education, legal rights, vocation, and recreation.

Examples of tasks of equal but less tangible importance to independent living include:

- Dealing with grief or anxiety regarding body image, sexuality, or personal relationships.
- Challenging attitudinal barriers and channeling feelings of frustration or anger related to the stigma of disability.
- Learning assertiveness and self-advocacy skills.

Many of these issues can most profitably be addressed in peer groups where the peer counselor and several clients at a time can share feelings and information, and offer each other support.

The peer counselor can function in practically every helping role. As one peer counselor commented, "You're the OT [occupational therapist], the PT [physical therapist], the doctor, the social worker, and the wheelchair repairman." This peer-of-all-trades definition has led to controversy regarding the limitations of the role of peer counselor.

An important part of the peer counselor's training must be learning to recognize when referral to a professional is appropriate. The need for medical or legal intervention is usually, but not always, obvious. For example, sometimes a professional is better able to resolve a bureaucratic snag in obtaining services. And just as there are times when peer support is crucial, there are times when the perspective of an able-bodied professional is needed.

Different peer counseling training programs emphasize different skills and philosophies (Corn, 1977; Jackins, 1970).

The success of a program depends on many factors, including the appropriateness of the program to the client population and the skill and commitment of supervisors, peer counselors, and administrators.

Programmatic Issues

In any counseling plan there are programmatic concerns that must be identified and discussed. Any program must justify itself both to funding agencies and to its potential constituency. Conducting a needs assessment survey is a way of documenting the need for the program and at the same time making it visible to relevant communities. Among the most important data to be collected are the numbers of potential clients in the geographic area, the numbers of people seeking various counseling services from other agencies, the success or failure of other agencies or approaches in serving these needs, and the prevalent concerns of local consumers and their desire for peer counseling services.

The needs assessment survey can take the form of a questionnaire or an interview and can be distributed to both consumers and professionals through local vocational rehabilitation agencies, hospital or custodial care institutions, and disabled student's centers.

Financial issues are important to the survival of any program, but can have special organizational implications for a peer counseling program. In particular, the question of whether peer counselors are volunteer or paid can be difficult to resolve. The obvious advantage of volunteer peer counselors is that the project saves money. However, drawbacks include volunteers' tendency to be less committed and, therefore, less dependable than workers who are paid. They cannot, as a rule, be expected to do substantial record keeping. Being paid often affects how one is viewed by clients and staff alike: free services are often devalued. Thus wherever possible, it seem advisable to pay peer counselors. The implementation of a salaried peer counseling program may necessitate the sometimes arduous process of rate setting negotiations with the state bureau. Unfortunately, few pay scale guidelines exist in this realm. A range from minimum wage to $20 per hour has been noted by this author.

The training and supervision available to peer counselors probably define the quality of a program to a greater extent than any other factor. There is considerable variation in this realm among the many programs in existence. Factors that determine the nature of the training program and supervision systems include the degree of formality; the program emphasis and defined objectives; the resources, including budget allocations; and the availability of counseling trainers and consultants.

An individual's disability alone does not qualify that person as a peer counselor. Screening criteria and procedures must be developed to locate the type of individuals sought by the program. The screening process can be initiated through an open introductory orientation meeting. Here the program's philosophy, goals, and activities can be discussed and the required commitment can be clarified. Such a meeting can allow persons to self-screen when the program does not meet their expectations, thereby saving the staff considerable time. Following the meeting, individual interviews can best assess the readiness of applicants. Other ways to do this include telephone interviews, group interviews, or accepting the recommendations of referring professionals.

Most peer counseling programs have at least three minimum prerequisites: that applicants have experienced a physical disability (or chronic disease) and can demonstrate adequate adjustment to this, that applicants have a desire to help others, and that they are willing to make a commitment of time and effort to the program during and after the training period. Other commonly included criteria are that applicants can demonstrate relaxed, caring interaction with others; can provide sustained attention; and are willing to share and explore their own feelings regarding their disability and other personal issues. Some programs, such as the Boston Self Help Center, request a commitment of a specified length of time or may require an additional investment of time to do practicum counseling sessions during the training period. A number of programs, one being the

Berkeley Center for Independent Living, require applicants to
have undergone formal training and/or to have an academic degree in counseling, psychology, or a rehabilitation-related field.
     The screening interview alone may be inadequate for de-
termining applicants' qualifications. Individuals with less well
developed interpersonal skills may be unprepared for counseling
in such areas as sexual adjustment or grieving but may be very
effective in teaching skills necessary for wheelchair maintenance.
The Boston Self Help Center has developed a selection process
which alleviates this problem. All applicants to the peer counseling training program are required to initially join one of several
groups—for example, a personal growth group, creative expression group, or couples group. This allows the applicants to demonstrate their commitment to the program and enables the staff
to become familiar with each applicant's interpersonal skills. In
this way the individuals' particular strengths as potential peer
counselors are identified and possible weaknesses can be worked
on. Applicants' eagerness to "rescue" or "mother" other disabled persons can be identified and dealt with before those people begin to function as peer counselors.
     A major objective of peer counseling is the establishment
of a genuinely empathetic relationship between client and counselor. Most peer counseling models used today are based on or
similar to Robert Carkhuff's model (1973), in which, simply
stated, the counselor facilitates an atmosphere of trust and gen-
uine respect, so that the client can express feelings without fear
of judgment from the counselor. It is assumed that clear thinking and decisive action will result after the client has had the opportunity to openly ventilate fears, anger, grief, and other emo-
tions. The principles of this "client-centered" counseling are
simple and readily learned by most individuals. The most important skill peer counselors must acquire is effective listening or
the ability to offer sustained, interested attention. It is assumed
that maximum growth occurs when responsibility for life decisions are made by the client. Therefore, peer counselors are generally discouraged from offering personal advice.
     A significant component of the training program is the
clear delineation of the nature and limitations of the peer coun-

selor's relationship to clients. Generally, a peer counselor is expected to meet regularly with each client to provide a climate in which the client may discuss ideas, express feelings, set goals, obtain information, and learn skills. Peer counselors are *not* expected to solve their clients' problems, socialize with their clients, or attempt to meet their clients' personal needs. Peer counselors must be trained to determine the difference between those life issues which are manageable in the peer counseling context and those which are not. For the latter, the client needs to be referred to an appropriate professional.

Adequate supervision is essential to maintaining such standards. The objectives of peer counseling supervision can include monitoring client progress, coordinating services with other programs within and outside the agency, monitoring documentation, providing on-going peer counseling skill development, and providing support for the peer counselor's experience of the counselor role. Supervision sessions can occur on a weekly or monthly basis, in group or individual meetings. The major focus of these sessions should, of course, be the needs of the client and accountability to the goals of the program. However, as in any kind of human services program, personal support for the staff can greatly enhance the quality of their services. Peer counselors are in the position of frequently confronting with clients issues which the counselors may not have fully resolved themselves. Such emotion-laden issues as physical loss, discrimination, or sexual difficulties may touch off feelings in the peer counselor. That the peer counselor reacts to such issues does not mean that he or she is unqualified for the role. Thoughtful intervention by the supervisor will benefit the peer counselor, the client, and the program as a whole. Qualifications for supervising peer counselors include commitment to and understanding of the peer counseling philosophy and familiarity with the training curriculum and the client population. The supervisor must be an effective communicator, flexible and open to a wide range of skill levels and able to model clarity with respect to disability issues. People in the supervisory role should have regular access to consultation.

As for the specific training curriculum, a number of peer

counseling manuals are available (Arkansas Research and Training Center, 1981; Arter and others, 1979; Saxton, 1981). Many of these blueprints can be adapted to a variety of settings and populations. For example, the Boston Self Help Center found it necessary to develop a peer counseling training program for disabled women that emphasized women's sexuality and the double discrimination of sexism and "able-bodiedism." Peer counselors can be trained to become more aware of their own value systems or cultural biases so as to not impose them on clients.

Peer counselors in any program must become familiar with issues related to cultural discrimination against people with disabilities because they will repeatedly confront such issues with their clients. In training sessions, trainees can share experi- ..es and explore insights into prevalent cultural attitudes auout disability and how they impact on the individual. Trainees can gain experience through the use of a "hands-on" approach to these issues in training sessions, which allows for immediate feedback and the exploration and expression of trainees' feelings and reactions to the counselor role. Longer practice sessions involving pairs of trainees, scheduled outside of training sessions with reports at the next meeting, can allow trainees to experience the client role. This greatly enhances the peer counselors' appreciation and understanding of the task of counselors and further accelerates the trainees' skill development. At the same time, personal understanding is broadened, which will help peer counselors when their clients reveal such feelings as self-blame, not "fitting in," being a burden, feelings of ugliness, or the need to overcompensate. If they have clarified issues of discrimination for themselves, peer counselors will be able to model clarity for clients and help them become aware that such attitudes about oneself are often the result of internalizing myths and stereotypes.

Finally, evaluation of peer counseling should be built into the program as an ongoing component. Regular feedback from clients about the effectiveness of the peer counseling relationship and its impact on their goal attainment can be obtained using questionnaires or interviews, conducted by persons other than the clients' regular peer counselors. Referring agencies and family members of clients can be requested to provide feedback on their observations of program effectiveness. Other chapters in this volume offer a more in-depth treatment of program evaluation.

Advantages of Peer Counseling

The population of persons with severe disability is considerably underserved by mental health professionals. Factors that contribute to this state of affairs include inadequate professional skills training, physical inaccessibility of programs, and attitudinal barriers on the part of mental health professionals. A comprehensive study to obtain substantive data (previously lacking) on the needs of persons with both physical and psychiatric disabilities is now underway at the Research and Training Center at Boston University (Spaniol, 1981). Although the picture is changing, particularly with the increasing attention to the problems of disabled persons, the current gap in services can profitably be addressed by paraprofessional and nonprofessional programs.

Peer counseling is often regarded as a less expensive alternative to traditional therapy. However, to justify its use solely on this basis is to regard peer counseling in a very narrow light. Disability professionals and program planners need to be aware of the unique benefits of peer counseling: benefits which define it as a social movement as well as a therapeutic paradigm. There is increasing awareness even among professionals that such peer helping is often the more effective. In *The Skilled Helper*, Gerald Egan writes: "There is a growing body of opinions and evidence that helpers with extensive training in psychological theory and a variety of academic credentials do not necessarily help, the that the para-professional helper, if properly trained in helping skills, can become very effective even without extensive training in psychological theory" (1975, p. 9).

The basic distinction between peer counseling and professional counseling cannot be ascribed to the depth, intensity, or content of the counseling. The difference lies in the *nature of the relationship* between helper and helpee. The common assumption that the term "peer" implies an inexperienced or less well trained helper does not hold up across the range of peer counseling programs found in this country. While some programs require an academic degree for their peer counselors, others offer on-going, nonacademic training and supervision commensurate to professional levels. The dilemmas facing the field of peer counseling are similar to those of the professional field: a necessary reliance on subjective evaluation methods and the need for innovative ways to ensure quality service delivery.

The presence of a disabled peer counselor on the rehabilitation team creates a valuable direct channel for consumer input into the rehabilitation process. The peer counselor can provide concrete information on the service needs of clients on a continuing basis. Rehabilitation professionals are not immune to patronizing attitudes toward their clients. Including disabled practitioners on the rehabilitation team encourages the able-bodied staff to see disabled people as peers rather than as mere recipients of services, thus challenging attitudinal barriers that may hinder the professional–client relationship. It must also be remembered that many individuals in this culture attach a considerable stigma to the traditional therapist, psychologist, or social worker. Some of these individuals may find it more acceptable to enter a helping relationship with a peer.

Intervention by a disabled peer can significantly accelerate the transition to independent living for a severely disabled client. For the client, the most readily identifiable benefit is the realization that the peer counselor has had to confront similar issues, feelings, barriers, and experiences and can, therefore, readily empathize with what the client is going through.

This common experience allows a greater sense of safety in sharing feelings and identifying personal issues. The client is less likely to feel judged by a peer who has experienced feelings of vulnerability, shame, grief, or fear which to an able-bodied person might seem excessive or remote. At the same time, the client's excuse, "I can't do it," is unlikely to be accepted by a disabled peer counselor—living proof of what the client *can* do. As a role model, the peer counselor demonstrates not only that he or she can function independently and lead a fulfilling life in the community but also that a disabled person can go on to become a helper for others.

A disabled person is just as likely as an able-bodied person to harbor negative stereotypes of disabled persons. These stereotypes are often perpetuated by the social, if not physical, isolation which most disabled persons experience. The only other disabled people the newly disabled person is likely to encounter are fellow patients. For the developmentally disabled person leaving an institution, disabled friends were fellow inmates. In both cases, disabled peers were patients, and patients, in our culture, are classically viewed as dependent and powerless. The role of the peer counselor counteracts this stereotype and the relationship that develops between counselor and client can profoundly alter the sense of isolation that the disabled client may feel. Counseling groups are particularly powerful in challenging the feeling that "no one else feels this way." The members of such groups are also in a position to offer practical information based on first-hand experience, whether it be tips on getting a wheelchair into a car, suggestions for dealing with one's personal care attendant, or snappy retorts to a discriminatory remark.

To act as a peer counselor can be a powerful learning experience for a disabled person. Peer counselors often develop new interpersonal skills which they can apply to other areas of their lives. Helping others increases one's sense of self-worth. A peer counselor may find herself in the position of working with a client who is experiencing feelings of despair, isolation, or powerlessness similar to those she herself once confronted and has since been able to transcend. Being in the role of helper encourages the peer counselor to take on a greater degree of objectivity. One peer counselor working at the Boston Self Help Center said: "I have been made more aware that there are others who face many of the same issues and frustrations that I grapple with. This has lessened my feelings of separateness from the mainstream." Another put it this way: "I get so much out of it [peer counseling]. I hear my own thoughts and feelings said in so many ways, but each person says something new for me to learn about. I wish every disabled person got the chance to be a peer counselor. They'd look at their disability in a different way."

Disability is most often viewed by our own culture as a

tragedy, something that should never have happened. The popular literature frequently romanticizes disability as an inspirational experience, while at the same time our medicalized culture focuses on some possible future cure. These views of disability are useless to the individual whose disability is a daily fact of life. The experiences and insights of the peer counselor, however, are very valuable to the client. That someone else can benefit from one's own experience serves to increase the value of that experience. In this light, disability can be viewed as a natural part of human development and of the continuing confrontation with human vulnerability.

11

Skills Training

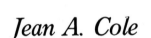

Jean A. Cole

Of the seventy-two independent living programs known to exist in the United States in 1982, 90 percent have indicated that one of their most important services is teaching independent living skills (Frieden and Widmer, 1982). In addition, as the influence of the Independent Living Movement has grown within the field of rehabilitation, a number of other types of facilities and agencies have also begun to offer independent living skills training to their clients. Such facilities and agencies include medical rehabilitation facilities, programs serving mentally retarded persons,

Note: My thinking about independent living issues has been shaped to a large degree by experience in the Cooperative Living, New Options, and Independent Living Research Utilization projects at the Institute for Rehabilitation and Research (TIRR) in Houston, Texas. A number of colleagues have provided valuable support and assistance, including Mary Ann Board, Lex Frieden, Laurie Gerken, Barbara Holden, Laurel Richards, William Spencer, Jane Sperry, and David Stock. The opinions expressed here are my own.

vocational facilities, colleges and universities, and public agencies such as home extension services.

The term *independent living skills training* is used to refer to a wide diversity of actual services. The purposes of this chapter are to identify what is meant by independent living skills within the Independent Living Movement, to describe alternative ways in which such skills are currently being taught, and to examine how the acquisition of independent living skills constitutes an important part of the overall rehabilitation or habilitation process.

Self-Direction: The Key Issue

An understanding of what *independent living skills* means can perhaps best be reached by examining the concept of independent living. Various definitions of this concept have recently been reviewed by Rice and Roessler (1980), with particular emphasis on those developed by Pflueger (1977) and by Frieden and others (1979). Despite minor differences, widely accepted definitions of independent living have two predominant themes in common: self-direction and control over their own lives for handicapped individuals and full participation by handicapped people in the life of the community, including both the responsibilities and the benefits shared by all citizens.

These two central principles of the independent living movement profoundly shape the ways independent living skills are conceptualized and taught, in contrast to skills historically taught to handicapped persons under the rubric of activities of daily living (ADL) or community living skills. The fundamental difference is that independent living skills are skills for self-direction, rather than task-oriented behavioral capabilities. This distinction arises from the basic expectation within the Independent Living Movement that handicapped individuals are capable of managing adult responsibilities. In contrast, the tacit expectation of the recent past has been that handicapped persons need to be taken care of as wards of their parents, appointed guardians, or public institutions. The role of ward does not require capabilities for self-direction; in fact, independence of mind is often strongly discouraged in handicapped persons who have been cast, either officially or tacitly, into the role of ward.

Skills for self-direction include the following types of capabilities typically expected of adults in our society:

- communicating effectively with others to acquire information, express viewpoints, and have needs met
- identifying and learning to use resources
- identifying and comparing choices
- making decisions and setting priorities
- making commitments to long-term goals and following through on a course of action until desired outcomes are attained
- developing sequential plans so that activities and efforts have a cumulative effect in leading to a long-term outcome
- assessing risks, anticipating consequences, and developing judgment about risk taking
- managing crises such as medical or financial emergencies
- solving problems

These capabilities seem ordinary enough, and most adult citizens are assumed to have them. Yet many handicapped persons have never learned or practiced self-direction because they have been hindered in doing so by their disabilities or by their environment, including not only the physical surroundings but also the social expectations and actions of influential persons such as parents or teachers who did not permit or foster independent functioning.

Many members of the handicapped consumer movement feel that self-direction by the handicapped individual is not a working goal of traditional programs serving handicapped persons, even though it is usually a part of the stated philosophies of such programs (Varela, 1979). The tendency of some traditional programs to foster dependence rather than independence has also been observed by rehabilitation professionals (DeJong, 1979; Trieschmann, 1980).

To understand how skills for self-direction are taught in independent living programs and how such training differs from traditional skills training, it is perhaps useful to compare how specific subjects such as attendant management are taught in both types of programs. In teaching attendant management, medical rehabilitation programs tend to emphasize tasks, focusing on techniques for catheter care, bowel programs, skin and nail care, and similar physical self-care tasks. In contrast, independent living programs consider attendant management training to include recruitment, hiring, and training of attendants; negotiation of working agreements; interpersonal relationships and styles of interaction; conflict resolution; discipline and termination; and payment for attendant services. Similarly, although many work adjustment programs at vocational facilities offer task-oriented financial training (for example, making ꞏnge and writing checks), they seldom address such personal financial management issues as long-term budgeting, tax planning, or self-advocacy in interacting with agencies and programs that provide financial benefits to handicapped persons.

In one sense, it is not surprising that, historically, the major emphasis has been on task-oriented approaches. No doubt the expectation that handicapped persons would be dependent on others contributed to that emphasis; there was no apparent need for them to learn self-management skills. In addition, task-oriented skills are simply easier to teach because they are concrete, observable, and procedurally oriented, and they are convenient for the rehabilitation practitioner to document. The methodological neatness of task-oriented training offers advantages in maintaining records of client goals and in measuring client progress, both of which may be required by sponsors of services, as is the case in independent living programs supported by Title VII funds.

However important and useful the performance of such physical tasks as "emptying pockets before doing laundry" (Van Soest and others, 1979) or "going to the mailbox and getting mail" (Walls, Zane, and Thredt, 1979) may be, it is indeed a misnomer to call them independent living skills if the philosophical premises underlying the Independent Living Movement are taken seriously. As Heumann states, "Independence is a mind process" (Pflueger, 1977, p. 1). This mind process is more difficult to translate into an operating program, document, and teach than are specific behavioral capabilities. Consequently, most traditional rehabilitation programs, at best, seek only to reinforce previously existing capabilities for self-direction when they occur in their clients.

The purpose of this discussion is not in any sense to criticize the teaching of physical tasks that have traditionally been referred to as activities of daily living or community living skills. They are clearly very important. Rather, the point is to clarify that something more than task performance training is needed by many handicapped persons and to stress that independent living programs have sought to provide that something more—namely, skills and capabilities for self-direction.

Assessing the Need for Independent Living Skills Training

Independent living skills training is widely offered by independent living programs to clients who have had previous rehabilitation or special education skills training. This practice gives validity to the premise that a substantial population of handicapped persons need to learn skills for self-direction and can benefit from such training. One program has referred to these clients as "less ready" for independent living responsibilities than the college student population originally served by the first independent living programs (Brown, 1978, p. 28). Indeed, as experience has been accrued in independent living programs, it has become clear that there are several different types of persons who may have difficulty with self-direction. These include mentally retarded individuals who may have cognitive or memory impairments (Sigelman and Parham, 1981), head-injured persons who may have sound intellectual skills but lack memory or the ability to make cogent judgments, and persons with disabilities who have been dependent since childhood. Persons in the last group usually have never been exposed to typical social experiences or to making decisions; plans and problems in their lives have always been dealt with by other people in caretaking roles (Cole and others, 1979a).

Because of substantial differences in the development of capabilities among various groups of handicapped persons, careful assessment of the individual's specific need for skills training is essential. Sometimes an individual has already mastered typical responsibilities of adults in our society and may only need to learn to exercise these responsibilities using aids such as a wheelchair or cane. For such persons, traditional rehabilitation programs—such as those provided by most medical facilities, training programs for mentally retarded persons, programs for blind or hearing-impaired persons, and vocational facilities—are sufficient because they address the largely task-oriented physical skills that must be mastered to attain independent functioning. Assessing a person's need to learn such task-oriented skills can be quite readily accomplished through systematic observation and the use of organizing tools such as a behavioral checklist (Walls, Zane, and Thredt, 1979) or standardized evaluation methodologies for physical or occupational therapy.

Much more difficult is the assessment of a person's capability for self-direction, which, as indicated above, is the central aspect of independent living that distinguishes it from more traditional programs. Such assessment can be done in part through careful interviewing about the individual's past experience and by asking for responses to hypothetical situations. A more accurate evaluation can often be obtained by observing actual performance as the individual encounters situations that require self-direction skills.

A few tools have been developed to assist in the systematic assessment of self-direction skills. For example, a series of standardized hypothetical situations that are likely to confront a handicapped individual in the community has been used in a study of individuals in the New Options Transitional Living Program (Sharp, 1980). Solutions the subjects offered to these hypothetical problems were evaluated by three persons who were familiar with the problems. Some functional assessment tools currently being developed attempt to identify and document difficulties with specific self-direction skills and to assess the individual's need to upgrade these skills (Crewe and Athelstan, 1978; Harrison, Garnett, and Watson, 1981). These functional assessments identify such self-direction skills as judgment, persistence, memory, consistency of behavior with rehabilitation goals, accurate perception of capabilities and limitations, and effective interaction with people as important factors that influence the individual's ability to function as a full member of society.

In assessing a person's need to learn self-direction, it seems particularly important to recognize subtle differences among people and to avoid making assumptions that certain capabilities are present or absent based on a person's type of disability or medical diagnostic label. For example, careful assessments of brain-injured persons can ascertain what specific parts of a given task they can do and what parts they find difficult; this is in sharp contrast to assuming that the entire task cannot be performed. Such distinctions apply not only to persons who may have difficulty with actual mental functioning but also to people whose previous life experience has prevented them from learning specific aspects of self-direction. For example, some persons may have grown up almost totally isolated from typical growth experiences and responsibilities, whereas others, who may have followed a typical developmental path with respect to managing shopping and financial affairs, may be extremely naive only with respect to social relationships such as dating.

In independent living programs that teach self-direction skills successfully, some form of written agreement is developed to document what is to be taught and what the responsibilities are of various persons who will be involved. Arriving at such an agreement may require negotiation if the handicapped individual and the person who is teaching have different views of what skills the handicapped person needs to learn. This type of discrepancy occurred quite often in the New Options Transitional Living Program (Cole and others, 1979b). For example, program participants often preferred not to learn such financial management skills as budgeting and planning ahead for contingencies because they viewed these subjects as boring and because, often, they had no way of judging how essential such knowledge would be to them later in a more independent living arrangement. Such an issue can cause an important philosophical dilemma for program staff who feel that the client should learn these crucial skills and who, at the same time, are committed to the program philosophy granting choice to the handicapped individual.

It is important that differences of opinion about the necessity of learning certain skills be resolved, because clients will not learn new skills if their potential usefulness is not perceived. One method of resolution is to have program clients make fundamental choices with the understanding that once those choices are made, other things follow automatically. (This has been likened to a person electing to have a particular type of surgery. Once the decision has been made to have the surgery, the selection of lab tests, preliminary procedures, and surgical techniques is not left to the individual; such decisions are considered to be necessary concomitants of the original choice.) In other cases, it may be preferable to begin with an agreement to work on a limited number of skills initially, with the expectation that the individual will recognize the need to learn other skills as he or she approaches situations that will require them. It has also proved valuable in a number of programs to have peer counselors or other handicapped individuals talk with clients to authenticate the need for certain skills. The opinion of a peer may be far more acceptable to the client than the advice of an able-bodied professional with whom the client cannot easily identify. Whatever process will achieve a pretraining agreement, having such an explicit understanding seems essential to assuring commitment and to avoiding misunderstandings about the expectations and responsibilities of all parties.

A written agreement delineating a course of study is useful not only in assuring clear interpersonal expectations but also in maintaining systematic client records. As has been pointed out previously, teaching task-oriented skills is attractive in part because behavioral objectives are easy to develop and progress can be documented in simple terms. Behavioral objectives can be formulated for the more abstract self-direction skills as well, although these often require more creativity and imagination to develop. A substantial literature exists on developing behavioral objectives in which concrete behaviors serve as indicators for more abstract capabilities (see, for example, Mager, 1975). In devising behavioral indicators for abstract self-management skills, the central issue seems to be whether behavioral tasks are merely ends in themselves or whether they are carefully selected to serve as indicators of more abstract self-management capabilities. (See Frieden, 1980a, on adapting individualized written rehabilitation plans to independent living.)

Methods of Teaching Independent Living Skills

Methods of teaching independent living skills range from an informal coaching relationship between a single client and a peer counselor to relatively formalized group courses on relevant topics. Two widely known independent living programs will serve to illustrate approaches that have been used successfully. The first of these programs is the New Options Transitional Living Program in Houston, Texas, which operated as a research and demonstration project from 1976 through 1979. In New Options, a six week live-in program, a curriculum of independent living training modules was developed on the basis of extensive interviews with handicapped persons who had already attained a variety of independent lifestyles. The training modules included attendant management, consumer affairs, financial management, functional skills, living arrangements, medical needs, mobility, sexuality, social skills, time management, and vocational and educational options. Each module was composed of five or six sessions selected to meet the needs of a particular group of program participants. Modules were taught by active handicapped persons from the community who were selected to represent a variety of solutions to the problems that typically confront handicapped persons seeking to live independently. Module leaders, called staff associates, were paid on a per-session basis for their work. Associates were recruited, trained, and supervised by a full-time coordinator. Field trips were used extensively in each module to give participants an opportunity to practice new skills in a variety of community settings. Individual counseling was important in helping participants develop goals, make plans, and identify skills and information they needed to reach their goals. Extensive information on New Options, including curriculum outlines for each module session, is available in several publications (Cole and others, 1979a, 1979b; Board and others, 1980).

At the Center for Independent Living (CIL) in Berkeley, California, a primary teaching method is one-to-one coaching of individual clients by peer counselors. Rather than spend time in a transitional living environment, CIL clients typically seek to establish an independent living arrangement directly in the community, with the program staff providing advice and assistance on an ongoing basis. One of the key functions of the peer counselor is to help clients anticipate potential problems in their new environment and refer them to specific supportive services of the center when such assistance is needed. There is a firm commitment to a coaching relationship in which the client retains control over his or her own goals, and the peer counselor plays a supportive and advisory rather than a directive role (Heumann, 1979).

Peer counseling is frequently chosen by independent living programs as a primary method for teaching independent living skills. Peer counselors are deliberately selected to serve as models with whom clients can identify because they have successfully resolved many of the problems clients themselves face in establishing an independent lifestyle. In some programs, a range of models is selected so that clients can observe directly that there are alternative ways to resolve problems. Modeling as a principle for teaching new skills and changing behavior depends not only on demonstration of the skills required to accomplish certain outcomes but also on demonstration of the rewards the learner can attain by acquiring a new skill. Effective modeling, in other words, affects motivation as well as skills acquisition (Bandura, 1966).

In addition to acting as models for their clients, peer counselors frequently function as coaches. In this capacity, they can offer advice about the effectiveness of various strategies chosen by the client and also provide feedback on how well the client is performing as he or she attempts to use new skills. As coaches, peer counselors can facilitate the problem-solving process by asking leading questions that help clients address solutions they might not otherwise have considered. A recent publication of the Institute on Rehabilitation Issues, *Peer Counseling as a Rehabilitation Resource,* summarizes many of the current issues in the field (Pankowski and others, 1981).

In contrast to the one-to-one modeling and coaching of peer counseling relationships, independent living programs frequently give formal group courses on topics of common interest to many clients. In some cases, a preplanned curriculum is used (Cole and others, 1979), and in other cases, such courses are encouraged to evolve on an ad hoc basis as problems are articulated within the group (Saxton, 1981). Group leaders for these courses are sometimes called peer educators to emphasize that their function is to educate rather than to counsel (Schatzlein, 1978). In selecting such teachers, it is important to consider philosophical commitment as well as personal capability. In programs that employ peer counselors as teachers, the counselors are selected because their handicaps are similar to those of their clients and because they have successfully resolved certain issues in developing their own independent lifestyles. It is also important that successful teachers have thorough knowledge of the subject they are expected to teach and that they be able to relate well to others in any teaching situation. Perhaps most important of all is a fundamental commitment to the independent living philosophy of self-direction and full integration into the community. This means that the successful teacher of independent living skills must be able to let clients make their own choices, practice new skills without being overprotected, and find their own solutions to problems. Frequently, this requires much more creativity and patience on the part of the teacher than would be required for them to solve the same problems. It requires a commitment not to rescue the handicapped person who is experiencing difficulty but who needs the opportunity to learn by working through the problem. Commitment to the independent living philosophy is frequently easy to voice but difficult to uphold in actual practice.

The principle of encouraging persons to learn through

practical experience and gradually to assume new responsibilities is based on a fundamental tenet of the Independent Living Movement, the right of all individuals to take risks and to fail. This principle contrasts with the overprotectiveness of many handicapped persons' upbringing as well as with the service philosophies of many agencies that serve handicapped persons. Yet, many of the issues involved in fostering autonomy and allowing persons to develop judgment by taking risks and experiencing the consequences of their actions are discussed in the body of popular literature on effective parenting. Such material is useful for both parents and rehabilitation professionals who must learn to let go in response to the emerging capabilities of the handicapped individual.

The Independent Living Movement's commitment to full integration into the community shapes the way self-direction skills are taught to the handicapped person. Practice within a special and isolated setting such as a rehabilitation facility frequently does not transfer to actual community situations. Most independent living programs are strongly committed to having their clients learn new skills within the community environments they will need to negotiate later on their own. This may be accomplished by peer counseling and coaching within the client's own living situation or by the use of field trips that give clients direct experience in a variety of settings.

Incorporating Skills Training into the Rehabilitation Process

The Independent Living Movement aims at self-direction and full participation in society for handicapped persons. Teaching handicapped persons the skills needed to function as autonomous and responsible adults in our society is an important part of the process. This method differs radically from the traditional expectations that shape handicapped persons to become dependent wards or, alternatively, superstars who are never supposed to make mistakes. The Independent Living Movement argues that the American ideal must be full citizenship for all handicapped persons and that all agencies serving handicapped individuals must be challenged to examine what they are preparing their clients for. Often, the actual effects of a program will be quite different from stated goals.

This contradiction raises the important issue of who can best teach independent living skills and how such training can best be incorporated into the developmental process of each handicapped individual. The answer, of course, must depend on the characteristics of the particular individual and on the array of support systems available in his or her community.

Originally, independent living skills training—that is, training for self-direction in a community context—was developed by independent living programs. There are several basic types of independent living programs, including nonresidential centers for independent living, short-term, live-in transitional programs, and long-term residential programs (Frieden and others, 1979). Different programs characteristically use different methods for teaching independent living skills. Nonresidential centers for independent living—of which Berkeley's CIL is a prototype—place heavy emphasis on peer counseling and the use of modeling and individual coaching. Some centers also offer group classes on such subjects as attendant management. Examples of this kind of center include Access Living in Chicago, Holistic Approaches to Independent Living (HAIL) in Denver, and the Houston Center for Independent Living. Short-term transitional programs, such as the New Options Program in Houston, the Worchester Area Transitional Housing Program in Massachusetts, and the Boston Center for Independent Living, emphasize a group teaching process and a relatively organized curriculum for teaching independent living skills. They place heavy emphasis on peer educators as teachers, models, and coaches and on extensive field trips as a means of practicing new skills in the community rather than in specialized settings. Residential independent living programs generally seem to place more emphasis on providing support services such as attendant assistance or transportation than on teaching new skills, but many residents of such programs have used the capabilities acquired in group residential settings to move on to other living arrangements in the community. Such programs are exemplified by Creative Living in Columbus, Ohio, and by the Cooperative Living Project in Houston. (See Chapter Four for a fuller discussion of program models.)

Earlier in this chapter it was mentioned that a number of other rehabilitation agencies are finally starting to offer independent living skills training. Although in some cases this training may simply be a new name for traditional services, many such facilities and agencies have indeed developed impressive programs of independent living skills training based on the principles of self-direction and active community participation by the handicapped individual.

Craig Hospital in Englewood, Colorado (in its Community Re-Entry program), and TIRR in Houston (in its Rehab III program) have developed substantially new methods of service delivery as a component of the overall medical rehabilitation process. Other medical rehabilitation facilities such as the University of Minnesota in Minneapolis and Tufts New England Medical Center in Boston have added peer educators or peer counselors to their medical rehabilitation teams to help clients prepare for an independent lifestyle in the community.

Programs that serve mentally retarded persons have also seen major efforts to foster maximum self-direction in various independent living arrangements, including individual as well as group homes. The citizen advocacy movement in this field emphasizes independent living goals for its clients, and in many communities citizen advocacy programs have successfully used individual coaching to teach independent living skills to mentally retarded clients. An extensive bibliography on citizen advocacy programs for mentally retarded persons has been developed by Rude (1979).

In some communities, the public education system has made substantial efforts to offer independent living skills training as part of the general programming at elementary, secondary, junior college, and adult education levels. The impetus behind this development has increased substantially since passage of the Education of All Handicapped Children Act in 1975. Methods used in such skills training programs have been documented in the literature on career education for handicapped persons (see, for example, Brolin, 1980; Brolin and Kokaska, 1979; Clark and White, 1980; Gillette, 1981). A comparative study by Frieden and Frieden of European and American programs (1981) indicates that several other countries have made more substantial progress than the United States in incorporating independent living skills training for handicapped persons into the public education system. Still, it is noteworthy that many colleges and universities in this country developed active disabled students programs in the late 1960s and early 1970s, many of which became the forerunners of independent living programs in their communities. Although independent living skills training per se is not often named as a major service of disabled students programs, in actual practice such training is provided to many disabled students through counseling services (President's Committee on Employment of the Handicapped, 1977).

In reviewing programs that offer some form of independent living skills training, the question arises when and how such training can be best provided in the course of the individual development of a handicapped person. As the independent living and educational mainstreaming movements gain momentum in this country, and as more and more handicapped persons seek to live as full citizens, the need for such training will grow substantially. Ideally, in the long term it will be preferable for disabled children to learn independent living skills in the same way their nondisabled counterparts learn them, through natural experiences and gradual assumption of new roles and responsibilities at home and at school. For persons who become disabled later in life, the initial medical care and rehabilitation would ideally include careful assessment of their existing capabilities for self-direction and offer opportunities for upgrading those skills as needed, using the teaching principles of independent living programs.

Until some future time when handicapped persons are included as full members of society and methods of cultivating skills for self-direction are commonplace, it will continue to be necessary to compensate for the negative experiences of handicapped persons who have been kept in institutions or isolated at home. For the foreseeable future, there will continue to be adults who have never handled even simple responsibilities such as shopping for their own clothing or selecting their own attendant, and these persons will need training and practice in self-direction in order to reach their full potential as independent persons. This training can best be provided by independent living programs, disabled students programs at universities, adult education programs, citizen advocacy programs, and similar programs that are firmly committed to a philosophy of self-direction and autonomy for handicapped citizens.

Independence and Interdependence

The goal of teaching self-direction skills to handicapped persons raises the fundamental question of how to teach those individuals who, because of genetic errors, birth trauma, and injury or disease that affects the brain, do not have the innate capability to analyze choices and make decisions, assess risks and develop judgment about the consequences of their behavior, or resolve problems that occur in daily life.

Perhaps the best way to address this issue is to analyze the relationship between an individual and the support system on which he or she relies. All humans are dependent to some extent on family members, friends, social organizations, workplace, and community services. The way dependence is organized and managed depends on the domain, capabilities, and personal preferences of each individual. Generally, handicapped persons have had much less choice in managing dependency than have nondisabled persons whose needs are more typical and for whom a wider array of solutions is possible. For example, there are many more car mechanics than wheelchair mechanics.

The crucial issue is how the dependency is managed. Who is in control? In almost all cases, the relationship between the handicapped person and the support systems on which he or she depends can be altered to give a greater measure of control to the handicapped person.

This suggests that there are *degrees* of independence and dependence for each person. It further suggests that for most handicapped persons a greater measure of self-direction could be attained if the person's support systems were designed to foster choice and self-direction and gradual cultivation of his or her capabilities. The concept of *relative independence* is often used in discussing independent living for persons with impairments that affect the basic capability for self-direction, such as persons who are mentally retarded or head injured (Sigelman and Parham, 1981). This concept places clear responsibility on providers of support services to handicapped persons—whether formal service providers, family members, or friends—to uphold the independent living principles of self-direction and full community participation. This is particularly true for persons who have difficulty with self-direction, for they themselves may be unable to advocate or negotiate for a relationship in which they have greater control and choice.

It remains a major challenge to develop more innovative ways of providing support services to persons who need help with self-direction. The citizen advocacy movement in the field of mental retardation has been able to establish a few exemplary community programs through which assistants provide mentally retarded persons with help in planning, decision making, and problem solving. This support is analogous in many respects to the physical help needed on a daily basis by a physically disabled person. Cultivating more such means of fostering autonomy, choice, and self-direction is a subtle and difficult task.

Goodman (1967) addresses the idea of relative independence in a wide-ranging study of the concept of individual autonomy in the literature of anthropology, psychology, and sociology. She quotes from Gordon Allport's classic work *Becoming* (1955) as follows: "Up until now, the tug of war between free will (or autonomy) and determinism has been marked by naivete. . . . Our previous considerations fall short of solving the problem of freedom. They urge us, however, to forego naive solutions. That there are upper limits to the possibilities of growth in each life no one can deny. But it seems likely that these limits are movable by virtue of the capacities for reflection, for self-objectification, and to a degree by breadth of education, and by the effort an individual may put forth. From the ethical and theological points of view the stretching toward this limit, whatever it is, is as much of a triumph for a life of slight potential as for a life whose potentials are great" (Goodman, 1967, pp. 6-10).

12

Accessible Transportation

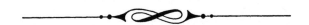

Frank Bowe

Accessible transportation serves both as a practical necessity and as a philosophical basis for independent living. Without means of transportation to educational, vocational, cultural, recreational, and commercial facilities in the community, it is virtually impossible for most severely disabled people to live outside an institutional environment. Thus, in a very real sense, transportation is a key to independent living. Its availability expands the disabled individual's horizon: access to transportation means access to cultural and recreational opportunities, to training that qualifies the individual for employment commensurate with his or her abilities, to life-support functions and services including medical care and daily sustenance, and to employment remote from the place of residence.

Note: This chapter is an extensively revised and expanded version of an article that appeared in the October 1979 issue of *Archives of Physical Medicine and Rehabilitation.*

Ideally, transportation sustains the philosophy of independent living by providing handicapped people with the same services and facilities available to able-bodied people, for the same price. In practice, however, transportation often is simply not available in any form for physically handicapped individuals. In no city in the United States is transportation as accessible to disabled as it is to nondisabled persons. That fact points to a central obstruction to independent living in the 1980s: if one cannot get around, how is one to live independently?

The problem has been recognized for some time. Over the past two decades, the United States Congress and various executive agencies have discussed the disparity between the availability of publicly supported transportation and its accessibility to people with physical impairments. The concept of independent living and the related problem of transportation were raised repeatedly in testimony presented to Congress during consideration of vocational rehabilitation legislation in the early 1960s. In 1970, language linking transportation and independent living was embodied in PL91-453, the so-called UmtAct amendments, when Representative Mario Biaggi of New York succeeded in attaching to the House bill, and retaining during the House-Senate conference, the following statement: "It is hereby declared to be the national policy that elderly and handicapped persons have the same right as other persons to utilize mass transportation facilities and services; that special efforts shall be made in the planning and design of mass transportation facilities and services so that the availability to elderly and handicapped persons of mass transportation which they can effectively utilize will be assured; and that all Federal programs offering assistance in the field of mass transportation (including the programs under this Act) should contain provisions implementing this policy" (section 16(a), 84 *Statutes at Large* 962, Urban Mass Transportation Assistance Act of 1970). Representative Biaggi described the section as guaranteeing "that equal rights to transportation facilities are extended" to elderly and handicapped persons and as stating congressional opposition to separate services as an alternative to equal access because such separate services "would further serve to segregate the elderly and handicapped" (116 *Congressional Record* 34180f).

The UmtAct was ahead of its time in a number of ways. It defined independent living, without using the term itself, as appropriate for senior citizens, physically disabled persons, and retarded individuals. It stressed the importance of access to mass transportation services at a time when disabled and elderly people were restricted almost exclusively to segregated special services. And it tied independent living directly and inseparably to transportation. Today, almost a decade and a half after the 1970 UmtAct amendments, we find ourselves just about where we were then: "special efforts," as vague and unenforceable now as then, remains the standard. Accessible public mass transit facilities and vehicles can be found in only a few metropolitan areas. The key to moving ahead is provided by the history of efforts to make public transportation accessible—and by the story of one particular effort, the Transbus program.

When four disabled students at the University of Illinois moved from a nursing home to a barrier-free apartment in 1969, and when several mobility-restricted students at the University of California at Berkeley began an equipment repair and peer counseling program in 1970, they were expressing a desire that was at the time rather startling. People with disabilities, long regarded as "sick" and as "patients," were insisting on their similarity to people who were not disabled—and on their right to live lives like those of ablebodied people. It is not surprising, given the climate of the times, that this nascent movement, like so many others, began on college campuses. From the outset, transportation formed a crucial component of the students' vision of an independent life. For vehicles, they looked first to vans, such as those Volkswagen manufactured at the time. They modified the vans for transporting electric wheelchairs by adding small lifts, wheelchair restraints, and hand controls and by removing rear seats and sometimes part of the front seats.

The beginning made by the students in Illinois and California soon spurred the formation of similar programs in Boston, Houston, and many other cities nationwide. In 1972, the pending amendments to the Rehabilitation Act of 1973 carried recognition of the emerging Independent Living Movement in the form of authorization for a program of activity. President Nixon vetoed the bill. In 1973, Congress dropped the independent living program from the bill that later became law (PL 93-112).

Meanwhile, the federal Department of Transportation (DOT), acting on PL91-453 and the 1974 National Mass Transportation Assistance Act (PL93-503), funded a number of projects to demonstrate dial-a-ride services, which offer door-to-door transportation for eligible disabled individuals. DOT also funded experimental design projects intended to develop what it called Transbus, "the bus of the future"—and instructed the manufacturers participating in the projects to make these experimental vehicles accessible to disabled and elderly persons.

Then, in 1977 and 1978, a convergence of events seemed to set the stage for explosive growth both in independent living and in transportation. First, DOT secretary Brock Adams announced on May 19, 1977 that all standard-sized urban mass transit buses purchased with federal financial assistance must be accessible Transbuses. The decision seemed to close the door at last on the segregated special services Biaggi had disparaged in his comments during the House debate on PL 91-453. A few months later, Congress began drafting what was to become PL 95-602, the Rehabilitation, Comprehensive Services and Developmental Disabilities Amendments of 1978. This legislation included specific authorization for independent living, which was for the first time called by that name in a piece of legislation signed into law. And it was good. Congress intended for the nation's eighty-four state vocational rehabilitation agencies, many of which served only blind and visually impaired clients, to coordinate a broad program of independent living rehabilitation services. Funds were to be provided through these agencies to independent living centers throughout the nation.

Disabled advocates found the combination exhilarating. At last it would be possible in any large urban area anywhere in the country to combine such independent living services as peer counseling and housing assistance with accessible mass transportation services. Severely disabled people could take public buses from their apartments and homes to independent living centers, to job training courses, and anywhere else they wanted to go—at the very low public transit fares charged others in the city's population.

Then, just as quickly as it had surfaced, the bubble burst. The federal executive agencies charged with implementing the 1978 Rehabilitation amendments interpreted the independent living program language to specify not a nationwide program but a series of small projects. Congress implicitly accepted this interpretation when it provided only $2 million in appropriations to carry out the program. This was so little that it meant it would be possible only for a few communities to support small independent living centers. And Adams was forced to back down from his Transbus mandate by the ineradicable opposition of bus manufacturers and mass transit operators. As a result of these events, it is the exception today rather than the rule for any given community to feature both an independent living center and an accessible mass transportation program. To understand what went wrong—and how similar setbacks can be avoided in the future—we must examine the Transbus story in depth.

Transbus was to be the bus of the future, the first entirely new design in standard-sized buses in a generation. In Washington, DOT officials prepared a lengthy list of specifications describing exactly how large, how heavy, how fuel-efficient, and how fast the bus would be. The specifications were so detailed that they included requirements in window size and shape, air conditioning and heating plant characteristics, and even rearview mirror size. DOT's primary objectives were to reduce running time, the time required for a bus to complete its route, thus lowering labor and equipment costs, and to increase the appeal of buses for urban populations, thereby increasing ridership and reducing urban congestion caused by cars. A secondary objective, one that did not become important until fairly late in the nine-year history of the project, was to satisfy the accessibility requirements contained in Biaggi's UmtAct amendment.

DOT expended $27 million in contracting with three

manufacturers to produce Transbus prototypes. General Motors, the dominant force in the industry, Flexible, GM's main competitor, and small AM General, a division of American Motors, participated in the project.

The federal government had reason for optimism about Transbus. A new bus was long overdue. The current version of standard-sized buses, dubbed the "advanced design" bus, was generally understood to be inadequate to meet America's urban mass transportation needs: the bus broke down frequently, had poor gas mileage, and was unpopular with riders. Knowing that 80 percent of all mass transit customers ride buses, with only one in five using subways or other urban systems, and recognizing the urgent need to contain urban pollution and traffic congestion, DOT had high hopes that Transbus would lead the way to affordable, attractive, and environment-aware public transit for the 1970s and beyond.

Meanwhile, disabled advocates who had been suing individual local transit operators for failure to provide accessible transportation had a stroke of genius: instead of going after the operators, they would attack the major source of funding for urban mass transportation, DOT itself. The reasoning seemed sound. DOT paid 80 percent of the purchasing costs and half of the operating costs of almost all buses used in urban mass transit, and set the rules by which these buses were made. If DOT could be pressured into requiring accessibility, the advocates argued, the manufacturers would have no choice but to build accessible buses and the operators no option but to buy them. So in 1976, twelve organizations of disabled people, led by Disabled in Action (DIA) of Pennsylvania, Paralyzed Veterans of America (PVA) and the newly formed American Coalition of Citizens with Disabilities (ACCD), filed suit against DOT's Urban Mass Transportation Administration.

Soon after the Carter administration took office in the early spring of 1977, DOT secretary Adams ordered a full-scale review of the Transbus project. Convinced that it was right, he announced on May 19, 1977 that DOT thereafter would provide federal funds only for the purchase of such vehicles. DIA, PVA, and ACCD dropped the suit upon Adams's announcement, which for them was a total victory.

Then the unraveling began. In retrospect, the essential weakness of the entire Transbus effort is readily apparent: it rested on an attempt by federal bureaucrats to dictate the course of a commercial endeavor. DOT, not the private manufacturers, decided what kind of bus would be constructed. And DOT, not the local operators, decided what kind of bus would be purchased for use in the nation's cities. Disabled advocates made the only sensible decision given the course of events—they went after the real decision makers, the bureaucrats in Washington. So everything turned on the federal government; Transbus would succeed or fail depending upon how well DOT performed its task.

The bus manufacturers were the first to attack DOT. Their initial concern was more political than engineering in nature. GM, in particular, resented strongly Washington's efforts to dictate bus manufacturing. This posture was similar to the company's outlook on other regulatory issues, such as seat belts, pollution controls, and the like. Being a major employer as well as a top Fortune 100 corporation, GM had a lot of political clout to apply to this political battle—and it used it. During the summer of 1978, the company succeeded in attaching to a pending bill, the Surface Mass Transportation Amendments of 1978, an amendment requiring Adams to "reevaluate" his Transbus mandate. Under considerable pressure from GM, Congress took the amendment seriously. Disabled advocates counterattacked fiercely, knowing that if the amendment stood, all was lost. Finally, congressional leaders invited GM to bring its bus design prototype to Washington for a demonstration, hoping that this would help resolve the increasingly vitriolic battle between GM on the one hand and disabled advocates on the other. The demonstration proved one thing: GM's version was inadequate. Its lift did not work properly, the boarding and disembarking time required for persons using wheelchairs was unrealistically lengthy, and the running time for the bus to complete its route was too long. Congress dropped the amendment from the bill that later became law.

GM may have lost that battle, but it won the war. It did so because the local transit operators, through their association, the American Public Transit Association (APTA) joined forces with GM to attack DOT directly. APTA's concern mirrored that of GM: they did not like having Washington dictate what kind of buses they would have to purchase and use. They were concerned, too, about the whole idea of disabled people riding on their buses. The operators' fear was that such riders would be unsafe for bus drivers to transport, that boarding and disembarking these riders would slow running time, and that able-bodied riders might start shunning buses were severely disabled people to start using them. The APTA leaders charged in public testimony on DOT's pending section 504 regulations, which featured Transbus as a centerpiece, that Adams's mandate was "absolute nonsense" (Crosby, 1978). Through a nationwide public relations campaign, APTA and GM convinced many in the media that the regulation was "rule-making gone amok," as Crosby put it in his Washington *Star* story headlined with a front-page screamer, *Mass Transportation's Emotional Block-buster.* Columnist Neal Pierce, picking up on APTA's theme, urged President Carter to "cease and desist" in the administration's attempt to force accessibility upon the nation's bus manufacturers and operators (Pierce, 1978). New York City Mayor Koch, who just eighteen months earlier, as a representative from Manhattan, had been one of Congress's strongest supporters of section 504, testified that DOT's section 504 rules "would literally bankrupt us." Transit spokesmen from Chicago claimed that the regulation would cost $910 million in that city alone and pointed out that this sum would exceed the total amount invested in Chicago's transit system since 1890. Privately, city officials admitted that they were guessing; no one had actually calculated the costs on a station-by-station, vehicle-by-vehicle basis. Nevertheless, the huge numbers had their intended effect: DOT relaxed its requirements. When DOT tried to salvage the situation by letting a contract to build the first set of Transbuses, all three manufacturers flatly refused to bid. When no foreign manufacturers accepted Adams's request to submit bids, Transbus was dead.

　Disabled advocates seeking accessible mass transportation in the future will have to use different tactics. The story of the ill-fated Transbus shows that Washington alone cannot effect accessibility. The advocates will have to enlist at least one manufacturer and at least a half-dozen local operators on their side. This the disabled advocates did try during the Transbus battle. They enlisted support from the transit authorities in Miami, Los Angeles, and Philadelphia—the three cities that formed a consortium requesting bids from the manufacturers for the first series of Transbuses. And the advocates sought the involvement of John Z. DeLorean, a sports car manufacturer, as a builder of Transbuses when the three established firms declined to bid for the consortium's business. But it was too little too late. The manufacturers knew they could ignore the three cities' request because few other transit authorities were prepared to order Transbuses, and DeLorean, beleaguered by problems in getting his sports car manufactured, never did make a firm commitment to build buses.

The final nail in the Transbus coffin was driven in by the hammer of the Court of Appeals for the District of Columbia when it granted APTA relief from DOT's section 504 regulation, sought by the association on behalf of its members. The Court's 1981 decision ruled that the regulation was overly burdensome to operators and exceeded the department's mandate from Congress. Another secretary of transportation might have appealed the decision in order to save the regulation, but not President Reagan's DOT secretary, Drew Lewis. Moving swiftly, Lewis responded to the court decision by rewriting the regulation in far weaker terms, saying that the revision represented an example of how President Reagan would keep his campaign promise to get government off the backs of the American people and to reduce the onerous burdens of federal rulemaking on private enterprise. The rewritten rules removed the requirement to purchase Transbus and substituted language requiring only "special efforts" by transit operators to accommodate disabled people in some way not specified in the rules. DOT had taken a giant step backwards to the same requirement that had proved so unsatisfactory a decade earlier.

While the dream of a nationwide network of independent living centers and of Transbus providing inexpensive accessible transportation using standard-sized buses has not been realized, progress still can be made by concerned individuals and advocates. Experiences of several transit authorities across the nation provide examples of what might be done.

Kinston's Independent Transportation for the Elderly (KITE) in Kinston, North Carolina, offers a way for disabled and older citizens in this city of twenty-six thousand to gain access to transportation. In Kinston, the only public transportation available is the taxi service offered by eight independent companies. Qualified disabled and elderly persons can buy ticket books from KITE that entitle them to taxi service at half price. A $4 book, for example, is good for $8 in service. There are no restrictions on use other than that the subsidized fares are good only within city limits. DOT's Urban Mass Transportation Administration supports the project with a three-year, $193,000 grant.

In San Mateo County, California, where the population is six hundred thousand, a different approach is taken. The San Mateo Transit District (SamTrans) contracts with a private company to offer a special transportation service to mobility-impaired residents of the county. The service, called Redi-Wheels, is a demand-response system that offers transportation within three zones in the SamTrans service area. Twelve 16-passenger lift-equipped buses owned by SamTrans provide about 145 one-way rides each day. Trips on Redi-Wheels must be requested twenty-four hours in advance; each trip must take place entirely within one of the three SamTrans zones. One-way fares are $.25 each, but the actual cost to SamTrans for each one-way trip is about $6. The subsidy that permits the low user fares is provided by the California Transit Development Act through the Metropolitan Transportation Commission.

A third example is offered by Atlanta's MARTA (Metropolitan Atlanta Rapid Transit Authority). Atlanta is one of the few urban centers in the country to have an accessible subway system. (Washington, D.C. and the San Francisco Bay area are others.) Many disabled and elderly persons use this fixed-route mainstream system, as do many other Atlanta residents and visitors. In addition, MARTA offers special bus services, one for disabled persons (the L-Bus, for Lift) and one for elderly citizens (the E-Bus, for Elderly). L-Bus service began on May 16, 1977 with twenty lift-equipped buses. It is a subscription service that offers fixed-route transportation for persons who subscribe. Each subscriber must use the service regularly, typically once daily or once a week, although other intervals are permitted. The L-Bus route is built around these scheduled routes. About thirty-five people use the service daily, with some 250 person-trips made each week. While the actual cost to MARTA for each such one-way trip is $19, users pay a flat fare of $1 for each trip. The subsidy is provided through general transit revenues. Bus service usage has declined since the accessible subway was introduced.

   Atlanta's experience has been exceptionally good in comparison with that of many other cities, notably Denver, Houston, and Los Angeles, where battles routinely are waged between transit authorities and local organizations of disabled people. MARTA's success may be traced, in large part, to the establishment, in early 1975, of an Elderly and Handicapped Advisory Committee. The fifteen members of this committee meet monthly and are involved in the development of transportation alternatives for disabled and elderly Atlantans. The subway system, for example, was accessible from the start at the committee's insistence. This was not true of San Francisco's Bay Area Rapid Transit (BART), nor was it true of Washington, D.C.'s METRO. Clearly, having a committee and listening to what it has to say helps a local transit authority avoid controversy while improving service.

   In areas where mass transportation is inaccessible, disabled and elderly people tend to rely on their own privately owned vehicles, particularly standard-sized cars and small vans. The Braun Corporation, of Winamac, Indiana, is an example of a manufacturer that provides modified vans for severely disabled persons. DriveMaster Corporation, of West Patterson, New Jersey, is another. Small buses are made by such companies as Bluebird Body Company, of Fort Valley, Georgia; Chance Manufacturing Company, of Dallas, Texas; and Skillcraft Industries, of Venice, Florida. Many disabled persons will purchase a regular van, such as those manufactured by Ford and Chevrolet, and modify it to meet their special needs. Wheelchair lifts, ramps, and securements may be purchased separately and installed on such vans. ABC Enterprises, of Mentor, Ohio; Electro Van Lift, of St. Paul, Minnesota; and Ricon Corporation, of Sun Valley, California, are examples of firms making lifts for small vans and buses. I am aware of only three manufacturers of van and small bus ramps in the United States: Collins Industries, of Hutchinson, Kansas; Handi-Ramp, of Mundelein, Illinois; and Medicab, of Yonkers, New York. Wheelchairs may be secured in vans and buses by means of belts, wheelchair holders, T-bars, lateral grab bars, frame locks, and other devices.

In some areas, private and public efforts are coordinated to enable disabled persons to achieve access to transportation. In Brockton, Massachusetts, for example, DIAL-A-BAT (DAB) offers a subscription service and a dial-a-ride service. The subscription service operates daily from 7 A.M. to 6 P.M. while the dial-a-ride service is in operation from 8 A.M. to 6 P.M. Individuals using the dial-a-ride service pay $1 for each one-way trip; people using the subscription service pay $.50 per one-way trip. Brockton's two systems allow disabled persons three choices: their own vehicle, a subscription service at low cost that requires regular use at prearranged times, and a dial-a-ride service that responds quickly to calls and provides door-to-door service. The coordinated approach seems to work. Brockton has been successful because its two main services meet the varying needs of the people who use them. In addition, BAT, the Brockton Area Transit Authority, is a recipient of DOT funds and can use these federal dollars to pay 80 percent of the costs of the vehicles used in the programs. BAT is also eligible for federal operating funds, which provide 50 percent of the operating deficit BAT incurs in the program (most transit authorities operate at a deficit, rather than at a profit). DAB, which contracts with BAT to offer the two services in Brockton, gets more vehicles at lower costs than otherwise would be the case because of BAT's federal assistance. DAB is also able to ensure that all drivers are fully trained in working with disabled and elderly persons. Finally, Brockton is successful because BAT recognized that large buses and commuter rail systems would be inappropriate for meeting the needs of the area's disabled and elderly citizens, many of whom use their personal vehicles for most transportation but rely upon the subscription service or the dial-a-ride service for special needs, much as the average person uses a car for daily shopping but depends on buses or trains to get from home to the central city for business purposes.

A similar approach is being taken in Florida, where the state legislature has required that transportation services be coordinated. That Florida leads the way in mandating coordinated transportation should not be surprising; it has the nation's highest per capita population of elderly citizens and one of the highest populations of disabled persons. Accessible transportation long has been an urgent priority in Florida; recall that Miami was one of the first three cities to place orders for Transbus. In June 1979, after the Transbus order produced no bids, the Florida legislature passed a bill (FL79–180) establishing a coordinating council on the transportation disadvantaged to coordinate the planning of state and federal funds available for transportation of disadvantaged persons, including those who are disabled and/or elderly, and to support the development of coordinated community transportation systems. The Florida Department of Transportation is the lead agency in implementation of the program. The council consists of the state DOT secretary, the secretary of health and rehabilitative services, the secretary of community affairs and education, and representatives of elderly and handicapped citizens appointed by the governor, as well as the president of the Florida Association of Community Action Agencies. The law's force comes from its provision requiring that no funds be expended unless provided for in the annual program of the Department of Transportation's Five Year Plan for serving transportation-disadvantaged persons.

The success of the Florida program suggests that future advances in transportation for disabled persons will be designed and implemented at the state level. Florida clearly benefited from Atlanta's demonstration of the importance of involving consumers in the design and development of accessible transportation services. It also learned from Massachusetts' Brockton

Area Transit Authority that coordination of services was vital. That state legislation may be the route of the future is suggested by the fact that California quickly followed Florida's lead—and that the federal Department of Transportation's new section 504 regulation requires such coordination of services on the state and local levels.

Leaders of independent living programs need not despair of realizing the concept of mainstreaming in transportation. As Florida is showing, access to regular transportation services is possible even without Transbus, and that is important. It indicates that advocates must continue to emphasize the design (where possible) and the retrofit (where necessary) of mainstream fixed-route transportation systems to meet the needs of disabled and elderly people. Alternative segregated special services, by contrast, restrict the range of choices available and, consequently, limit the disabled person's ability to live independently in the community. They also take disabled people out of contact with able-bodied persons, thus violating the entire spirit of independent living.

Yet, progress is likely to be slow. The 98th Congress is faced with the necessity of planning not for expanded and improved public services but for an era of reduced federal involvement—in transportation, as in other areas—due, in part, to reductions in revenue resulting from the 1981 tax cuts. Still, advocates will find that transportation remains a key to independent living—and a crucial element in the nation's program to cope with massive funding difficulties. With accessible transportation, many disabled and elderly people can work and many others need fewer social services. These people can turn from being tax users to being tax payers.

An agenda for action is beginning to take shape. Advocates need to work on the state and local level to become involved in transportation planning processes. They can point to successful programs in Florida, Brockton, and elsewhere to show that accessible transportation is an achievable goal and that government—as well as citizens—benefits when disabled people use accessible transportation to live independently in the community.

13

Specialized Housing

Stephen F. Wiggins

Housing has always been a fundamental issue in the Independent Living Movement. It is central to anyone's achievement of independence. Yet most communities have few, if any, housing alternatives for disabled adults. Lack of funding and expertise are the most common reasons behind this shortcoming.

This chapter will examine housing and its relationship to the Independent Living Movement. It has been drafted as a handbook for individuals or organizations concerned with the development of barrier-free housing. This chapter will not address the institutional approach to meeting the housing needs of disabled adults. Rather, the discussion will center on housing alternatives for independent living.

As executive director of a nonprofit corporation involved exclusively with the development of housing for elderly and disabled adults, my observations are naturally influenced by experience. The six housing projects we have developed for disabled adults are all different. Each project draws on the lessons

219

of its predecessors. With this in mind, I have chosen to concentrate on the following subjects: housing needs, elements of the development process, project feasibility, design principles, financing, and marketing.

Housing Needs

Housing options for the disabled are as varied as individuals. The types of disabilities to be served greatly influence the development process. In our development work, it has proved useful to separate disabled individuals into two categories: the self-supported and the system-supported independent disabled person. The self-supported independent disabled person has the ability to care for himself or herself, while the system-supported independent person needs daily support services. An example of the self-supported disabled person would be a paraplegic with a spinal cord lesion in the lower back, who would need a barrier-free environment but might not need any additional services. This person would be able to feed himself or herself, to drive an automobile with adaptive equipment, and to carry out most or all daily household functions. Statistics for the Midwest indicate that a majority of the disabled population in that region can be categorized as self-supported.

No generalizations can be made regarding the best approach to housing for self-supported persons. Our experience has shown that these individuals want a diversity of options available to them. The obvious alternatives are apartments (either newly constructed or rehabilitated units), scattered-site shared units, and single-family homes.

Self-supported persons have historically been given many more housing opportunities than system-supported individuals. They were first among the disabled population to be served by the housing industry, through the development of high- and low-density subsidized apartment buildings. This has been a good market for private developers. It involves no commitment to provide additional in-home services, and market entry is relatively uncomplicated.

During the late 1970s, many entrepreneurs and investors took advantage of this situation. Government money was targeted for use in barrier-free housing, and developers lined up for a share of this low-cost, subsidized financing. In many cities, developers attempted to serve large numbers of disabled persons in one project. High-density housing projects are always the most appealing to the profit-motivated developer. Yet the results are not always favorable. Many disabled people object to the semi-institutional settings of such subsidized housing and have come to refer to high-rise development as the ghettoization of the disabled population. The controversy has highlighted the need for small-scale responses as part of the overall solution to the housing needs of disabled people.

Overall, there has been a major improvement in the availability of barrier-free housing. Options not available five or ten years ago now exist in many metropolitan communities. In spite of the fact that there is still considerable variance between housing availability in different cities, most metropolitan areas have begun to respond to the needs of the self-supported independent disabled person.

A critical limitation on housing choice for both the self-supported and system-supported disabled person is financial status. The first issue is whether potential occupants are competitively employed or must rely on public assistance for financial support. The experience of many developers has shown that the market for condominiums, cooperatives and other forms of owner-occupied housing is practically nonexistent among the disabled. Those disabled individuals with sufficient resources have usually purchased a single-family home and adapted it to their needs. In any case, our research shows that few would even consider purchasing a unit in a building inhabited only by disabled adults.

The vast majority of disabled adults can be categorized as low-income. It is necessary, therefore, to determine the maximum amount of rent that can be afforded by a target population of handicapped people. Over the past ten years, it has become increasingly difficult to develop rental housing without charging disproportionately high rents. The inflated cost of building materials, labor, and financing has forced rents on new construction units far above the rents charged on older units. Because of this differential, there has been little demand for privately developed, market-rate rental housing. Most developers of apartment buildings who were active in the late 1960s and early 1970s have redirected their energies into the condominium market. Coupled with the increase in conversions of rental units to condominiums, this has strained the rental market in most urban areas, making it difficult even for the able-bodied renter to obtain housing. As a result, it is no longer feasible to build new rental housing for disabled people without charging extremely high rents. Because of the income limitations of most handicapped people, there is a need for subsidy assistance from the federal Department of Housing and Urban Development (HUD). Federal rent subsidies, called section 8 subsidies, are available to low-income people whose income does not exceed 80 percent of the area average. A tenant typically pays 25 percent of his or her income toward the rent obligation, and the federal government pays the remainder.

There is no single solution to the housing needs of disabled adults. This is especially true for the system-supported independent disabled person. By system-supported, I mean an individual who is dependent on more than just a barrier-free structure to achieve independent living. For the purpose of this discussion, the term will be limited to the nonretarded disabled person, defined as someone who has the intellectual capacity to achieve self-reliance, yet needs support services.

Unfortunately, very few housing models exist for this population. While unique models have been developed in Boston, Atlanta, San Francisco, and Minneapolis, other cities still lack any housing alternatives that include support services.

Most states have limited options when it comes to providing in-home services. Probably the most significant deterrent to the development of more system-supported independent living settings is the fact that most state welfare plans do not provide for in-home personal care services. Federal guidelines governing Title XIX expenditures allow states to provide in-home personal care services. However, it is left to the discretion of the state whether or not to include them in its welfare plan. The financial difficulties facing most states lead to a guarded state welfare plan, usually excluding in-home personal care. Exclusion is a simple cost-containment measure. As a result, system-supported persons are usually faced with the choice of living in an institution or moving in with family members.

In addition to in-home personal care services, there is also a need for publicly reimbursed cooking and cleaning services. In most cases, Title XX funds are used for these homemaker services. Anyone seeking to develop housing for system-supported individuals should inquire with county governments to find out whether such programs exist.

Like other disabled persons, most of those who are system-supported have low incomes. Therefore, it is also necessary to ensure the availability of section 8 rent subsidies for this population.

Groups considering development of housing for the system-supported must also determine the size and the precise needs of the population to be served. Will personal care services be needed? Will homemaker or chore services be needed? Will supervisory services be needed? What is the income level of the potential residents? What types of disabilities will be served? How big should the project be? Will the units be shared or separate? Will meals be provided centrally, or will tenants fend for themselves? Answers to all these questions are needed before starting a development project.

Once the needs and appropriate responses have been determined, many development strategies can be used to create the housing project. In most cases, the developer in question is a nonprofit organization. Health care or health-related organizations are often the most appropriate developers. The next sections will describe the various elements of the development process and give suggestions on financing techniques. The emphasis of these sections is on developing physical facilities. Other chapters of this book provide information and ideas regarding service programs. However, any development group should take an integrative approach that combines service development with facility development.

The Development Process

The process of developing barrier-free housing involves a complex set of decisions. Key decision agents include the landowner, the developer and/or group undertaking the development, and the consumer; other decision agents include realtors, financiers, and public officials. The development of a site occurs in discernible stages, the sequence of which usually follows a fixed pattern (O'Mara, 1978).

The first stage involves determining *whom* the housing is for. This may seem a simple question to answer. Yet a church or synagogue might view housing needs differently from a nursing home or a neighborhood block association.

The next step is to examine the developing group's assets and liabilities. This exercise will help prepare the group for the tough questions that will be asked by a potential lender, a zoning board, a state health official, a health agency representative, or a member of its own board.

A good track record in delivering services to the disabled community will give a group a considerable advantage over its competitors. Experience is important, and experience involves more than merely visiting or associating with members of the disabled community. Experience may mean owning or managing income-producing real estate that serves the disabled community; owning or managing a health care facility; organizing and operating a center for independent living; providing financial assistance to disabled people, for example, through fund drives; coordinating service activities with other community organizations; or having financial management experience, particularly in health care or housing. However, lenders and government agencies may not feel that experience alone is enough: They will want to see *success* in providing services to the disabled.

Tangible assets such as cash, securities, or possession of valuable land may make it easier to begin a major development effort. Unfortunately, most groups responding to the need for barrier-free housing lack the financial capability to develop such projects on their own. Building an independent living facility of any kind requires ready cash—meaning a savings account, marketable bonds such as notes or debentures, land, or stock.

There are many forms of financing that will give one the bulk of funds required to build, but it takes cash even to make a loan application. Such expenses as architectural fees, legal fees to form a corporation, or even travel expenses to attend a meeting must be met. This basic cash requirement is commonly referred to as seed money. Later in this chapter, I will provide a list of alternative sources of seed money.

Frequently, the support a project receives from community groups already serving the disabled is crucial in enabling it to get off the ground. It is important for a development group to take time to identify individuals and organizations who may be of assistance in the development of its project. These might include community organizations with similar interests in developing housing or services for the disabled and those that have been successful in doing so; members of the local zoning and planning board; political and community members in the town, city, county, or state; banks with whom the developer has a good relationship; governmental agencies that will have regulatory authority over the project, such as health systems agencies, departments of health, and HUD area offices; and organizations or businesses that might have something to offer the project, such as land, financial assistance, or advertising—these would include chambers of commerce, Jaycees, and church and civic groups.

Establishing goals is an evolutionary process that continues as a group learns more about itself, the community and its needs, and the feasibility of reaching its goal. A goal can be categorized either as a *general goal*—for example, improving the human condition of the disabled in a certain community—or as a *specific goal*—for example, the development of a twenty-unit barrier-free housing project. Once a specific goal is developed, it is advisable to test any proposal both in relation to community need and in relation to financial viability. This will help to ensure program success. In the field of barrier-free housing, many projects are not tested in a methodical way at the outset. Large sums of money are frequently spent on projects that subsequently must be broken off, owing to oversight or lack of testing. Noncompliance with zoning laws and lack of need for barrier-free units are typical impediments. For this reason, a group must next determine whether its ideas make sense and can be turned into reality.

Project Feasibility

Planning a facility always involves much discussion of whether a project is feasible. Development groups are required to provide a feasibility study to a lending institution or to HUD before a mortgage, loan, or mortgage insurance can be approved. A feasibility study analyzes demographic and other data to determine whether a need for a particular service exists in a given community and, if so, whether that need can be met with available financial resources.

There are several approaches that can be taken in determining the feasibility of a project. One can carry out an in-house analysis, or one can make use of community resources or professional consultants. Most groups pursuing the development of barrier-free housing take the in-house approach. In this regard, the resources of a group's planning committee or board of directors may prove valuable. Many groups have provided sufficient documentation of an existing need for barrier-free housing simply through the expertise and knowledge of their own membership. In most communities, interested organizations and government agencies can provide data documenting the need for a particular service. They may also be able to provide insight into financial alternatives for financing the project.

Professional consultants can also be a key resource in determining the needs of the community, as well as in providing pertinent financial management information. Such professionals include market researchers, financial analysts, rehabilitation specialists, architects, and engineers.

To determine the need for a project in a community, one should start with an evaluation of available demographic or population statistics to determine how many people in a community are disabled and what percentage of the total population they make up. One must also determine what their general health status is and what the predominant disability types are. Another important piece of background information is the median income or range of income for those individuals who would seek the type of housing one's group is proposing. This information should be compared to national statistics.

Once the universe of potential clients is determined, one must consider the kinds of housing that are already available to the disabled. Does the community have existing barrier-free housing projects? If it does, it is important to determine how many units are available, where they are located, what services are provided, and what income groups they serve. Occupancy rates or waiting lists at existing housing projects should also be taken into account. If possible, one should obtain these lists and inquire of the people on them whether they would consider a project such as the one being planned.

As part of the analysis of available housing and services, it is important to talk to local government officials. The local HUD office, health systems agency, and housing authority often perceive a need for services and housing that is substantially different from needs identified by a nonprofit development group.

Health systems agencies and housing assistance plans can also be important considerations in determining the need for a project and the existing regulatory climate. A health systems agency (HSA) is a quasi-governmental body whose purpose is to avoid costly duplication of services by health care organizations in the region. HSAs issue certificates of need that are required before major capital expenditures (for example, a new building or a CT scanner) can be made. They were created in 1976 through PL93-641. The law is still in place, but it may be repealed in the current deregulation effort. If there is a health systems agency plan for the area, and if it indicates a shortage of independent living alternatives for disabled persons, then the HSA can be a valuable ally in the development process. The local housing assistance plan, if there is one, may provide similar information. (Housing assistance plans are written annually by local governments to define the needs of low-income families and other needs for special housing in the community.) The regulatory climate will also determine whether section 8 rent subsidies are available to the disabled or what the likelihood is of those subsidies being available in the foreseeable future.

The purpose of a financial feasibility analysis is to formulate a basis for making decisions. Feasibility analysis requires a systematic evaluation of all relevant data in a form consistent with the project under consideration. The degree of sophistication needed to make a decision on a project varies. In some cases, a development group will have to acquire data from consultants at considerable expense. In other cases, the development group may have all the data necessary. In whatever form, the purpose of a financial feasibility analysis is to ground abstract ideas in hard numbers.

Cost and revenue estimates, however, are subject to varying degrees of error. The most critical factor is time. Projections made today about what will occur one month from today will probably be more accurate than similar projections one year later. In a feasibility analysis dealing with market conditions four or five years in the future, one must expect a high degree of error. A good analysis recognizes this problem; projections are labeled best estimate, subject to revision. A frequent failing of development groups is to ignore new data when such figures become available. Both cost and revenue figures will rise over time. Inflation in the construction industry is a critical factor, because construction costs have risen faster than the general price level. Balancing this to some extent has been an even greater increase in real property values. Using a national index to project cost increases is not sufficient, because different regions of the country differ dramatically from the national average. It is highly advisable to conduct a periodic review of all estimates that project beyond two years.

Knowing what financing options are available is critical to the accuracy of a feasibility study. A rental project may have the potential to support a mortgage loan over a thirty-year period, yet such a long-term loan may not be available. Thus, careful evaluation of financing alternatives is essential. Later in this chapter, specific financing options will be discussed.

The participants in a development project are another critical element. Barrier-free housing development is no different from standard housing development in this regard. In the past, the development process was often viewed as a set of operations rather than as a process requiring constant analysis. Roles of interested parties were narrowly defined and development was divided up into neat chronological stages. This traditional method is no longer workable in typical residential housing development and is particularly unworkable in the development of barrier-free housing. The increased size and complexity of development, in addition to greater participation of the public and of government agencies at all levels, necessarily complicates the task of building. Consequently, each step has to be thought out, weighed, and incorporated into the framework of the entire development process.

This makes it imperative for experts in various disciplines to participate in the early decision-making phases as well as in succeeding ones. A development group should not assume at the outset that it has all the necessary knowledge. There is always a need for a development team. Economic, political, financial, esthetic, medical, legal, and accessibility experts have become increasingly important to the success of any contemporary barrier-free housing development. In cases where a service program is planned, experts capable of working with complex welfare regulations should also be retained.

Most groups find it necessary to engage professional assistance far in advance of any determination of feasibility. It is rare that a group working alone can both determine the need for a project and assemble the financial resources to respond to that need. Depending on the project's complexity, the following team members may be required: attorney, planner, engineer, medical specialist, architect, landscape architect, financier, banker, realtor, and contractor. The proper execution of a development plan requires input from all these professions, although not necessarily at every stage of development. Project analysis is a repetitive process of increasing refinement, in which all the factors must be reweighed at each stage. It is best to have the development group perform as much of the initial analysis as possible and rely on experts only as the complexity of the project increases.

Design Principles

Effective barrier-free design responds to specific needs. Therefore, a development group must first determine the physical parameters of its target population before starting the design process. How disabled are the prospective residents? How do their disabilities bear on access to transportation, shopping, and other community services?

Once the level of physical functioning of future residents is determined, the next decision is the appropriate scale of the project. Density is an important issue in any development, and particularly so in independent living projects. As we have mentioned, private developers prefer the high-rise developments that disabled people characterize as handicapped ghettos. However, public financing programs have come to recognize the drawbacks of high-density, barrier-free development. For example, the section 202 program, which was authorized under the Housing Act of 1959 to grant loans for housing construction, now ʹ ʹts the number of units allowed in a development for handicapped persons.

Project density usually depends in part on goals established during the feasibility stage and in part on the types of disabilities to be served and the levels of those disabilities. Independent apartment units have been the most common mode of development, while in recent years, smaller group housing has become a popular method of responding to more specialized needs.

In designing an independent living environment, selection of the project architect is extremely important. The Washington-based National Center for a Barrier-Free Environment provides information on architects with prior experience in barrier-free design as well as on design principles. Good barrier-free design is really the art of accessories. Small, seemingly insignificant design details can make a world of difference to the disabled person. Product inventory catalogues and state-of-the-art barrier-free design publications are thus useful resources for the architect. One such publication is the *Product Inventory of Hardware, Equipment, and Appliances for Barrier-Free Design*, published by the National Handicapped Housing Institute in Minneapolis.

Most sponsors of independent living developments will have a more acute perception of the needs of their target population than any hired professional. Since the field of barrer-free design is still in its infancy, development groups should not discount their own design ideas.

Financing

Finding capital is often the toughest hurdle in the development process (Greendale and Knock, 1976; Star, 1975; Wilner, Pease, and Wallgren, 1978). As an ongoing concern, it is never very distant from the decision-making process. The funds to pay for all of the projects that individuals and organizations wish to undertake obviously do not exist. Development groups compete among themselves and with other users of capital for available resources. The supply side of the capital market is diverse; it includes individuals with only a few dollars to lend and corporations and government agencies with millions. The challenge is to find the right source, at the right price.

Nonprofit corporations such as the one I work for usually try to avoid equity participation by private individuals or institutions so that we retain control of decisions about the project. Instead, we seek seed money from foundations, government agencies, or private donations. Any successful project depends on this seed money to pay for the expertise needed to develop a project that will be acceptable to the lender, the community, and the disabled people who will benefit from it.

Loans and grants can also be obtained for these expenses from HUD, state housing finance agencies, private foundations, fund drives or special donations, sponsoring organizations, or equity syndications. Because seed money funds are so important, I will discuss a few of these sources here.

HUD provides interest-free seed money loans to nonprofit sponsors under section 106(b) of the Housing and Development Act of 1968 in order to stimulate construction of low- and middle-income housing. Loans of up to $50 thousand are available for up to 80 percent of the development costs incurred by a development group in planning and in obtaining financing under section 202 of the Housing Act of 1959. (Section 202, a direct loan program, will be discussed in more detail later in this chapter.) Although section 106(b) funding was originally made available to nonprofit sponsors developing projects under several HUD programs, it is currently limited to sponsors of section 202 housing. The process works as follows: A nonprofit developer applies for section 202 funds, and when the proposal is accepted, monies are "set aside" for the development. The direct loan is not granted until all plans and budgets have been assembled by the development group and approved by HUD.

To be eligible for a seed money loan, a sponsoring group must be an incorporated, private, nonprofit organization and have an approved section 202 fund reservation. The organization or group must demonstrate that not less than 20 percent of total estimated development expenses is available.

Section 106(b) funds are not easy to obtain, even if all program requirements are met. A large percentage of those who apply for section 202 loans also request section 106(b) assistance. However, the additional paperwork required for participation in the 106(b) program often discourages developers from completing the application. Standards used to determine eligibility for section 106(b) funding differ somewhat from those used to evaluate section 202 direct loan applications. The area office, which is responsible for the evaluation of both proposals, bases its selection of recipients of seed money assistance on the availability of monies in the 106(b) revolving fund as well as on criteria deemed essential in the successful sponsorship of low- and middle-income housing. These criteria include

* serious motivation to provide housing for low- and middle-income elderly and handicapped individuals
* demonstrated ability to assume responsibility for the sponsorship of such housing, including development and management of the project
* roots in the community and the capacity to communicate effectively with residents of the neighborhood to be served
* freedom from influence or control by any party seeking profit from the development of the project
* existence of an adequate market for the proposed units
* evidence that the development group has obligated or expended its share of the required funds

An archdiocese, synod, regional or national fraternal organization, health care corporation, community action agency, or other sponsoring organization may be an additional source of seed money. Many of these groups have discretionary funds available for projects they deem worthy. Our organization has found that the best way to identify potential sponsoring organizations is to determine what we can offer other organizations. Good will, good public image, management contracts, and experience are all legitimate benefits accruing to the sponsoring organization. It is up to the nonprofit development group to identify which of these incentives is most appropriate and to point them out in discussions with potential sponsors.

Equity syndication is a technique by which the tax loss (tax shelter) in a real estate project is sold to those who can benefit from it. The proceeds resulting from equity syndication are a principal source of seed money or equity for a development group. By and large, the rules for syndicating a government assisted housing project and a conventional project are the same, although the details of the two types of transaction may be quite different.

A tax shelter is just what the term implies; it is a legal means of lessening one's tax liability. The Internal Revenue Service recognizes the depreciation of real estate as a legitimate business expense to an owner. Therefore, an owner can deduct from income the annual depreciation on his property. Because depreciation is only an accounting transaction and not a cash expense, it may allow the owner to claim a net loss for tax purposes, even when an actual loss has not occurred.

In general, the federal government allows even nonprofit development groups to enjoy the benefits of equity syndications. The following example applies to either a nonprofit or a profit-motivated developer of a barrier-free housing project:

1. A site is selected for the proposed project.
2. An option or purchase agreement is entered into.
3. Approvals are gained in such matters as zoning, environmental impact, and utilities.
4. A nonprofit development group recognizes the need for equity yet wants to retain control of the project. The group determines that an equity syndication is appropri-

ate, with the nonprofit group acting as the general partner and the investors acting as the limited partner. (Partnerships will be discussed in greater detail later.)

5. Architectural plans and specifications are prepared.
6. Detailed financial projections are prepared; particular attention is paid to the tax benefit projected during and after construction, since this is what will be sold to investors.
7. Tentative financing arrangements are obtained and a builder is found.
8. At this point, the development group interests investors in forming a limited partnership in the project and seeks their cash investment to get construction underway. Usually the nonprofit group retains only a small part of the ownership, as it does not need the tax shelter.
9. The liability of the general and limited partners is restricted to the value of the property itself and excludes other assets of the individual partners.
10. Construction begins.

This arrangement can be a good source of seed money. To the syndicate or partnership, it has tax value. This tax value often is paid to the nonprofit sponsor, thus providing it with the necessary seed money.

Syndication is more common in a proprietary venture than in a nonprofit venture because of the tax-exempt nature of nonprofit organizations. If, however, a nonprofit developer lacks sufficient capital for the project, a venture can be structured to contain both a proprietary and a nonprofit partner.

Barrier-free developments have been financed using both private and public sources of funds. The latter include government programs such as the Farmer's Home Administration direct loan or the public sale of tax-exempt bonds. Private finance refers to any nongovernmental source of long-term capital, such as conventional mortgage loans, gifts, public or private taxable bonds, tax-exempt revenue bonds, or state housing financing agencies.

Private financing permits maximum flexibility, because it

can be tailored to meet the particular financial needs of the project. In addition, it is the quickest of all financing techniques and can frequently be implemented in two to four months, avoiding delays that can substantially increase construction costs. Because of their increasing use in independent living projects, some of the more popular long-term financing vehicles are worth considering in greater detail.

Conventional lenders include savings and loan associations, mutual savings banks, life insurance companies, commercial banks and pension funds. Each and every lending institution varies in its approach to loan applications. Typically, conventional lenders will not exceed a 75 percent loan to value ratio. This means that only 75 percent of the total project costs can be covered through the conventional loan.

Part of the funding for any construction effort must be in the form of nonborrowed money, or equity. Because this can amount to as much as 50 percent of the project cost, it is important to determine how this amount can be raised. Very often a development group obtains these funds through the solicitation of gifts from its membership. Gifts or donations are critical to a capital expansion effort, and it requires a great deal of an organization's time and talent to sustain and develop them.

Private placement of taxable bonds has not been widely used by the Independent Living Movement; however, it is worthy of consideration. It works as follows: An investment banking firm or institutional bond house underwrites a loan to the developer. The underwriter then distributes the bonds to private investors, such as bond funds or pension funds. The underwriter charges an *underwriting spread,* which is taken in the form of a discount when the bonds are issued. Traditionally, underwriting guidelines for taxable bonds have been very restrictive. As the percentage of financing is usually held to less than 60 percent of the total project cost, this method is not feasible in very many cases. Moreover, the term of the loan is short, often fifteen to twenty years. This frequently requires refinancing of the unamortized balance of the loan. This can be a disadvantage because of the uncertainty of credit markets fifteen years in the future and the fact that the borrower must pay financing fees all over again.

There are many costs associated with a taxable bond issue which can make the transaction more burdensome than other financing vehicles. Public taxable bonds differ from private taxable bonds in distribution. Public bonds are sold on the open market and in smaller denominations. Private bonds are sold to far fewer investors and are not sold on the open market. Savings associated with private, as opposed to public, placement of taxable bonds occur in such areas as smaller sales commission, reduced printing costs, fewer feasibility study requirements, and waiver of the bond rating.

Tax-exempt revenue bonds have gained a great deal of popularity in recent years as more and more states pass enabling legislation. Because the interest earned on these bonds is exempt from federal income taxes, investors are willing to receive 1½–2 percent lower return on their investment than they would on similar taxable issues. These bonds may be issued by a state or municipal authority, by a county or city, or directly by a nonprofit corporation. Internal Revenue Service guidelines stipulate that a nonprofit corporation may issue bonds only if it gives a beneficial interest in a facility to the municipality, thereby ensuring that the property subsidized by tax-exempt funds will always be used for purposes that contribute to the public good.

Tax-exempt revenue bonds allow for the highest ratio of financing. Many facilities are able to finance up to 100 percent of their project costs, in addition to financing expenses and interest during construction and refinancing existing debt. Moreover, this method allows for an extremely long maturity of thirty to forty years, which reduces the annual debt service.

A group developing barrier-free housing should recognize that bond financing can cause them to borrow more funds than other methods of financing would. This is due to expenses such as underwriting discounts, legal and printing costs, the bond reserve fund, and capitalized interest during construction. Processing time can also be prolonged because of the involvement in the transaction of third parties such as a public authority or municipality and because of the work required on the documentation and the need for a detailed feasibility study. Altogether, the preparation and placement of tax-exempt bonds frequently take longer than any other nongovernmental approach to long-term financing.

On the positive side, interest payments on a tax-exempt revenue bond can be capitalized during construction, easing cash flow needs. Existing debt can usually be refinanced with this type of issue, and it is well suited for joint financing in combination, for example, with direct loans from the federal government.

State housing finance agencies are authorized by individual state legislation to provide financing and technical assistance to nonprofit and limited-dividend sponsors of low- and middle-income housing. These agencies were formed to encourage development of housing within each state. Their given names vary from state to state, and often several agencies in a state share the responsibilities for these tasks. Many of these state agencies designate some funds specifically for housing for handicapped individuals.

State housing finance agencies have state-wide powers to finance housing through the sale of notes and bonds in tax-exempt markets. Typically, a state housing finance agency can provide construction and long-term financing (for multifamily housing), seed money loans at an interest-free rate, and technical assistance. Many also have their own loan insurance programs. These programs operate in a fashion similar to the Federal Housing Administration mortgage insurance programs in that they provide insurance to a private lender. To determine whether your state has a loan insurance program and to find out additional information about your state housing finance agency, arrange for a meeting with the agency's officials to discuss the program they offer, the requirements and processing steps of those programs.

There are a number of governmental programs for the development of projects serving the disabled. Public financing, ranging from small grants to direct loans and mortgage insurance, is offered by the Farmer's Home Administration, the Federal Housing Administration, and the Veterans Administration, to name a few. A big difference between public and private financing is the smaller amount of cash necessary to develop a program with public financing. Because of this, the processing of an application can involve an awesome amount of time and many stages of approval.

HUD has been instrumental in providing low-interest loans, mortgage insurance, and technical assistance to groups interested in meeting the housing and health care needs of disabled adults. Although HUD was established in 1965, its housing policies and assistance programs date back to the National Housing Act of 1934 (Betnun, 1976).

HUD programs undergo periodic changes, and any group considering development of an independent living alternative should review the current programs. Some of the most popular HUD programs include section 213 (cooperative housing), section 221(d)(3) and (4) (conventional rental housing), section 202 (rental housing for elderly and handicapped persons), section 234 (nursing homes), and section 236 (rental housing; interest subsidy).

Over the years, the most popular program for the development of barrier-free housing has been the section 202 program. Section 202 was authorized by the Housing Act of 1959 to provide private, nonprofit sponsors with direct loans with which to build housing for the elderly or handicapped. These projects may be in the form of rental or cooperative housing and may contain related facilities such as a central dining room, community spaces, and commercial areas. Sponsors may also make use of section 8 rent subsidies for low- and middle-income handicapped persons.

It is this piggy-back element of the section 202 program that makes it so popular. Most groups trying to develop housing for disabled persons quickly realize the need for rent subsidies. Most disabled individuals are unable to cover the cost of a rental unit and must rely on some type of government support. For this reason, the section 8 rent assistance program becomes an almost essential factor in most development projects serving the disabled. The section 8 program was authorized under the Housing and Community Redevelopment Act of 1974 to assist low-income families in obtaining rental housing that adequately meets their physical and financial needs. Section 8 does not provide for the financing of a project but rather offers housing assistance payments, or rent subsidies, to qualified families and individuals to offset monthly rents on units of their choice. In recent years, section 8 has become perhaps the most widely utilized of HUD's programs. The availability of section 8 allocations in a particular locale depends on the housing assistance plan submitted by the local government for that year. This plan defines the housing needs of low-income families, including the disabled, and in turn establishes goals for the provision of new and rehabilitated housing in the community.

One of the restrictions of the section 202 program is that projects for the physically handicapped are limited to a maximum of twenty-four units, while a twelve-person maximum per site is placed on section 202 projects for the developmentally disabled.

Section 202 is one of the few well-funded and well-protected programs. In addition, it can provide 100 percent of financing, making it a popular and competitive program. The program is also known for being political, in the sense that local nonprofit groups will often urge their congressman to actively support a section 202 project.

Most groups developing barrier-free housing would prefer to work alone. When they do take on private partners, it is assumed to be for the purpose of raising needed capital. There are three types of ownership entity: direct ownership, partnership, and corporation. They differ in legal and tax consequences, rather than in substance.

A nonprofit development group, private individual, or other community organization that has direct ownership of a project is legally entitled to all profit and all tax benefits and is personally responsible for all liability. Direct ownership ensures control over the direction and management of the project and affords the opportunity to receive the greatest benefit from successful development. It also has the burden of unshared risk. Direct ownership is the simplest kind of equity participation in development. It is generally limited to small projects where equity cash needs are not great and where tax benefits are limited, as would be the case, for example, in a section 202 project.

Partnerships encompass many forms of organization, including syndications, joint ventures, and any other unincorporated association of two or more persons. A partnership is an entity under the law and as such can own and develop property in its own name. A partnership's primary function is to serve as a conduit. Money flows from the partners to the organization to buy and develop land. Benefits flow back to the partners in the form of tax losses. This transfer is the major activity of the partnership. Partners receive and declare profits and losses based on the proportion of their share in the partnership's holdings. Two forms of partnership exist, general and limited, but both forms may be combined in one entity. Few nonprofit development groups choose the general partnership approach when developing barrier-free housing. The most significant feature of a general partnership is that each partner is personally responsible for all debts and liabilities. To the extent that a project is successful, a general partner profits according to the proportion of his or her share. To the extent, however, that a project is unsuccessful, a partner could carry the burden of the whole. One general partner can bind the other general partners.

A limited partnership contains at least two members, one of whom is a general partner. The limited partner has a fixed interest in the project, and his or her liability is restricted to the amount of personal investment as spelled out in the partnership agreement. Actions of the general partners do not affect these liabilities.

Limited partnerships are the most widely used form of real estate ownership for both conventional and barrier-free housing developments. Their greatest strength is that they combine a transfer of all tax losses with limits to liability. Taken together, these two aspects are a great draw to investors who seek the tax benefits of real estate investment but who desire a passive and relatively trouble-free role in the development and/or management side of the project. In most barrier-free developments, a nonprofit organization and perhaps a major active financing agent will be the general partners, and the investors, frequently many more in number, will be the limited partners. A partnership is a very flexible tool for generating equity capital. The specifics of such deals are too complicated to be discussed here. This section merely identifies the opportunities available to development groups through partnerships. If a group intends to use a partnership to generate equity capital, the services of a tax attorney or a tax accountant will be necessary.

A real estate corporation, like any corporation, is a legal, taxable entity with rights and liabilities compared to those of an individual. It can sue and be sued, it pays taxes, and it lasts until it is terminated. Shareholders have no liability beyond the amount they have invested in purchase of the stock. Nor do they have the power to bind the corporation or change this liability. However, they can freely transfer their ownership interest.

Real estate corporations are rarely, if ever, used to develop barrier-free housing. A corporation's major advantage as far as potential investors are concerned is that liability is limited and transfer of investment easy. The disadvantage is that the corporation pays a tax on its earnings before paying them out to stockholders, who then must pay a second tax on their dividends. Of equal or greater importance is the fact that tax losses cannot be transferred to shareholders. The elimination of this tax loss potential has made real estate corporations an unpopular ownership vehicle.

This discussion suggests that limited partnerships are most appropriate for independent living projects. However, development groups should always take the approach that best fits their needs. Such a decision usually flows from the analysis of an organization's strengths and weaknesses. Success in development is often linked to financing, and financing problems are particularly challenging in the case of barrier-free housing. Construction costs are often higher in a barrier-free development than a standard housing development. This is usually a result of the unique features included in a project serving the disabled.

Creative financing has thus become a key to successful development of barrier-free housing. Many development groups combine two or three financing approaches to meet the needs of their project. Community development block grants, urban development action grants, and tax increment financing are popular elements of a creative financing package. Block grants and action grants administered through municipal governments can cover many costs that otherwise would be covered through mortgage funds. Tax increment financing can also be used in a variety of creative ways to lower development costs. With the continuing decline of government participation in housing projects, multi-faceted approaches to financing have become both necessary and commonplace. The successful development group should evaluate all possibilities, in order to identify the financing package that most appropriately meets its requirement.

Marketing

Any organization that has done its homework should have no problem marketing a barrier-free development. Demand for independent living alternatives should exceed supply for a long time to come. The challenge to developers of barrier-free housing is not finding enough applicants; it is finding appropriate applicants.

If the project is a typical apartment dwelling, one must look for individuals with the capacity to live independently. This may or may not include those dependent on personal care and other support services. Experience has shown that physical dexterity is not the only determining factor in a disabled individual's ability to achieve independence. Obtaining and coordinating in-home support services requires intellectual competence as well. Someone who has grown up in an institutionalized setting may not have learned such simple (but crucial) independent living skills as money management, grocery shopping, meal planning, cooking, or attendant management.

In the case of group homes, the challenge is to create a household of compatible roommates. The ability to communicate and take responsibility are usually good indicators of appropriate candidates. Probing interviews are thus an essential element in marketing a group home setting.

The best places to spread the word about a new independent living project include nursing homes, centers for independent living, rehabilitation departments of local hospitals, outpatient rehabilitation agencies, and existing providers of health care and social services to the target population.

Housing commands a central role in the Independent Living Movement, yet responses to housing needs of disabled adults have been slow and disjointed. Most communities have few, if any, available housing alternatives, and those that have responded to independent living needs have tended to focus their energies on only one segment of the disabled community.

Experience has shown that appropriate responses to independent living needs include more than facility development alone. Programs and services must often be integrated into the housing environment to create a viable alternative to institutional care. The varying types and degrees of disability highlight the need for a multifaceted approach to housing.

This chapter has been concerned primarily with development of physical facilities. Other chapters of this book provide useful insights into service programs and sources of reimbursement. The intent here has been to establish a framework for groups pursuing the development of independent living projects. I have highlighted the numerous alternatives available for developing and financing facilities that meet the varied needs of disabled persons. I have stressed that a careful analysis of needs, coupled with astute planning and creative use of resources, are essential factors in the successful financing of independent living projects. Yet this discussion should not be considered exhaustive. Development groups should explore all approaches and select project designs and financing vehicles that meet established criteria. A proposed development project must focus on a specific need, and each step in the development should be geared to meeting that need.

Development groups are finding it increasingly necessary to pursue creative methods of financing a facility. A combination of approaches has become the norm. Partnerships including individual investors and organizations are popular responses to the shrinking involvement of government and the increasing costs of construction projects. Nonprofit groups utilizing partnerships must continue to seek ways of arranging the partnership to meet the needs of both interests.

The housing challenges facing the Independent Living Movement are substantial. Effective responses are possible only through creative, cooperative initiatives.

14

Technology

Shelia Stephens Newman
John E. Schatzlein
Rayelenn Sparks

"The computer not only helps us organize or synthesize 'blips' into coherent models of reality, it also stretches the far limits of the possible. The computer can be asked by us to think the unthinkable and the previously unthought. It makes possible a flood of new theories, ideas, ideologies, artistic insights, technical advances, and economic and political innovations that were, in the most literal sense, unthinkable and unimaginable before now" (Toffler, 1980, pp. 193-194).

Toffler's words aptly apply to the role of technology in independent living. Technology's potential for positive impact on disabled people is staggering. Applications will continually evolve as people become more knowledgeable about technology and its place in society, as they become less fearful of it, and as they begin to see it as a means to maximize their potential for growth.

In the sense in which it is used here, the term *technology* can be broken down into three primary concepts (Thomas, 1971; Ayers, 1977). The first is *nontechnology*, which can most easily be defined as helping techniques, such as therapies or services. The second is *halfway technology*, which encompasses any product that substitutes for a loss in physical function due to disability. *Decisive technology*, the third concept, is the high technology of medicine. According to Ayers (1977), the thrust of decisive technology is largely preventive. Typical activities include development of vaccines and identification of interventions to prevent disabling conditions.

These concepts make it immediately clear why technology is too broad a topic to cover completely, even in the context of independent living. Therefore, this chapter will limit itself to an overview of technology as it applies to independent living. The chapter's main intent is to acquaint the rehabilitation practitioner with technologies in the areas of communication, activities of daily living, education, and employment. Without attempting to be exhaustive, it will try to familiarize practitioners with the ways in which appropriate technology can benefit disabled people. Finally, it will discuss general problems in the development and delivery of such technology.

History of Rehabilitation Technology

Regarded by many as a new phenomenon and an outgrowth of the Independent Living Movement and of recent advances in technology, rehabilitation technology began long ago when early man made wooden prostheses from tree limbs. Examples from later history abound. La Rocca and Turem (1978) cite Roger Bacon's 1268 description of framed optical lenses for reading; Franklin's invention of bifocals in 1784; Edison's phonograph in 1877 with its potential for talking books for the blind; the Pratt-Smoot Act of 1931, which appropriated money for services for the blind; and the teaching of independent foot-travel to blind and sight-impaired people in the 1940s. Parsons and Rappaport (1977) credit war with making the public aware of physically disabled people. According to them, the federal government in America began providing prostheses to veterans with amputations at the end of the Civil War. In 1917, the surgeon general of the army called limbmakers to Washington to consider the problems of World War I veterans with amputations. Technology for disabled people was almost entirely limited to prosthetics until the end of World War II. Late in 1944, the surgeon general of the army asked the National Academy of Sciences (NAS) to make recommendations concerning prosthetics for the thousands of returning World War II amputees. A conference organized for this purpose in 1945 attracted scientists, engineers, surgeons, and prosthetists. The result of the conference was the formation of an NAS research and development program, the Committee on Prosthetics Research and Development. This merger of the medical and engineering fields to study prosthetics paved the way for the application of technology to all types of disabilities. In particular, according to La Rocca and Turem, it marked the birth of the profession now known as rehabilitation engineering.

From 1955 to 1975, several federal agencies contributed to NAS rehabilitation engineering research (University of Virginia Rehabilitation Engineering Center, 1977). In 1970, the NAS Committee on Prosthetics Research and Development organized a conference that resulted in a plan for the conduct of research, development, evaluation, and education in rehabilitation engineering. Since then, twelve rehabilitation engineering centers have been established in the United States and three in Europe. The objective of these centers is to engage in research and development; to collaborate with laboratories and industry in the development of new devices; to exchange information with other institutions; to cooperate with other centers in clinical evaluation of devices; and to educate physicians, engineers, and other professionals about new devices and techniques (Parsons and Rappaport, 1977).

As rehabilitation engineering expanded, it became apparent that technologies developed in other fields could be applied to problems created by disabilities. For instance, a number of government agencies, university medical centers, and private corporations have come to recognize that knowledge gained from advanced aerospace research can be adapted to assist disabled people. Bell (1979) gives examples of such technology applied to the needs of disabled and elderly people. The list includes switches that operate by eye movement; breath-activated switches that operate television, lights, and door locks; rechargeable pacemakers; and many other products. In developing such devices, NASA's technology utilization program relies on engineers and others who appreciate the needs of disabled people. Aerospace research provides the most spectacular examples of technology transfer, but developments in other fields are of equal importance from the point of view of disabled persons. Even such simple labor-saving devices as electric can-openers and remote control switches have helped to increase the independence of disabled people. Perhaps the most vital advances have been made in four areas: communications, daily living, education, and employment.

Communication

Most activities of daily living require the ability to communicate with others. However, many people with losses of visual, hearing, speech, or motor function are not able to use common modes of communication.

Communication can be divided into two primary modes: the conversational and the graphic. Vanderheiden (U.S. Congress, 1980) shows that in both, the individual must be able to send as well as receive communication. The four populations of people whose communication needs are most affected by their disabilities are those who have hearing impairments, visual impairments, and speech impairments, and those with physical impairments affecting motor control. Members of each group are generally capable of operating independently in at least one of the four modes of communication (conversational input, conversational output, graphic input, and graphic output).

The hearing-impaired generally need no specific technology in the graphic input or the graphic output modes, as hearing impairment per se does not affect the ability to communicate in writing. However, many hearing-impaired people suffer from reduced linguistic fluency because they were unable to acquire language in the normal ways. More critically, many hearing-impaired people face handicaps in the conversational input and (for some) in the conversational output modes. In these cases, technological applications have proven useful. A wide variety of hearing aids, each with features intended to combat specific aspects of hearing loss, are available. Whether it is a question of simple amplifiers or of complex, surgically implanted electrode systems, hearing aid technology has greatly advanced from the ear trumpets of the last century. Unfortunately, as Hansen (1979) points out, these devices are only able to restore hearing in persons whose hearing loss is conductive, that is, caused by damage to the middle or inner ear; they cannot help individuals with a defective auditory nerve.

Other technologies provide a substitute stimulus when hearing is impaired. Sign languages, in all their forms, as well as cued speech (the system by which the sounds of speech are made visible as manual or electronic cues) fall into this category, as do devices that translate sound stimuli into visual or tactile stimuli. Telecaption technologies, which print information on a television screen, and the wide variety of signaling devices used by the deaf—doorbells, fire alarms, telephone-ringing signals, alarm clocks, and baby cry alarms, for example—also belong in this group.

Ironically, although the invention of the telephone came about serendipitously, in the course of Bell's experiments with hearing devices for the deaf, for many years the telephone was virtually useless to persons with impaired hearing. Finally, the adaptation of newsroom teletype equipment allowed hearing-impaired persons to converse. Typed messages were converted to electronic signals and transmitted over the telephone lines. Since the first bulky equipment, much innovation has taken place, leading to today's hand-held, calculator-like instrument with a light emitting diode (LED).

While many hearing-impaired people have intelligible speech, others might well be considered speech-impaired. The most common sources of speech impairment are the deterioration or the removal of the larynx, or other part of the vocal system, and the inability to coordinate muscle or breath control so as to form words.

Writing messages is a common and effective way of overcoming the conversational communication barrier, except among persons whose disabilities include severe difficulty with motor control. Sign language can also be used, but only if those being spoken to know the sign language. Other communication aids are available to those who cannot speak or be understood. Those who are able to use a finger or mouthstick to point can employ a simple communication board, on which is printed a grid with a number of useful words and phrases as well as an alphabet. The disabled person merely points at the words, phrases, or letters in the order that he or she wishes to communicate an idea. The listener generally repeats the utterance as it is being given, so that the disabled person will know whether or not the listener's interpretation of the message is accurate. Also available is a miniature hand-held electronic typewriter keyboard, with an LED read-out unit which can be attached to one's lapel, allowing for face-to-face conversation with normal eye contact. Research is in progress to develop speech clarifiers. A person with consistent but unintelligible speech would be able to program such a device to recognize his or her speech. The device would analyze words as they were spoken and repeat them in a more intelligible form. Technologies already exist to correct certain speech impairments. For instance, the electrolarynx is a device that vibrates the throat area to produce a sound that can be articulated for those whose larynx has been removed or is nonfunctioning.

For the visually impaired population, the ability to function in the conversational mode is not significantly impaired by lack of vision, even though the nonsighted listener cannot make use of additional clues such as speech (or lip) reading or awareness of gesture and facial expression. Most of the technological applications devised to meet the communication needs of the visually impaired focus on the graphic mode of communication, since that is the function most seriously affected by the disability. In particular, although visually impaired people can manipulate pencils, typewriter keyboards, or computer consoles, their inability to see what they are producing makes accurate output problematic.

Again, a wide variety of devices and products are available (and others are being developed) to facilitate written communication among the visually impaired. Early experimentation with raised print led to a general acceptance of the braille system, and since that time, technology for faster production of braille texts has been developed. Adaptations of the familiar electric typewriter have allowed individually brailled copies to be produced more efficiently, while computerized, electronic braille machines can create large quantities of brailled copy in a short time. Electronic braille machines record brailled text in digital form on cassette tape. The information is then replayed on a braille display controlled by the user. As much as 600 pages of braille can be recorded on a sixty-minute cassette tape.

Research on print-to-speech and print-to-braille technologies is still underway, although some devices have been made available. One such device is a reader that converts book pages or single sheets in any typeface into braille. Another, known as a Kurzweil machine, converts printed pages to speech, using a speech synthesis program.

For those with partial vision, a wide variety of magnifiers have been developed, from the simple hand-held glass to the highly sophisticated closed-circuit television reading systems which use high-powered close-up lenses and television monitors with magnifications ranging up to 50x. In addition, cameras that permit text to be displayed on cathode ray tube terminals and microfiche readers have been designed.

Moyer (1980) discusses sound recordings, which have long been a valuable means of providing impaired individuals with access to books, magazines, and journals. The Library of Congress began producing records for this purpose in the 1930s, through its talking book program. Now the more convenient cassette tapes are used. Condensed speech, and variable speed controls provided the option of speed listening for those who desired it. This technology was later improved by the advent of compressed speech, which sped up the rate of speech without altering the pitch of the recorded voice.

Persons with limb damage or mobility impairments affecting motor control and grasp are generally not handicapped in the conversational mode, but may require assistance in order to produce written communication and, in some cases, to read. Simple appliances have been designed which make it easier for those who can use pencil and paper. Pencils with built-up handles, and wrist-strapped writing utensils provide greater control of the writing process at very little expense to the user. The typewriter can facilitate writing for those people who cannot easily handle a writing instrument. Adaptations for the typewriter keyboard include templates placed over the keyboard to provide more stability to a person with spastic movements and mouthsticks designed to allow those with no manual agility to type. When reading, those who cannot hold books or turn pages can use an automatic device designed for these tasks.

The question remains, What of those whose handicaps are multiple, or so extensive that a number of functions related to communication are impaired, making the technological applications already examined inadequate? Increasing awareness of the needs of severely disabled people has prompted new interest in providing technological solutions to some of the problems posed by severe or multiple disabilities. For those who are both deaf and blind, a telecommunication device for the deaf (TDD) is available with a braille printer instead of the hard copy paper printout or light emitting diode of standard equipment. Signaling devices (telephone ringing signals, doorbells, or baby cry alarms) can be used to activate a small fan which disturbs the air enough to alert the deaf and blind person.

The field of nonvocal communication technology has developed rapidly in the past decade. A number of communication aids are based on the communication board. One electronic device, for example, uses a scanning technique on an otherwise standard communication board, allowing the user to select alphabetic characters with only a minimum of physical movement (U.S. Congress, 1980). Another electronic system has two buttons which can be operated by a mouthstick—a dot and a dash. The disabled person inputs a message in Morse code, which the machine translates and displays on a screen. For people who lack even enough mobility to manipulate a mouthstick, a number of eye-gaze powered technologies are being developed. Many of these involve having a person gaze at a word or letter on a communication board until it prints out on an accompanying screen. While this technique has some problems, especially for severely handicapped people who have ocular motor problems, it shows great potential for further development.

Activities of Daily Living

Independence in the basic activities of daily living is necessary before such activities as getting an education or gaining employment are possible. Technological products and systems can help to compensate for functional loss and increase physical independence. Self-care, mobility, transportation, and housing deserve particular discussion. In these four important areas of daily living, technology is making advances, both in products such as assist devices and labor-saving equipment and in systems such as training programs and counseling opportunities.

Self-care is a broad term, encompassing food preparation and eating, personal health care, grooming, and bowel and bladder care. While some people may require aids to perform some of these functions, others may require only individual training to understand these aspects of self-care and to perform them regularly.

Many technological solutions to self-care problems require neither expense nor engineering expertise. A foam hair curler wrapped around the handle of a spoon gives better grip and friction to a person with limited hand function. The rubber grip from a bicycle handlebar can serve a similar purpose. The creative, innovative mind can devise any number of effective and durable aids from simple household materials. More sophisticated devices are available from a wide variety of manufacturers. *Aids to Independent Living* (Lowman and Klinger,

1969) lists hundreds of items, including eating and drinking devices; toilet transfer aids; tub, shower and bath aids; aids for care of hair, teeth, nails, and skin; and dressing aids. Many of these products are available to the general public as labor-saving devices, while others have been designed particularly for the specific needs of disabled consumers.

Mobility is another area in which disabled people find that technology can provide needed assistance. Mobility is a central concern of those persons whose impairments require lower limb prostheses and of those who use canes, walkers, crutches, or wheelchairs. A different set of mobility problems is faced by those with vision impairments.

The thirty-six-inch hardwood cane is a simple and familiar device, but in analyzing the balance and support needs of people with various mobility impairments, technology has made it possible to produce canes with better traction and distribution of weight. The so-called crab cane, for example, stands on a tripod base to offer secure contact on uneven ground. Another cane has a curved design that puts the person's weight on the actual center of the cane, providing greater balance and control. Crutches and walkers, too, come in a variety of designs, each offering specific features of comfort, control, and support to the individuals who require their use. Technological advances have even affected the contour and material of crutches' protective pads. Physicists and medical personnel have analyzed the motions involved in walking, and can offer gait training to those who are learning to adapt to crutch, cane, or walker use.

Lowman and Klinger (1969, p. 192) assert that "a wheelchair should provide the patient with maximal comfort, safety, maneuverability, and independence." A number of standard wheelchair models are available, but custom-made chairs, or customized features, are available for those who need them. Whether manually operated or battery-powered, whether controlled by hand, joy stick, sip and puff mouth switch, or voice control, modern wheelchairs have helped to open up the possibilities of independent living for many disabled people.

For people with visual impairments, mobility training with white cane or guide dog is still a standard practice. However, other methods of aiding mobility are now available or are being developed. A small device that hangs around the neck can give a blind person auditory clues as to physical barriers in the path ahead. The narrow-range night vision caused by retinitis pigmentosa and other ocular diseases can be partially relieved by a small machine that the user holds up to the eyes, rather like binoculars.

Transportation and housing are two other major necessities which can pose problems for people with disabilities. Automobile travel, at one time considered nearly impossible for the severely disabled, is now a common occurrence. Devices are available that allow a driver who has a mobility impairment to enter a car or van and operate the vehicle. Such devices make it possible for some individuals with high-cervical spinal cord injuries to drive. Hand controls substitute for brake, clutch, and accelerator functions, and the hand controls can even be modified in such a way that people with limited hand function can operate motor vehicles.

Public transportation is also making strides in assisting disabled consumers with both short- and long-distance travel. The advent of the so-called kneeling bus, which lowers to curb-level a wheelchair-sized platform at the vehicle's entrance, has opened up transportation possibilities in those areas where they are available. Many airlines and train companies are using up-to-date technological advances to allow disabled passengers safer and more convenient transport.

Accessible and comfortable housing is equally important. Fortunately, many adaptations required by disabled persons demand neither extensive renovation nor great expense and, in fact, can make the dwelling safer and more functional for all who live there.

Lowman and Klinger (1969) identify eight housing features of specific concern to mobility-impaired individuals. They are: site; entrances (doors, stairs, garage); floor plan (space for maneuvering); details (doors, windows, floors, walls); furniture; heating, air conditioning, electrical systems; lighting and wiring; and plumbing. Certain disabled persons may require specific adaptations for other housing needs; for example, deaf people may need alternate doorbell, smoke, or fire alarm signaling systems.

Education

The American view of education is that every person has the right to develop to his or her highest potential. However, legislation had to be enacted in 1975 to ensure that disabled children received appropriate education. PL94-142 and the accompanying individualized educational program may force school systems to use technology more effectively. Withrow (U.S. Congress, 1980) argues that without technology, it is unlikely that the mandates of the individualized educational program can be met.

Educational technology operates in three ways: to compensate for the limitations imposed by disability; to enhance students' learning; and to assist research, management, evaluation, and administration.

Many of the aids that compensate for sensory or functional limitations are discussed elsewhere in this chapter. Devices such as ramps or writing aids for the mobility impaired, microphone and FM radio systems for the hearing impaired, or reading devices for the visually impaired are just a few examples of the application of technology to the classroom setting. In addition, aids such as talking slide rules or adapted science laboratory equipment are being developed primarily for use in educational facilities.

The more technology is used to enhance the learning process, the more likely it is that a disabled student can benefit from the educational program. Not only are physical barriers removed, but also compensation can be made for learning disabilities or communication disorders. For example, mentally retarded students can practice the same exercise over and over on a computer terminal, without trying the patience of the teacher, or slowing the progress of other students. Computer-based instruction, and other similar technologies can be easily brought into severely disabled students' homes through the telephone.

Use of audio-visual media in the classroom can directly

enhance student learning. Both disabled students and nondisabled students benefit greatly from the application of this bourgeoning field of technology to education. The potential for reinforcement of printed or spoken information is clear. The opportunity for immediate feedback, a concept important in the learning process, is provided by the instant playback capabilities of both audio- and video-tape units. For many students, greater interest and motivation to succeed are demonstrated when performing for a camera or recorder, and attention spans may be significantly increased. Cable and closed-circuit television allow a great variety of experiences to be brought into the classroom, thus enhancing students' contact with the world in which they live. Videodisk, electronic games, and teleconferencing are related technologies with potential to aid disabled students.

In this country, educational research relating to the handicapped has traditionally been supported almost entirely by the federal Bureau of Education for the Handicapped, now called the Office of Special Education. According to the Council for Exceptional Children (1977, p. 271), the "interpretation and dissemination of research results from the disciplines of medicine, biology, and genetics" will be of major importance over the next decades.

Evaluation is another systematic technology that is increasingly pursued in educational settings. According to the Council for Exceptional Children (1977), evaluation of the cognitive, motor, self-help, and personal and social skills of disabled people has two objectives: classification and program development.

Information sharing is a key to improved management of learning resources. A number of data bases and other formal information systems are available to help educators learn about appropriate learning technologies—information systems appropriate for schools, better classroom methods, and better ways for children to learn. Commercially available devices that help to overcome performance losses caused by physical disability are being developed. People in rehabilitation engineering centers are being trained to act as intermediaries between the data base and its users (National Rehabilitation Information Center, 1981). In addition, information management systems that allow educators to evaluate, track, and assist students is available. Cost-effective microcomputer technology, with its vast range of applications, contributes to all three of these areas of educational technology: aids or products that compensate for the limitations imposed by disability, technologies that directly enhance students' learning, and technologies of research, management, evaluation, and administration.

Employment

While most people in our society are expected to work, disabled people have, historically, been excused from this rule and often have not been adequately informed about the world of work. Until very recently, there have been more reasons for disabled people not to work than to work. These disincentives are slowly being eliminated by legislation, changing attitudes, and technology. While federal and state laws are encouraging employers to take affirmative action in hiring disabled people, technology is creating the means by which they can competitively enter the labor market. In turn, these actions are creating more positive attitudes and making the work world accessible to even the most severely disabled people.

Technological advances in systems and products have reduced reliance on physical function to perform many tasks, thus increasing the work potential of many physically disabled people. The computer age has opened career opportunities in industry and government that put physically disabled people on an equal basis with other workers because they rely more on education and training than on physical labor.

Another factor that has been influenced by technology and has affected the employment of disabled people is the trend toward home-based employment, which Alvin Toffler (1980) sees as the return of cottage industry. Prior to the industrial revolution, many people worked out of their homes or in neighborhood workplaces. With mass production and industrialization, the workplace changed and people began leaving their homes to work in large plants. Now, several large companies have begun identifying work tasks that can be performed in the home, thus reducing space costs for the company and transportation problems and costs for the employee. This is particularly beneficial to those disabled people who cannot get to the workplace. In addition, flexible work schedules and employment policies such as job sharing can greatly increase job possibilities for those with limited physical stamina.

Obviously, these phenomena do not solve all the employment problems of disabled people. Those who prefer or must have traditional, full-time employment at the workplace face problems, many of which, however, have technological solutions.

The same technological aids and devices that increase communication, educational opportunities, and activities of daily living can be transferred to the workplace and can increase employment opportunities. Other technological systems and products are specific to the workplace. Sale (1977) identifies several processes or systems that have aided the employment of disabled people in recent years, including selective placement, reengineering, job modification, and job restructuring.

An example of reengineering is the replacement of foot controls with hand controls for paraplegic machine operators. An example of job restructuring might be to break assembly line jobs down into individual tasks that retarded workers can learn by repetition. The same tasks are done, but only one task is performed by each person. According to *Rehabilitation Engineering* (Study Group on Rehabilitation Engineering, 1979), job site modifications can be as simple as raising a desk on blocks or as complex as providing innovative computer-entry processes, using eye movement sensors or sip and puff switches.

Selective placement programs usually use a work evaluation and job analysis system to solve problems that could prohibit employment for disabled persons. Many publications that identify technological solutions to problems caused by functional limitations also discuss problems related to employment. One such publication is the *Rehabilitation Engineering Sourcebook* (Institute for Information Studies, 1979).

La Rocca and Turem (1978) discuss a number of projects that have demonstrated how technology can help disabled people perform jobs and tasks that would otherwise have been impossible. Projects with Industry is a nationwide program jointly sponsored by the federal government and private corporations. It utilizes the latest systems technologies of work evaluation, job training, and job placement to place severely disabled people in industry. The Cerebral Palsy Research Foundation Center of Kansas is a rehabilitation engineering center that concentrates on employment. This center is developing a support package of engineering modifications, manufacturing techniques, and manufacturing engineering methodologies to enable severely disabled people to be placed in competitive employment. The job development laboratory at George Washington University uses work evaluation and job analysis to place clients (Mallik and Sablowsky, 1975). The National Technical Institute for the Deaf provides technical and professional education to deaf students and helps them develop personal, social, and communication skills, utilizing every applicable technology. The Optacon Fund works to open employment opportunities for blind people through the acquisition and development of sensory aids and the American Association for the Advancement of Science, among its other functions, serves as an advocacy and information resource for disabled professionals and students of science. This list is by no means exhaustive; La Rocca and Turem also mention, for example, the contributions of advocacy groups conferences, and awareness training seminars that promote the employment of disabled people.

Vocational rehabilitation has long claimed to be cost-effective. In order to continue to make that claim while serving an increasing number of severely disabled people, it must do more to place them in competitive employment. Rehabilitation professionals must become familiar with technology that can increase productivity, and use it to meet the goal of cost-effective rehabilitation and the goal of disabled people to live independently and support themselves through employment.

Problems of Technology

Hardly a person exists who cannot identify how his or her life has been improved through the application of modern technology. As the previous section of this chapter indicates, some improvements through technology in devices, systems, and information have enhanced the quality of life for some disabled people. However, considering the enormous potential of technology, current technologies have actually had little impact on the majority of disabled people.

Despite the examples of individuals whose lives have been improved, the evidence indicates that the application of technological advances to the problems of the disabled has so far been inadequate. This is most clearly illustrated by the continued underemployment and unemployment of disabled people. A report of the National Research Council of the National Academy of Sciences (1976, p. v) states: "Only a very small fraction of the country's scientific and technological capabilities have been effectively utilized to aid the physically handicapped. Few devices commonly used by the handicapped show the influence of current technology at all; many devices such as wheelchairs, which are produced by a multimillion-dollar industry, have been virtually unchanged for decades."

In 1965, long before the National Research Council's report was published, Mary Switzer, former Commissioner of the Vocational Rehabilitation Administration, wrote in the Foreword to a research and development grant "The time has arrived to apply the new knowledge that is becoming available, if the benefits of research are to reach the people who need them" (Rehabilitation Services Administration, 1975). Since the time of Switzer's comments and the National Research Council's 1976 report, many disabled individuals and organizations have worked diligently to improve this situation. Conferences have been held, awareness papers have been written, and reports have been made to committees and subcommittees of Congress. Still, many problems remain unsolved and large gaps in the application of technological developments to the problems of disabled people exist. Why, one wonders, are the existing technologies not being better utilized to benefit the thirty-five million physically and mentally disabled people in the United States?

The question has been explored many times since Switzer made her recommendation in 1965. Government, private industry, service providers, and consumers offer similar answers that can be generalized to (1) the market, (2) lack of financial incentive in the development and distribution of technological products for the disabled, (3) inadequate technology transfer, (4) lack of coordination among the relevant disciplines, (5) no mechanism of dissemination of information, (6) no evaluation or standards for products, and (7) lack of training related to rehabilitation technology. All of these reasons are closely related.

The Market. One of the most important issues is the market. If each technological rehabilitation product could be used by all thirty-five million disabled Americans, manufacturers might be more willing to develop and disseminate these products. However, the thirty-five million is divided into populations of specific disabilities and a variety of resulting problems. In dition, technologies must be highly specific even within disability groups. Recognizing a limited market, manufacturers fail to see a financial incentive. They are also aware that because the majority of disabled people are underemployed, and therefore have limited buying power, they are not a target population for many products. Another problem is that even when manufacturers do produce products and recognize a profit, they have a captive market and little competition to worry about. Thus, there is often little incentive to improve the product, to be responsive to consumer needs, or to price the product competitively. La Rocca and Turem (1978) point out that many of the approximately 400,000 American wheelchair users are dissatisfied with their wheelchairs. Despite the multimillion dollar revenues, manufacturers have not significantly changed the design of the wheelchair since the 1940s.

Financial Disincentives. Few rehabilitation products offer manufacturers the financial rewards that the wheelchair does. The design, development, evaluation, marketing, and servicing of most new technologies are viewed as being too costly to be entered into competitively.

The problems to be resolved by technology must be clearly identified by an interdisciplinary team of experts since the problems are often specific to one disability population, or even one person with a special problem. The expense of this type of product design and development is enormous as compared to product design and development based on the needs of an average population.

Evaluation for safety, durability, and reliability presents problems in that potential users must be identified and the evaluation may be conducted in a hospital or clinic, thus adding to the costs of development. Product liability insurance is also high. In addition, most manufacturers are not willing to solve the marketing problems encountered with disability products. These include the inability to exploit the usual advertising sources and the requirement that some products be prescribed by a physician. Manufacturers trying to be competitive find that there is no existing marketing system and that it is difficult to collect accurate information on the market. Another problem to be faced is that the manufacturer is often expected to provide modification, maintenance, and repair of products. This includes the training of sales and service personnel, and represents an unrealistic investment in light of the limited market for many of the products. Clearly, costs on the one hand, and market size on the other, minimize the profit potential for private manufacturers.

Technology Transfer. A third issue is the inadequate transfer of technology from other fields. As we have seen, technologies created for other purposes can be utilized to serve disabled people. Parsons and Rappaport (1977) list equipment, moving vehicles, instruments, computers, and communications as the main areas of technology transfer. Just as many technologies designed for the general public can be used by disabled people, products developed for disabled people often help the general public. The typewriter and the telephone are instances of devices originally invented for disabled people. Clearly, some mechanism is needed to expedite transfer of the many existing technologies from one field to another. Such a mechanism would require a coordinated effort among industry, government, and the diverse groups involved with disabled people. The NASA Technology Utilization Program, described earlier in this chapter, represented one such effort. More programs that rely on the initiative of engineers and managers in the private sector who recognize the problems created by disabilities, and are willing to invest capital to solve them, are needed.

Coordination. Juhr and others (1979) identified six basic groups who determine disabled consumers' needs for technological products: private inventors, university researchers, research staff of private manufacturers, the biomedical application division of NASA, the rehabilitation engineering centers of the federal Rehabilitation Services Administration, and disabled consumers. Other interested parties include consumers' families, service providers, administrators, educators, and legislators. At present, there is no means to coordinate the efforts of these diverse groups, and coordination is needed before optimal technological utilization can be achieved. Most critical is the cooperation of the public sector and the private sector. Ayers (1977, p. 29) states that neither sector alone can "marshal the full range of efforts required for effective and efficient development and application of technology to benefit handicapped persons."

Information Dissemination. A coordinated effort of the many disciplines involved cannot be achieved until there is an effective mechanism to disseminate information. Juhr and others (1979, p. 1) identify ineffective communication channels as a major reason for the lack of progress in the application of technological products and systems to the problems of disabled people: "Systematic access to reliable information concerning the availability of these devices and their applicability to the rehabilitative process is enjoyed neither by rehabilitation agencies, nor by the handicapped consumer, nor by third party payers who could through reimbursement facilitate the purchase of assistive and restorative technology." No formal mechanism exists for the dissemination of rehabilitation engineering research to potential manufacturers. Designers, doctors, therapists, third-party payers, counselors, other practitioners, and consumers need information on available products. Consumers also need a means to let all of these people know their needs. Designers who lack such information spend time developing unneeded products and duplicating existing products.

Evaluation and Standardization. Closely related to lack of coordination and information dissemination are lack of evaluation and standardization. Although expensive, product evaluation is greatly needed. Durability, reliability, safety, and appropriateness must be objectively determined by consumers and professionals. Standardization is a problem because of the enormous number of technologies.

The variable needs of the individual consumer make the development of standardized devices difficult. In many cases, individual needs (even among those who share similar disabilities) require unique technological solutions. It is nearly impossible to mass-produce or mass-market such devices. Devices are developed on a problem/solution basis and cannot be standardized. As Kornbluh explains: "Existing devices, systems, and equipment for the handicapped, serving essentially the same purposes, may have different timings, different electronic requirements, basic operational differences, different materials composition, and dissimilar safety and health features. Further, compatible accessories for aids and standard interfaces which allow devices manufactured by different firms to be used interchangeably, are not always readily available. Moreover, standard training materials, methods, and programs to show how to properly use the devices, systems, and equipment that are marketed may be inadequate or simply unavailable" (1980, p. 9).

Training. Even before a product can be developed, rehabilitation engineers must be trained. According to the Urban Institute (1975), there were only 50 rehabilitation engineers in the United States in 1975. Despite estimates of the number needed (250 then, and 2,000 by 1985), there are no graduate training programs in rehabilitation engineering in the United States. In addition to rehabilitation engineers, members of related professions require training. Usually, a product reaches the disabled person through one of many rehabilitation professionals. These professionals must have the technological information necessary to appropriately aid disabled consumers. They must know not only what products and systems are available, but also be able to train disabled people to use them.

Recommendations

Attempts are being made to solve the problems outlined above. Congress's commitment to help, for example, is outlined in the joint committee print, *Application of Technology to Handicapped Individuals* (U.S. Congress, 1980). Advisory panels made up of consumers, clinicians, engineers, representatives from consumer organizations and government research and development executives were established in 1977 and 1978. These panels emphasized the need to focus research and development on human rehabilitation. Their deliberations helped spur the creation of the National Institute for Handicapped Research. According to the congressional report, the mission of this organization is to promote research aimed at improving the lives of disabled people. The Interagency Committee on Handicapped Research and a National Council on the Handicapped have also been established. The National Science Foundation has been trying to establish a program to carry research through to implementation. Parsons and Rappaport (1977) relate that the biomedical application division of NASA has given attention to these problems and to the interaction between federal and other public agencies. A number of other federally mandated agencies geared to product design, development, and delivery have also come into existence in the past decade.

At the federal level, the Department of Education sponsored workshops on the education of disabled people and proposed that a technology transfer agency be established (Telesensory Systems, Inc., 1979). The Rehabilitation Services Administration tries to stimulate the development of technologies and coordinates information from its rehabilitation engineering centers to determine priorities for new technologies. Parsons and Rappaport (1977) trace the involvement of the Veterans Administration in rehabilitation engineering research. Also, the Department of Housing and Urban Development, the Department of Transportation, and the Rehabilitation Services Administration fund projects bringing technology to disabled consumers.

Training programs for rehabilitation professionals are being developed. The University of Virginia master's program in electrical, mechanical, and bio-engineering is heavily oriented toward rehabilitation. Other universities are considering incorporating a rehabilitation engineering option in their engineering programs.

Despite these and other attempts, many problems remain. If technological products are ever to become widely utilized, they must be produced in quantities that will make them available and affordable to consumers. Production technology itself is no longer a stumbling-block. Getting products to the market is the major remaining obstacle. Companies are reluctant to manufacture products that show low returns on sales. On the other hand, consumers must be aware of and able to afford the product before sales will rise. Private industry will not be able to solve the existing problems alone, but must be given incentives to manufacture products for disabled people. There is a need for coordinated efforts among private companies, consumer groups, nonprofit organizations, and federal, state, and local agencies.

Information must be made available to the parties that need it: rehabilitation agencies, disabled consumers, their families, third-party payers, doctors, researchers, and others. An information network must be developed to inform potential manufacturers of new developments or to involve them in critical stages of design and development. This network would, in turn, help solve many of the other obstacles. It could provide manufacturers with a marketing system and it would further enhance the necessary coordination among the many disciplines involved. Information on existing products could be better disseminated, thus paving the way for product standardization.

Awareness training for manufacturers and technological specialists in other fields is needed to facilitate technology transfer. Likewise, consumer training in use of existing products is needed.

It appears that all of these problems will be solved only through costly backing of research, design, development, production, and dissemination. Currently, it does not seem likely that the United States will follow Sweden's model, as outlined in the National Research Council of the Academy of Sciences report (1976). Sweden's government finances disability-related industrial research and development (on a pay-back basis) and purchases aids for disabled consumers that have been approved by Sweden's Institute for the Handicapped. Nor is it likely that private industry will bear the burden alone. The only real hope is for government, private industry, and public and private organizations to work together.

The following specific recommendations are offered with regard to the seven major problem areas:

- *The Market:* Funding is needed to subsidize research and to collect demographic information on the population, for the purpose of encouraging private production and developing delivery systems.
- *Financial Disincentives:* Money should be appropriated as authorized in the Rehabilitation Act of 1973 to solve problems of design, development, and distribution of technologies.
- *Technology Transfer:* The Technology Transfer Agency proposed by the federal Bureau of Standards should be funded.
- *Lack of Coordination:* A national organization and publication geared to all disciplines would be helpful.
- *Information Dissemination:* A nationwide information delivery system is needed.
- *Evaluation and Standards:* An appointed body to evaluate and set standards is needed.
- *Training:* More degree programs in rehabilitation engineering should be established and practitioners, disabled consumers, and their families should be taught about existing systems and products and their uses.

Kornbluh has this to say about the relationship of technology and independent living:

The picture of the development and application of technology to aid handicapped persons—from the point of view of handicapped people themselves and the researchers who work closely with them—seems to be one of pessimism and optimism. There appear to be many unsolved problems, unmet needs, and large gaps in technological knowledge. At the same time, however, there seem to be many creative and dedicated individuals and organizations determined to solve these problems, satisfy the needs and fill in the gaps. Actual and potential application of technology has shown considerable progress in preventing, curing, and ameliorating handicaps which afflict the Nation's citizens. Perhaps the central question to pose is one of value. Is the cost of developing and applying technology to aid handicapped individuals worth it—in terms of the single person whose mobility, productivity, and communication is improved (the micro perspective) and of society as a whole whose lost earning capacity and welfare payments could be decreased (the macro perspective)? [1980, p. 10].

Kornbluh's emphasis on the improved quality of life of individuals and the revenue returned to society through income taxes of employed disabled people is important. Yet the contributions to society that disabled people can make when given the opportunity must be considered of at least equal importance. These contributions can be greatly forwarded by appropriate technologies.

Part Four

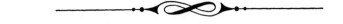

Achievements and Prospects

Chapters in this section are devoted to the need for and process of evaluating current achievements in independent living and to considering prospects for the future. The first two chapters present strikingly different approaches to evaluation. The first tells how objective, survey methodology can be used to enumerate the activities and quantify the results of services in IL centers. The second describes field research, a more subjective process that depends on direct observation to tap the insights of consumers. The third chapter demonstrates a blending of both approaches in its study of the disability rights movement in four states. Data gathering techniques including interviews, surveys, and site visits are used to examine the movement, both from the point of view of its leaders and from that of service providers, who are often targets of its actions.

Much information is still needed including strong cost-benefit figures and controlled studies of service effects. Nevertheless, the apparent progress of the IL movement, young though

271

it is, is undeniably impressive; the main question seems not to be whether it will exist, but in what form. Changes can be expected as a result of experience and growth within the IL movement. Other modifications will result from broader changes within the society as a whole. One of the final chapters considers the likely impact of the technological revolution on work, family life, education, and leisure for everyone, and how that may especially affect IL. But technology is not the only force that will shape the future. Human factors command the spotlight in the last chapter, for they, after all, will finally determine when, how—and whether—disabled people are allowed to take their rightful place as fully participative citizens.

15

Evaluating Program Methods and Results

Susan Stoddard

Independent living became a reality in California in 1970, with the founding of the physically disabled students program at the University of California at Berkeley. Two years later, the Berkeley Center for Independent Living (CIL) opened its doors. CIL was unique among early independent living centers. Other pioneer centers, such as the Boston Center for Independent Living or Cooperative Living in Houston, Texas, were residential programs, providing housing as a focus for service. CIL, however, was not a residential program but a program based on planning and coordinating the resources required for living and working in the community.

Note: The research on which this chapter is based was supported by evaluation funds allocated by the California legislature as part of the state appropriation for independent living centers under AB 204. The author would like to acknowledge the contribution of Fran Katsuranis, Linda Toms, Dan Finnegan, and Shirley Langlois, of the Berkeley Planning Associates, and Bruce Brown and Harry Greenblatt, of the California Department of Rehabilitation.

Innovation and expansion grants from the United States Rehabilitation Services Administration (RSA) were used by the California Department of Rehabilitation to fund a second generation of centers patterned after CIL (Brown, 1978). Like CIL, these new centers were consumer-controlled and provided a wide range of services either directly or by referral.

In 1979, the California legislature passed Assembly Bill 204, which authorized an appropriation of $1.8 million from the general fund to maintain and expand CIL and the system of second-generation centers. As a condition of funding, the legislature asked for a specific report on the activities and effects of these programs, including number and description of disabled individuals who receive services; range of problems presented by the individuals served and the services provided in response to those problems; number of individuals who moved from an institutional setting to a more independent setting, classified by type of setting; number of individuals who entered vocational rehabilitation or employment; impact of services on costs of other services (medical and supportive); impact of services on disabled individuals' participation in family and community activities; cost and savings to the general fund of providing the services; other sources of funding for independent living centers; and other information specified by the California Department of Rehabilitation.

While these questions address only some of the possible outcomes of independent living services, it is notable that the California legislature called for such reporting. Many IL activists had maintained that the IL system was too new to evaluate or that because client outcome was difficult to measure, the programs could not be evaluated by standard methods. The Urban Institute, in a nation-wide federally funded comprehensive needs study, had discussed possible evaluation models (Counts, 1978), but in general, IL programs around the country had not developed methods of systematic analysis.

The legislature wanted answers before consideration of the next fiscal year's budget. Consequently, the time allowed for the study was short. Moreover, the study was to be undertaken by an independent contractor. After the contract bidding process, only three and one-half months remained for the design and implementation of a study and the analysis and reporting of findings. This chapter presents the findings of that study, which was carried out by Berkeley Planning Associates (BPA).

Study Method

Four methods of collecting data were used by BPA: analysis of existing center and agency materials; client survey (by mail); site visits to each center; and interviews with community and state officials. This approach was selected so that information could be extracted from a variety of sources in the short time available. The combination of methods provided a check on the validity of findings and a richness of detail not possible with any one method.

An independent living research study of the state Department of Rehabilitation had gathered information about eight of the centers BPA was to evaluate. Some of these materials were made available to BPA. In addition, many of the centers had themselves prepared materials and reports. Analysis of these sources gave a preliminary picture of IL centers before the main field work began.

Information on clients' demographic characteristics and their use and assessments of center services was obtained through a mail survey of clients. BPA designed a systematic random method for centers to follow in selecting sample clients from service or case files. To ensure client confidentiality, the centers selected clients and mailed questionnaires to those clients, who sent returns to BPA. The questionnaires were brief (seventeen pages, forty-seven questions), and the items called for yes/no or multiple-choice answers. The overall response rate was 42 percent, with 368 questionnaires returned.

To collect information on service provision and on the centers' knowledge of their clients, BPA staff conducted site visits to each center. Short visits to six centers assessed the availability of information and probed the range of service models, as a preliminary to designing questionnaires and drafting field protocols. Full-scale site visits were made to eleven centers. These took either one or two days, depending on the size of the center, the availability of information, and the diversity of staff.

By telephone, BPA interviewed several persons in the communities served by the IL programs. Respondents included rehabilitation counselors, workers from county departments of social services, staff members of regional developmental disabilities centers, and mayors' or city councils' representatives.

Throughout the study, BPA discussed availability and interpretation of data with staff from the state Department of Rehabilitation and with an advisory committee composed of representatives from five of the centers. The site visits supported the survey data as reasonably representative of the total client population and operations of centers. Reviews of the survey data by the advisory committee and by state Department of Rehabilitation researchers conducting a parallel independent living research study also supported the validity of response patterns and absence of special bias in demographic characteristics.

Independent Living Services

Eleven of California's independent living centers designated for AB 204 funds participated in the study. Two other centers were originally designed for inclusion. One, the Adult Independence Development Center, near San Jose, did not lose its other funding to the extent required for AB 204 aid. The other, the Pasadena Center for Living Independently, could not be included because the center closed owing to labor problems.

These eleven centers are diverse in size and in the services they provided, as Table 1 shows. Two of the centers were substantially larger than the others, and except for the Center for Independent Living, all were four years old or younger at the time of the study. Two centers reported annual budgets of over $500 thousand, two reported budgets of from $251 thousand to $500 thousand, and five reported annual budgets of under $250 thousand. Three of the centers indicated that they typically served more than 200 clients per month; four served between 100 and 200 clients per month; and the remaining four reported fewer than 100 clients per month.

Table 1. Center Profiles.

Name	Location	Staff Size	Clients per Month	Budget	Age
Center for Independent Living	Berkeley	large	high	large	8
Community Service Center for the Disabled	San Diego	large	high	large	4
San Francisco Independent Living Project	San Francisco	medium	low	small	3
Community Resources for Independence	Santa Rosa	small	low	small	3
Disabled Resources Center	Long Beach	medium	low	small	3
Good Shepherd Center for Independent Living	Los Angeles	medium	medium	medium	3
Westside Community for Independent Living	Los Angeles	medium	high	medium	3
Darrell McDaniel Independent Living Center	Van Nuys	small	low	small	3
Resources for Independent Living	Sacramento	small	medium	small	3
CAPH Service Center	Fresno	medium	medium	medium	3
Dayle McIntosh Center for the Disabled	Garden Grove	medium	medium	medium	2

Staff Size
small: 0–15
medium: 16–40
large: over 40

Clients per Month
low: 0–99
medium: 100–199
high: over 200

Budget (in thousands)
small: $0–$250
medium: $251–$500
large: over $500

Age
Number of years center had
been operating at time of
data collection

Source: Stoddard and others, 1980, p. 4.

AB 204 specified that centers supported by funding under the act provide at least the following five services: peer counseling, advocacy, attendant referral, housing assistance, and other referrals. It also specified that they provide such other services as might be deemed necessary, such as transportation, job development, equipment maintenance and evaluation, training in independent living skills, mobility assistance, and communication assistance. Table 2 indicates the number of centers reporting a particular service as a *major* service of the center.

Table 2. Services Provided in IL Centers (for Ten Centers).

Service	Definition	Centers Reporting Service as a Major Service
Attendant referral	Referral of an individual to an attendant or referral of an attendant to a client in need of such services. The service may include training of the client in use and management of an attendant.	10
General advocacy	This may include activities directed not toward benefiting a single, identifiable client but rather toward groups of persons with disabilities. Activities may include public speaking, meetings with community organizations, development of new referral sources.	10
Peer counseling	May be one-to-one counseling or group counseling in areas not specifically defined below. It is to be provided by a person with a disability. (Note: several centers took exception, indicating that in some cases the peer may not be disabled; for example, parents of a disabled child would find a peer in another parent.)	10
Housing assistance	This includes referrals to accessible housing, home or apartment modifications and moving assistance. (Section 8 certification and landlord advocacy would be included under personal advocacy.)	7
Identification of accessible housing	Location of housing units that are accessible to persons with disabilities.	7

Table 2. Services Provided in IL Centers (for Ten Centers), Cont'd.

Service	Definition	Centers Reporting Service as a Major Service
Benefits counseling	Counseling one-to-one or in a group regarding benefits a client may be entitled to and how to apply for these benefits. Often includes and subsumes financial counseling, below.	7
Legal advocacy	Is provided on behalf of or with an individual during a legal proceeding or formal hearing.	5
Personal advocacy	Is provided on behalf of or with an individual in problems with other agencies or individuals, for example, direct interventions resulting from benefits counseling or legal advocacy.	4
Transportation	Arranging for transportation for a client with a transportation service or the provision of transportation by the center.	4
Employment preparation, job seeking skills, and placement	May include grooming, résumé writing, mock employment interviews, job development, and placement of an individual client. Services may be provided one-to-one or in a group.	4
Financial counseling	Counseling one-to-one or in a group regarding management of personal finances.	3
Special services for the deaf	Includes special services required by persons who are deaf to benefit from services at the center or in the community, for example, interpreter services.	3
Special services for the blind	Includes special services required by persons who are blind to benefit from services at the center or in the community, for example, reader services, brailling, and mobility instruction.	2
Vehicle access, repair, modification	Vehicle is defined as a wheelchair or a motorized vehicle (car/van/cart) used for purposes of mobility and/or transportation. Access may include assistance in researching appropriate models and purchase.	1

(continued on next page)

Table 2. Services Provided in IL Centers (for Ten Centers), Cont'd.

Service	Definition	Centers Reporting Service as a Major Service
Attendant training	Training of attendants in order to develop an attendant pool for use by center clients.	1
Substance abuse counseling	Counseling one-to-one or in a group regarding substance abuse either as an intervention or for purposes of prevention.	1

Note: Westside Center did not complete the data forms on which this table is based.
Source: Stoddard and others, 1980, pp. 17–18.

Centers were asked to make their own determination as to whether the service was a major part of their program. Consequently, only three of the five required services were identified as major in all centers: peer counseling, attendant referral, and general advocacy. Housing assistance was cited as a major service in seven centers. Other services are primarily forms of counseling, such as general peer counseling or legal, financial, or benefits counseling. Other services cited by several centers as major included certification for subsidized housing; independent living skills counseling, including goal setting and problem solving; TTY phone service; and interpreter provision or referral.

BPA found that the range of services provided by the centers is in part a function of center size, of center location in relationship to other service provision organizations, and of the needs of the local population. There is a great deal of variation in service patterns from center to center and in the emphasis placed on particular services in their overall programs.

The Clients

From discussions with center staff and review of center records, BPA estimated that as many as eighteen thousand individuals were served annually by the eleven centers. Two of the eleven centers account for more than half of this figure. The remaining nine centers reported the size of their client populations as anything between one hundred thirty and eighteen hundred persons. The site visits, record reviews, and survey data provide a composite portrait of these clients.

While independent living services were open to individuals with any type of disability, persons with a physical disability (especially of an orthopedic nature) were most likely to utilize such services. Frequently, other agencies in the community, such as regional centers, mental health centers, and community service centers, serve other disabled populations with specialized needs such as the deaf, the developmentally disabled, or the emotionally disturbed. The disabilities most frequently reported in the client survey population fell under the categories of "spinal cord injury" and "other orthopedic." Table 3 shows the distribution of disabilities in the survey sample.

Table 3. Prevalence of Disability.

Disability	Number	Percentage
Visual	23	6
Hearing	16	5
Arthritis	36	10
Muscular dystrophy	9	3
Multiple sclerosis	38	11
Spinal cord injury	64	18
Cerebral palsy	38	11
Missing limbs	7	2
Other orthopedic	64	18
Mental illness	6	2
Mental retardation	5	1
Other	45	13
Total	351	100

Source: Stoddard and others, 1980, p. 6.

Of the clients who responded to the mail survey, 194 (54 percent) stated that they used a wheelchair. Among individual centers, the proportion ranged from 33 percent (in two centers) to 70 percent. In seven centers, over 50 percent of the clients surveyed were wheelchair users.

At the time the survey was completed, the largest proportion of respondents (52.9 percent) could be classified as long-term disabled—that is, as having been disabled eleven or more years. The number of clients who were disabled fewer than three years was fifty-seven, representing 15.6 percent of the client sample. The remaining 31.5 percent reported having been disabled for three to ten years. Figure 1 illustrates the distribu-

Figure 1. Age/Sex Distribution of Client Sample.

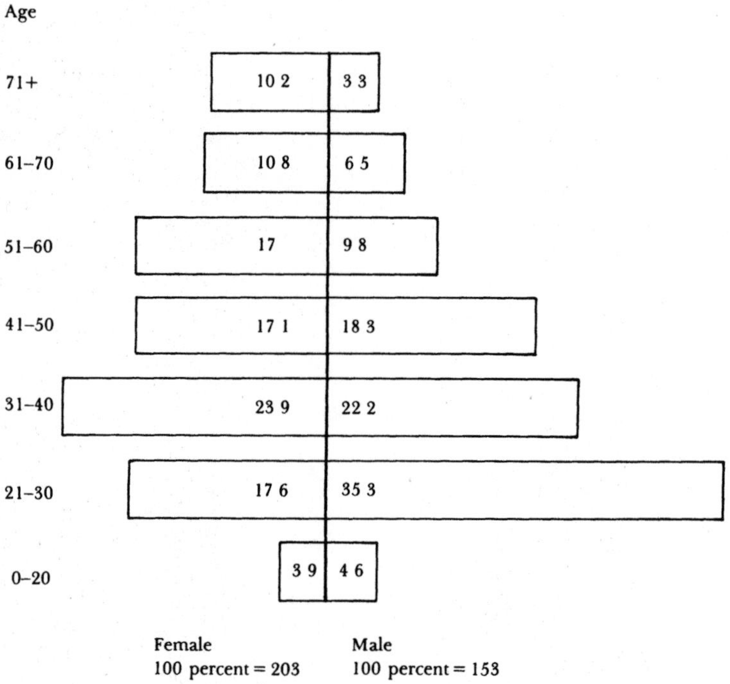

Age

Age	Female	Male
71+	10 2	3 3
61–70	10 8	6 5
51–60	17	9 8
41–50	17 1	18 3
31–40	23 9	22 2
21–30	17 6	35 3
0–20	3 9	4 6

Female
100 percent = 203

Male
100 percent = 153

Source: Stoddard and others, 1980, p. 7.

tion of the total client sample by age and sex. The mean age of this sample was forty-two years. This is slightly older than one would expect from center staff estimates of the age distribution of their client population, since eight of the eleven centers reported that eighteen- to thirty-four-year-olds represented the largest single age group served, making up more than half the clientele of three centers. The remaining three centers primarily serve an older population; two of these three estimated that 35-40 percent of their clients were over sixty years of age.

Staff at the centers estimated that the ratio of male to female clients was approximately equal—men slightly outnumbered women in four centers, and women outnumbered men in another four. This ratio is roughly comparable to that of the client survey population, in which female respondents accounted for 57 percent of clients sampled and males for 43 percent.

Patterns of Service Use

Clients of independent living centers present a wide range of problems. Patterns of client needs to some extent can be derived from analysis of data from the client survey. Table 4 shows the reasons clients gave for the first visit or call to the center. The most frequently cited reason was to get advice from a coun-

Table 4. Reasons for First Visit or Call to Center.
(N = 357)

Reason for First Visit	Number	Percentage[a]
To get advice from a counselor	107	29
To find an attendant	102	28
To find out about other places to get help	95	26
To talk to people with similar problems	90	24
To get help finding a new place to live	86	23
To meet people	80	22
To get help in improving housing situation	73	20
To get a ride	66	18
To get legal help	58	16
To get help finding a job or job training	56	15
To get help in dealing with the Department of Rehabilitation	51	14
To get help in dealing with an agency	49	13
To get or use a special device or piece of equipment	32	9
To get help in dealing with landlord	21	6
To get a piece of equipment repaired or modified	9	2
To get a reader or interpreter	9	2
To get help in dealing with an employer	8	2

[a]Since respondents could indicate multiple reasons for first visit, the sum of percentages will exceed 100 percent.
Source: Stoddard and others, 1980, p. 14.

selor; second was the need to find an attendant. It should be noted that many of the main reasons given for calling or visiting centers do not relate to specific problems, such as need for special devices or dealing with an employer. Rather, they tend to be general in nature and indicate the client's interest in finding people with similar problems to talk with, and in creating a personal social and information network. Also, there was no one predominant reason given for coming to the center.

Clients of California IL centers may receive several services as a part of a casework process in which a peer counselor assists the client in bridging gaps left by public agencies, or they may use the centers for only one service. One third of the clients completing the questionnaire indicated that they received only one type of help from the center, while another third received help in four or more service areas. Among multiple-service users, BPA found an interesting pattern of relationships among service needs. Figure 2 illustrates the relationship between the seven services most frequently cited by these clients. The arrows in the diagram indicate the direction of the relationship; the percentages illustrate the strength. For instance, of those clients receiving counseling, 52 percent indicated that they also received information about other places to get help, and 37 percent received help in meeting people. The reader should note the close relationship between meeting people, talking to people with similar problems, finding out about other places to get help, and counseling.

Finding an attendant, finding a new place to live, and getting a ride were often mentioned as areas where the center helped. Yet, in the diagram it is easy to see that these problems .y have been addressed independently of the counseling and socializing process of the center; in fact, fewer than half of those citing rides or attendants used any other one service. As to patterns of use over time, of those who received at least one service from the center, 35 percent were frequent users (twenty or more times), while 33 percent had used the center fewer than six times. Fifty percent of those reporting positive effects were clients (some of them center staff) who had used the center more than ten times. In fact, over one third of these clients reported use of 20 or more times.

Figure 2. Relationships Among Services (Seven Most Popular Services).

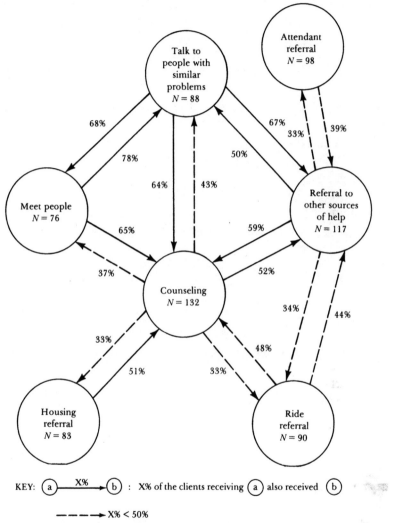

KEY: (a) —X%→ (b) : X% of the clients receiving (a) also received (b)

- - - - → X% < 50%

Source: Stoddard and others, 1980, p. 23.

Independent Living Outcomes

At the outset, the legislature posed several questions about
the results of IL services. In the study, since longitudinal tracking was impossible in the given time frame, clients were asked

two types of questions that would facilitate evaluation of services. They were asked to recall some details of their living and work status prior to receiving services, and they were asked to assess whether center services had had any effect on improvements that had taken place during the service period.

The legislature had asked specifically about movement of clients to a more independent setting. BPA found that at least two thirds of the centers' housing service efforts were directed toward *maintaining* disabled individuals in noninstitutional settings. Of respondents living alone when they first contacted the center, and who subsequently received assistance finding new ׳ ׳sing, 93 percent were still living alone at the time of the sur- v y, compared with 77 percent of those who had received no housing service from the center. During this same interval between first contact and the time of the survey, an average of 24 months, 29 percent of the respondents had changed their type of housing situation, resulting in a 10 percent increase in those living alone, a 28 percent decrease in those living with parents, a 47 percent increase in those living with roommates, and a 61 percent decrease in those living in institutions. Of the clients who reported that the centers had provided them with help in looking for a new place to live, 65 percent reported the centers had had a positive impact on their housing situation.

Another important IL outcome was client employment. However, employment services were a major service area in only four of the eleven centers. The employment situation for working-age clients improved slightly after contact with the centers, with 8 percent of those unemployed and not looking for work when they came to the center reporting full- or part-time work at the time of the survey. While unemployed clients not looking for work account for 60 percent of the clients in the sample, 25 percent of working-age disabled clients indicated that they were unemployed but looking for work.

The centers reported a strong relationship with the California Department of Rehabilitation. All the centers had at least one counselor from the department working regularly in the center, and over 40 percent of clients saw a rehabilitation counselor. Over 70 percent of those clients receiving employment-related service reported positive effects, such as help finding a job or help with an employer.

A further client goal identified by the legislature was participation in family and community activities. Evaluation of the centers' impact on client participation in family and community activities is difficult. There is no one ideal level of participation that applies to all clients. The appropriate level of participation depends on the wishes of the individual client and his or her own family and friends.

Most clients in the mail survey reported no impact on their relationships with family, friends, or the larger community. In all cases where such an effect did occur, however, the client reported it as positive. Thirty-seven percent of clients living with parents when first contacting the center, and twenty-six percent of those living with their family or a spouse, reported improvements in their relationships.

Overall, about one third of the clients responding indicated a positive effect on social relationships with friends and members of the community. Many clients included comments in their survey returns. One wrote: "This center gave me an opportunity to meet other disabled persons, successfully living independently, and helped me put my own situation and disabilities into proper perspective. In other words, it gave me a realization of all the things I *am,* not what I am *not.* I feel more confident about myself and am much more vocal in what I believe." Another client reported: "This center has helped me to get my self-respect. They have helped me to be useful. Helped me to be needed. They have helped me to build up my self-image so much that I feel free to ask a woman out for a date. I have only started dating within the last four years." And: "I am much more involved in the community more politically aware, And being involved in making political changes" (Stoddard and others, 1980, pp. 64-65).

These rough indicators did show client gain in key IL areas. However, the legislative questions that bounded the study had also limited the range of client outcomes to be explored. Furthermore, the short time frame of the study did not allow the kind of measurement and client tracking that would characterize a comprehensive evaluation. Nonetheless, within these parameters, the study showed that deinstitutionalization and employment services were *not* key programs to the extent implied by IL rhetoric and that maintenance of independent living settings and improvement of the quality of life for IL clients were the more central service goals of the centers. Studies are in progress to develop client-gain information in more detail (Heihle, 1981).

Cost and IL

The legislature had framed several questions regarding the cost-effectiveness of IL services. One question dealt with the impact of IL services on the costs of medical and support services. Medical and support services are those services that the severely disabled person needs in order to assume the role of an independent member of the community. While specific needs for support services vary according to the client's disability and functional limitations, BPA identified a core of support services that are needed to some degree by most severely disabled persons. This core includes attendant care, financial support, and other services such as transportation, equipment, and readers and interpreters, in addition to such medical services as hospitalization and physician visits.

Expenses to provide support services for those living independently proved difficult to estimate, owing to difficulty in capturing all the social costs of delivering publicly provided services and to lack of specific information on the expenses incurred by clients. It was possible, however, to observe some trends in the use of such services by those served by IL centers.

Comparing clients' current use of medical services with the use patterns of those clients before they came to the center, the study found a decrease of 47 percent in frequent hospitalization, little difference in the frequency of therapy, doctors' visits, and counseling, and a slight increase in the number of individuals stating that they used no medical services frequently. Although direct provision of health services is not among the list of regularly provided center services, 31 percent of clients reported that centers had a positive effect on their self-health care. These results indicate possible savings in both private and public medical costs.

Review of attendant utilization patterns before and after contact with the center shows an increase of 24 percent in the number of clients using an attendant and a reduction of 28 percent in those not using an attendant but looking for one. In addition, a net increase was found in the average number of attendant hours used. Sixty-nine percent of those receiving help in finding attendants reported that the center had had a positive effect on the quality of their attendant care. The increase in utilization may indicate a parallel increase in costs, since both the numbers of people using attendant care and the hours of care show an increase. This cost may be borne by the individual or by the public through various support programs.

The one financial support program that showed a substantial change after client contact with centers was Homemaker Chore, where there was an overall increase in the number of individuals using it as a source of income. Other income sources more frequently utilized by clients after contact with the center included job earnings and SSI and SSDI payments. Forty-eight percent of the respondents who reported current job earnings indicated that they had had no job earnings before. IL centers appear to have positively affected clients' abilities to get rides when needed and to get help from equipment or devices. The centers helped 83 percent of clients needing help in getting a ride, 86 percent of clients needing help with equipment provision, and 88 percent of clients needing equipment repair.

Almost half of all clients from centers that provided transportation reported positive effects in getting rides, compared with 29 percent from centers providing neither transportation nor referral. It is difficult to assess the possible cost implications of such service use. On the one hand, an increase in the use of already purchased equipment may mean an increase in the cost-effectiveness of such equipment and an increase in the client's ability to obtain jobs and pursue independent living goals. On the other hand, increased ability to get rides may mean an increase in transportation operating costs—an increase that must be borne by public agencies.

Nonetheless, the study concluded that public or private savings are indicated by a decrease in hospitalization costs, an increase in job earnings, and a small decrease in total costs for institutional care. Public costs are raised, however, by use of attendant care and other in-home support services, by increased use of transportation, and by increase in clients' abilities to obtain aid payments to which they are entitled.

Cost-effectiveness studies cannot conclusively demonstrate whether or not independent living for severely disabled persons results in a net saving to the state. There are many noneconomic benefits that must be considered, in addition to economic savings that might be realized. One client in the survey linked the economic and personal costs of unavailable transportation: "Without the transportation, I would have to use taxis which I could not afford. My visits to the Kaiser clinics would be abandoned. The health of people like me would deteriorate. We would perish before our time" (Stoddard and others, 1980, p. 55).

The eleven centers were supported by a variety of funding sources, with support in the study year alone totaling approximately $5.6 million. About half of this amount was reported as coming from a variety of programs administered by the California Department of Rehabilitation. This included funds from the state general fund and from federal programs of the Rehabilitation Services Administration. At the time of the study, almost one third of the budgets of the eleven IL centers were supported by the state general fund, through AB 204. In addition, many of the IL services clients receive are supported by the general fund under various state programs or as a result of state matching of federal funds. Altogether, public funds accounted for over 90 percent of the total income of the eleven centers.

Dependence on money that could end after brief contract periods presented centers with numerous fiscal problems; in the long run, a more stable funding base is sought. In the short run, continued funding depended largely on what was available.

Some centers were developing fee for service approaches to program support but reported difficulty in setting prices that cover cost.

Overall, California's IL centers have had a positive influence in facilitating the transition to independent living, in reducing hospitalization of disabled persons, and in increasing use of attendant care. The BPA study exemplifies the utility of carrying out such studies while a program is still developing, when it is most critical to identify key processes, separate fact from rhetoric, and keep funding sources informed. As the result of the study, directors and staff of the centers themselves learned more about the clients their centers served and about how those clients evaluated their programs (Stoddard and Brown, 1980).

As IL centers become more sophisticated, they should develop the capacity for self-evaluation. In its infancy, the IL movement was able to gain support on the idea alone. As IL centers move into their second decade, at a time of shrinking public funds, they will increasingly be required to demonstrate their effectiveness in terms that legislatures and budget committees will understand. With maturity comes the responsibility for demonstrating the fulfillment of promises.

16

Using Field Research to Gain Subjective Insights

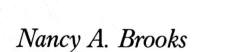

Nancy A. Brooks

Joseph Stubbins (1977) proposes that people with disabilities experience a reality that is not well understood by professionals. Professionals tend to seek general patterns that will lead to predictable outcomes expressed as probabilities. In contrast, disabled persons confront immediate personal and environmental dilemmas that cry out for practical solutions.

This gap between professional and consumer viewpoints needs to be closed, since problems investigated by professionals ᴵⱼy not be the same as the problems that disabled people wish to solve (Dembo, 1977). The complexities of independent living especially require investigation incorporating the disabled person's experience. Both the general, systematic overview of the professional and the unique, subjective insight of the consumer are needed as foundations for effective policies and programs. The purpose of this chapter is to introduce field research as a method which ties the realities of independent living to the need for valid research data. By adding direct observation to more traditional quantitative methods, researchers can provide insight into the living patterns of disabled people.

The Independent Living Movement has created an entirely new lifestyle, one which balances professional services with consumer initiative. DeJong (1979) suggests that this development calls for a new research paradigm that will correspond to independent living goals. Researchers are challenged to discover a set of variables that are most reflective of IL values. Attention to values such as consumer involvement, environmental modification, and comprehensive service provision to severely disabled people produces new understanding of disability and alters the traditional relationships among policy-makers, service providers and disabled individuals. If these new relationships are to be productive, solid information about the reality of independent living is needed.

It is important to remember that good intentions do not automatically result in sound policies. Institutions, for example, were originally built by those who assumed that a protected environment staffed by objective caretakers would lead to better lives for vulnerable people (Helsel, 1971). The detriments of institutionalization were not widely acknowledged for many decades, in part because such early institutions may indeed have provided better living conditions than were available in communities at the time. More recently, a precautionary note has been sounded in regard to deinstitutionalization of mentally disabled persons. According to Bradley (1980, p. 182), the recent, optimistic belief in community-based programs has proved naive. "The possibility of a better lot for mentally disabled persons outside institutions appears to have receded as evidence of the more unattractive realities of community-based care piles up." Given these experiences, it is apparent that researchers have a responsibility to determine the degree to which the actual living patterns of disabled individuals fulfill IL values. By giving systematic attention to the daily routine, social activities, and environmental surroundings of disabled persons, professionals will expand their understanding to "knowing" rather than "knowing about" IL experiences.

Because field research is based upon direct observation of

and interaction with research subjects and their environments, it offers a means of bridging the gap between professional and lay realities. Field research is defined as "an immersion by the researcher into an unfamiliar way of life in order to establish first-hand knowledge about selected aspects of the setting" (Shaffir, Stebbins, and Turowetz, 1980, p. 6). Observations and interviews generate qualitative data as distinct from quantitative data resulting from surveys or experimental studies. The perceptions of both researcher and subject are considered valid indicators of the reality experienced in the observed context. Detailed instructions for carrying out this form of research will not be ꞏꞏn here but relevance to IL settings will be elaborated. Special methods appropriate to conducting interviews and observations among severely disabled people will be suggested, and examples of IL field studies will be summarized. Since field research does entail certain difficulties in application to IL studies, problems of the method will also be discussed.

Relevance to Independent Living

Field researchers collect data through direct observation to document how people cope with their environments. The usefulness of this method has been demonstrated in studies showing how marginal groups manage to exist within the confines of mainstream society (Gans, 1962; Liebow, 1967; Stack, 1974; Whyte, 1943). The lessons of this work are applicable to IL studies since disabled people are not yet integrated into most social systems. Study of disabled individuals living in the community can lead to a greater appreciation for the variety of human efforts striving to come to terms with their surroundings (Glaser and Strauss, 1967).

With qualitative methods, researchers can begin to answer the question, What lifestyles are available to disabled individuals living in the community? To answer this question means that researchers must come into contact with the world they study and open themselves to the experience of managing attendants, locating accessible transportation, and practicing acceptable social roles in ordinary communities, all within the constraint of physical disability. Observers who subjectively experience unfamiliar social settings and translate that learning into comprehension of group life can communicate their awareness to other outsiders.

Field work is based on the assumption that what people actually do in their daily lives, and how they interpret their routine, follows observable patterns that can be understood by trained investigators. These patterns are important to the evaluation of IL settings, for they reveal the setting as it occurs, rather than as it might have been predicted.

Field research is especially suitable to the study of process. Unlike surveys and experiments, which are concerned with an instant of time, direct observation requires attention to sequence and schedule. Daily routines, social relationships, and critical incidents are observed over time, allowing the investigator to discover changes as well as stable patterns. Long-term observation in a social setting enables the researcher to understand how people construct and modify their understanding of their environment.

Many independent living programs reflect the assumption that disabled people will acquire independence skills and develop social roles that are as normal as possible. The qualitative approach is effective for investigating how consumers perceive program goals, what value they place upon achieving independence skills, and how IL goals are evaluated once achieved.

For example, an IL program may construct accessible housing to replace inadequate accommodations for severely disabled persons. Once the housing is occupied, however, residents may complain that accessible housing is less important than transportation. They may organize advocacy groups and lobby for more access to the public transportation system. Such a scenario would test the ability of researchers to comprehend whether the new housing was devalued by the residents or whether it functioned to release their time and efforts to solicit greater social participation. Careful study of daily schedules and extensive interviewing concerning residents' definitions of independence would discover the relationship between what consumers were saying and what they were doing. Regardless of whether an IL program is residential, transitional, or supportive, evaluation of the program benefits from understanding of the process by which disabled individuals change as they respond to their environment.

The nature of social interaction among disabled persons deserves thorough investigation, since the norms and values of disabled persons may determine group response to skill development and social participation. Field research methods are highly appropriate to such investigations. The interpersonal elements of mutual aid, referral, and pure social exchange can be studied as they contribute to or detract from independent living. Systematic observation may reveal, for example, that clients of an IL program avoid friendships with other disabled persons, preferring to seek social contacts with able-bodied persons. What sponsors may view as an excellent opportunity for social interaction may be perceived by consumers as stigmatizing.

On the other hand, social networks embody the values of independent living as they provide the means for disabled individuals to mold daily experience into an established lifestyle. Social relationships can fill service gaps, as when cooperative shopping and cooking groups develop to replace inadequate food services or when experienced consumers teach newcomers how to deal with community agencies. Furthermore, social interaction has a strong normalizing function when relationships between consumers and attendants, service providers, neighbors, and other disabled persons expand to include the full range of social roles.

External social forces such as service systems, community acceptance, and financial support programs are also part of the consumer's reality. Field investigators should be sensitive to the coping strategies employed by consumers in regard to these factors.

Observations of daily routines will provide evidence of consumer response to service systems. Field notes show how frequently services are utilized and how they are interpreted by consumers. It would be appropriate, for example, for observers to document whether consumers valued social interaction with personal care attendants more highly than accessible housing.

Similarly, observers can record the influence of community attitudes upon independent living. Having physical access to the able-bodied community does not necessarily guarantee positive experience. Being on the scene gives the field researcher opportunity to note whether customers in wheelchairs are readily served in shopping and recreation areas and whether able-bodied neighbors share frequent social exchanges with disabled residents. Both the physical and social environments must be hospitable before IL programs will achieve integration.

The research areas suggested above address the combined influence that consumers, social networks, and external factors have upon independent living goals. The techniques of long-term observation and interviewing have specific advantages in this endeavor. Because field research methods investigate everyday realities and the shared meanings of community settings, they facilitate understanding of human means for managing social and environmental conditions.

Observing IL Settings

As with all systematic study, field work focuses upon identifiable research problems such as those discussed earlier in this chapter. However, there are differences in the ways qualitative and quantitative studies identify questions and carry out investigations. It is not the purpose of this chapter to elaborate upon the theories and techniques of field research, which have in any case been thoroughly discussed in other contexts (Filstead, 1970; Glaser and Strauss, 1967; Lofland, 1971; Schwartz and Jacobs, 1979). Instead, the basic functions and limitations of field research and their application to IL studies will be considered. In addition, observing and interviewing disabled individuals raises certain questions regarding technique, ethics, and subject-researcher relationships that will also be addressed here.

A major property of field research is its reliance upon the inductive approach. Research procedures are organized so that observations determine hypotheses; observers discover research problems during the process of investigation (Babbie, 1979). Although a general interest sustains the initial inquiry, detailed questions emerge only after the observer has acquired a fundamental understanding of the subjects' way of life. For example, an observer might begin by asking how the need for personal assistance in daily activities such as dressing, eating, and toileting affects disabled individuals who are trying to live as independently as possible. Close observation of consumer–attendant relationships will tend to redirect the inquiry toward more specific matters. If recruitment, management, reimbursement, and termination of attendants were found to require considerable time and effort, then this process might become a study topic.

Field research, then, begins with an attempt to define the fundamental elements of a given situation. Observers record incidents that recur and have established meanings, distributions and frequencies of incidents and the populations involved, and social structure as revealed by expressed norms and ranking systems (Zelditch, 1971). From these data, researchers can identify specific problems and patterns that reflect "the ongoing stream of naturally occurring social activities" (Speier, 1973, p. 11).

A second feature of field research is intimacy to the subject. Regardless of whether researchers delve into the complexities of one setting or make comparative studies among several environments, they amass detail by means of close examination. Lofland proposes four approaches that will bring researcher and subjects into close relationship and produce the necessary indepth data: physical proximity, duration through time, sense of social intimacy and confidentiality, and reporting of extensive details (Lofland, 1971, p. 3).

Since IL arrangements take many forms, techniques for developing close involvement with consumers must vary with each environment. Frieden has identified four types of IL settings: the independent living center, the independent living residential program, the independent living transitional program, and the independent living service provider. Each program varies in service setting, service delivery, helping style, vocational emphasis, goal-orientation, and client type (Frieden, 1980b). The details of daily routine can be studied from many perspectives. For observational studies to be sufficiently intimate, researchers must conduct preliminary investigations to determine how the observations should be undertaken.

A third essential element of field research is its attempt to go beyond description, to reveal the structure of shared human experience. Merely reporting how people cope with their environments is not enough; consistent themes must be unveiled. To accomplish this, the observer must attend to what happens, what interpretations are given to events, what patterns of interaction occur, what established relationships are observed, and how coherent the entire setting is (Lofland, 1971, p. 15). The discovery, for example, that a setting is characterized by disorganization, fragmented relationships, and instability can promote understanding of human attempts to cope with such situations.

Learning how disabled persons construct shared lifestyles supported by IL programs will also advance understanding of their social roles in the larger community. For example, shared environmental and social conditions may affect disabled individuals' perceptions of themselves as working members of the community. Discovering how employment schedules mesh with IL routines, how employment is evaluated by disabled persons, and whether employment affects social relationships and social prestige among IL consumers will increase comprehension of the attitudes of disabled persons toward work. Moreover, although disabled people encounter many barriers to full social participation, they also share resources for contending with their disadvantages. The structure of these shared resources has yet to be adequately researched.

Perhaps the most important element of field research is researcher involvement. Researchers who employ subjective techniques in studying social environments usually employ a form of participant observation (Shaffir, Stebbins, and Turowetz, 1980, p. 6), either overtly gathering information as recognized investigators or covertly observing the scene from the vantage point of another role. In either case, participant-observation is defined as "being in the presence of others on an ongoing basis and having some nominal status for them as someone who is part of their lives" (Schwartz and Jacobs, 1979, p. 46). An advantage to being a known (rather than covert) observer is that subjects will instruct an outsider in the community's norms and social structure.

The observer's sensitivity is a primary feature of participant observation. Systematic records of the observer's subjective perceptions and emotional responses to the subjects and the environment become part of the research documentation. The personal log is added to field notes, tape recordings, photographs, and interview transcripts as a record of human response to the research setting. When observers document their own anxieties, pleasures, and surprises in response to the study environment they move closer to their subjects' experiences. Because disabled individuals respond to the IL setting on a subjective level, observers should participate in that experience by recording subjective as well as active experiences.

There is a valid need for sensitive and trained observers to relay disabled individuals' views of themselves and their environments to other groups. Finding out what daily living with a disability means to someone who is participating in an IL program will assist both the practical and the theoretical dimensions of IL studies.

Actual implementation of field research requires training. Formulating research questions, becoming deeply involved in the setting, discovering structure and patterns, and practicing introspective participant observation are standard, learned research procedures. Academic programs for anthropologists, sociologists, and community psychologists can train potential independent living field researchers. However, there are a number of special procedures for conducting research among disabled persons that require discussion here since they are unlikely to be taught in standard field methods training.

Special Considerations for IL Studies

Since field research often requires extensive face-to-face interaction between researcher and subject, the social competency of both parties will be tested. The business of starting, maintaining, and ending at least a minimal relationship must be managed. The very fact that the subjects are disabled, and perhaps severely disabled, introduces special considerations into the research relationship.

In the first place, it is likely that investigators will be able-bodied individuals. These persons may or may not have had previous experience interacting with disabled persons. If they are not experienced, their reactions to disability may interfere with communication. Nervous investigators may behave awkwardly, fidget, stand too far away, or lose eye contact with disabled subjects. Such behaviors are typical of initial able-bodied to disabled person interactions (Kleck, Hiroshi, and Hastort, 1966), but are not conducive to research relationships. It has been my own experience that new investigators require at least two days of casual meetings with IL subjects until the impact of disabling conditions diminishes and investigators can develop person-to-person communication. Explanations of subjects' physical conditions also have assisted my co-investigators' accommodation to subjects. Learning about the effects of cerebral palsy, spinal cord injury, or multiple sclerosis gives investigators a basis for interpreting what appear to be unaccountable behaviors or appearances. Preparation for entering an unfamiliar social environment can only benefit the research effort.

However, the entire responsibility for sustaining communication need not devolve upon the investigator. Even though subjects may have speech, hearing, or visual impairments, they will bring their own social skills to the communication effort and may assist the investigator who is learning how to manage social interaction with disabled subjects. Investigators can usually rely upon their subjects to repeat misunderstood words, employ writing when an investigator does not use sign language, or ask for assistance when it is needed. When able-bodied field researchers participate in a disabled person's world, researchers may very well require assistance from the disabled person.

In the second place, field researchers must be prepared to observe or partake in activities that are stigmatized by society (Goffman, 1963). Long-term observers of the severely disabled will learn about the daily business of managing catheters and leg bags, braces and respirators, spasticity and drooling, and through that learning they will become partly stigmatized themselves.

An extreme example of such learning is illustrated by the

following anecdote. When the investigator knocked at a subject's apartment door, she heard the occupant call "Come in." The investigator found no one in the living room but located the interview subject in the bathroom sitting on the toilet, where, she said, she had been left one half hour earlier by an attendant. Although the investigator offered to search for the attendant, the subject insisted on beginning the interview immediately. So, the first fifteen minutes of interview were conducted in the bathroom while the investigator sought to control her composure. Sustaining a conversation with a stranger who is sitting on a toilet is not a conventional social practice. However, severely disabled woman apparently was accustomed to a different value system, one which had very likely arisen from years of being assisted by others.

Many researchers find suspending everyday wisdom and entering the world of severely disabled individuals an uncomfortable experience, partly because they may feel parasitic knowing that they will report their observations to outsiders (Sanders, 1980). Investigators who operate in unfamiliar settings suffer the anxiety and uncertainty of people trying to live in two worlds (Shaffir, Stebbins, and Turowetz, 1980, p. 3). Nonetheless, it is important to affirm the subject's value system.

A third consideration in IL field studies is the ambiguity of researcher–subject relationships. All observers are likely to experience some role conflict as they perform research in the context of personal relationships, but deciding whether to act as a person or as a researcher can be markedly problematic when disabled subjects request aid from an observer.

To what extent should the outside observer provide information, advice, or physical assistance to fulfill the needs of disabled subjects? In resolving this question, observers must consider the effect of their actions both upon the subjects and upon the research. By giving aid, researchers directly influence the scene which they observe, so a judgment must be made as to the status of such requests within the given context. Accustomed to receiving help from able-bodied persons, disabled subjects may simply request assistance as a way of meeting needs and controlling their environment. Although field researchers are constrained to show some responsibility for subjects who are exposing their private lives to an outsider (Shaffir, Stebbins, and Turowetz, 1980, p. 16), there may be limits to the assistance disabled subjects can expect to receive. Even when researchers want to help, they may be limited by questions of liability if subjects request lifting, feeding, or transportation. Case-by-case decisions must be made regarding the urgency of the request, the alternatives available to the disabled person, and the consequences to the researcher–subject relationship. In my work, I have found that honest discussions with subjects usually satisfy both parties if help cannot be given. Otherwise, giving help not only reinforces the subject–researcher relationship, but also gives the observer insight into another dimension of independent living.

Last, some attention should be given to adjusting research procedures so that physical impairments will be accommodated. Both the schedule and the actual research techniques should reflect the subjects' capacities for speech and mobility. Because disabled persons may need relatively longer time for movement or speech, the project should allow for longer observation and interview periods than might be necessary for able-bodied subjects. Ordinary writing instruments should be avoided when the researcher is gathering life histories or personal accounts from severely disabled (and, of course, blind) persons. Tape recording and photographic flashes should be tested prior to use since audio recording may produce nervousness that disrupts speech and flashes may trigger spasms. Also, researchers should monitor their own interview styles to determine whether their anxiety about communicating with disabled subjects is causing them to ask leading questions. The tension of waiting for disabled subjects to accomplish physical or verbal tasks may goad researchers into dominating the scene. Patience and self-control, crucial to all field research, are especially necessary in IL field studies.

Just as special consideration should be given to research techniques applied to disabled subjects, care should be taken to report research findings in an ethical way. Since field researchers purposefully establish social relationships with their subjects, questions of suppressing negative information may arise. An investigator who absorbs the values of an IL setting may choose to protect that way of life by reporting only its positive elements.

Although selective reporting is not in keeping with standard research principles, investigators may perceive obligations to respect the reputations of subjects who have opened their entire lives to scrutiny. Especially when the group being studied is seeking an improved way of life, researchers may become sensitive to the implications of their work. Observers who discover socially unacceptable conditions in the research setting face the question: "Is revelation likely to produce enough long-term benefit to warrant any immediate damage to persons or programs?" (Fichter and Kolb, 1970, p. 269). Because field work gathers behind the scenes information, it has the potential for exposing unexpected data that might have serious impact upon policies and programs.

In what is the tradition of the profession, field researchers are likely to report inadequacies discovered in powerful groups (Glazer, 1972). But ethical questions may appear when researchers discover that dependent populations misuse the services they receive. If researchers were to uncover such collective behaviors as unreported income-producing activities that might affect financial benefits, or abuse of prescribed medications, they might be tempted to suppress their results in order to protect the subjects.

When researchers decide how to report their findings, they may wish to judge how much society needs data that would be detrimental to people of low status, for even those whom society considers unrespectable deserve respect from scientists (Fichter and Kolb, 1970, p. 269). Although researchers' first obligation is to present accurate findings, they also have a tacit agreement with subjects, incurred during frequent face-to-face interaction, to behave responsibly when exposing these people. Neither whitewashing nor muckraking will be beneficial to science or to subjects.

The issues of ethical reporting are associated with other

limitations of field research. As compared to other methods, field research makes no attempt to limit or direct the stimuli which may influence subjects. Thus, these methods are considered unsuitable for determining cause (Labovitz and Hagedorn, 1971). Campbell and Stanley (1963) criticize the "one-shot" case study for lacking comparison groups or making implicit comparisons to undetermined groups, thus rendering it unreplicable. Furthermore, because subjects may behave differently and modify social relationships to accommodate the outsider, the validity of observation may be negated in some instances (Babbie, 1979, p. 228). Because of these difficulties, field research has often been confined to exploratory work. Researchers have assumed that case study findings were not generalizable.

Criticisms of field research do not tell the full story. In their own defense, field researchers would argue that validity is not a major concern since subjects are more constrained by group expectations than by the presence of an observer (Shaffir, Stebbins, and Turowetz, 1980, p. 14). Furthermore, the importance of an outside constraint should be diminished by the sheer volume of data accumulated in such a study, which draws on many more sources than do surveys or experimental studies. Finally, field workers can confirm subjects' reports through observation or checking with other informants (Shaffir, Stebbins, and Turowetz, 1980, p. 14). As for replication, since substantially systematic field methods have been developed, comparative studies have become increasingly replicable (Edgerton and Langness, 1978).

Concern about the scientific credibility of qualitative data should extend to quantitative techniques as well. Researcher bias can appear in quantitative work during problem selection, sampling, or analytic procedures. After reviewing the literature on multiple regression analysis used in rehabilitation research, Bolton (1978) concludes that appropriate use of statistical analysis requires human judgment and subjectivity, and a thorough understanding of the available knowledge of each and every analytical tool. Field research deserves the same study and respect.

Case Studies

Direct observation has already been employed in several studies of IL settings. Providing comprehensive and detailed views of independent living, these studies demonstrate the strengths of field research. Following are summaries of three case studies which illustrate the realities of independent living.

Houston, Texas. As a part of a larger study of the cooperative living transitional residential program for severely physically disabled young adults, Stock and Cole (1971) investigated the impact of environment on consumer in several accessible residential settings in Houston. Using interviews, direct observation, and residents' diaries, investigators recorded daily routines and documented residents' evaluations of apartments, dormitories, or nursing homes as housing facilities. Findings showed that each setting developed a distinct social character and that the activities and social contacts of disabled residents varied among different environments. Moreover, comparative observations showed that these conditions changed over time. As social stratification and division of labor evolved, IL residential programs provided experiences in role modeling and peer counseling that contributed to residents' social competency. Program success was found to relate to residents' abilities to manage social and financial affairs and to utilize community resources. Experiences gained in the various IL settings resulted in different outcomes, but in each case, the prevailing social environment influenced emerging lifestyles.

The findings of this field study have implications for program development and management. The investigators concluded that because social environments vary between facilities and also change over time, service providers should be prepared to supply a range of housing and service options that suit the social as well as the physical needs of individual disabled consumers.

Wichita, Kansas. The Urban Residential Center (URC), a housing and service-providing facility for severely physically disabled adults, was observed by Brooks and Hartman over a ten month period (Brooks and Hartman, 1979). During that time,

URC housed twenty-seven residents, most of whom had been disabled since early childhood by cerebral palsy. The purpose of the study was to describe the URC lifestyle from the point of view of residents and to identify social skills contributing to success in a facility that sought normalized life experiences.

Lifestyles at URC were found to be relatively active and diverse, considering the severity of disabilities observed. The daily routine filled a long day, from 4:30 P.M. to 10:00 P.M., and included activities ranging from work and school to church and organized sports. Social interaction among residents was intimate, even communal, since the residents shared rooms, meals, transportation, and, occasionally, employers.

In keeping with the participant-observer approach, the investigation evolved as shared values and definitions were offered by the residents. The following skills were reported by residents as attributes of a successful URC resident:

- Able to establish and maintain social relationships.
- Active in a variety of social relationships both within and outside URC.
- Accepting of URC program, staff, and residents.
- Experienced and capable in employment.

These characteristics illustrate the importance of social competency to the URC social system. Although social relationships outside URC were considered desirable, successful residents were also expected to conform to the URC program. This finding raises interesting questions about IL residential facilities which house the same population for relatively long periods of time. Providing accessible housing and other supporting services may not be the complete answer to community integration if the pressures of communal living require residents to accept enduring social structures.

Berkeley, California. Lifchez and Winslow (1979) chose the psychosocial interview to probe the individual living styles of severely disabled adults seeking independent living outside of an organized program. The Berkeley community provides a network of referral services to locate housing, attendant care, and related services, resulting in a collection of unique adaptations rather than an organized program of services. The study presents profiles of thirteen informants who explain their individual living styles as arrangements of physical, social, and service components. Each account of the process of putting together adequate support services, accessible housing, and full social networks reemphasizes IL values such as self-determination. Independent living emerges as a continuing process of identifying choices and creating personal solutions.

The field studies summarized above examine implementations of the IL model from the consumer's viewpoint. Each demonstrates how the combination of accessible environments and comprehensive services is interpreted and utilized by disabled persons either at individual initiative or within organized programs. Each contributes to a fuller picture of IL programs by reporting consumers' response to policies and service systems.

Studies of other vulnerable populations show other ways of providing deinstitutionalized services. Specifically, studies of alternative living environments for aging persons and community-based housing for mentally retarded persons have implications for IL research. These programs also provide appropriate environments, supporting services, and community integration for previously segregated populations. Field studies of these settings extend understanding of the consumer experience.

Edgerton and Langness (1978), for example, report success in establishing supportive, enjoyable research relationships among mentally retarded residents of community living facilities. These relationships were productive in revealing residents' daily routines and experiences of managing social roles in the community. Through the use of rather complicated methods including multiple observers, long-term study, mapping, and both audio and video recording, investigators found that retarded persons are capable of more independence and flexibility than sponsors usually assume.

Similar conclusions were reached by Perkinson (1980). In her study of a retirement community, she found that the aged do not necessarily lose accustomed social roles but instead adopt new social patterns more in keeping with the facts of aging. Data from open-ended interviews and existing documents showed that community solidarity assisted the transition from middle-age norms to the norms of age. Shared symbols, ceremonies, and interdependence networks and the common living environment of a retirement community facilitated interpretations of aging as a legitimate process. Aging persons were found highly capable of managing an alternative living setting.

There is an increasing demand for the social sciences to contribute solutions to social problems (Prewitt, 1981). According to Glaser and Strauss (1967, pp. 232-239), systematic ideas generated from observation are especially appropriate to applications that meet social needs. Theories grounded in everyday reality are intelligible to lay persons, can be generalized to ever changing daily situations, and provide a sound basis for prediction. Theories that easily translate into action are of great benefit to anyone trying to solve social problems.

Field studies can determine, for example, whether there are routines in independent living comparable to the colonizing, apathy, rebelling, conversion, or "playing it cool" that inmates develop as responses to institutional authority (Goffman, 1960). Distinct IL lifestyles may also be found within the major IL program types. Furthermore, IL programs themselves may exhibit life cycles that influence consumers' experiences; consumers who enter new IL programs may encounter different opportunities than those who join long-established programs.

That severely disabled persons now live in ordinary neighborhoods where they receive the benefits of accessible environments and reinforcing social services is an unfamiliar social and personal development which raises valid questions of community acceptance, engineering feasibility, and personal adjustment. In order to test whether it is workable in its many social, environmental, and personal ramifications, in-depth and long-term research is needed. Since it is the intent of IL programs to improve the quality of life for severely disabled people, research methods should reflect concern for the consumer experience.

The ultimate contribution of field research will be to show whether or not IL lifestyles produce lives that are as normal as possible for severely disabled persons. Deinstitutionalization policies require thorough evaluation, and the consumer viewpoint should be included in that examination. Better understanding of such normalized living environments will then be generalizable to other programs serving vulnerable populations, such as community-based facilities for mentally retarded persons, alternative living programs for aging individuals, and transitional housing programs for mentally ill persons. The theories and policies that have opened institution doors affect individual lives just as much as funding procedures and legal processes do, and deserve equivalent examination.

17

Organizing
Disabled People
for Political Action

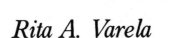

Rita A. Varela

The disability rights movement has been largely ignored by social scientists. Most disability research deals with medicine, physical rehabilitation, special education, and behavior modification. Most research portrays disabled persons as clients. An exception to this was a project begun in 1977 by the American Coalition of Citizens with Disabilities (ACCD), a three-year study of consumer involvement in rehabilitation. As coordinator of the project, I enjoyed a unique opportunity to study the disability rights movement from the vantage point both of its leaders and of the rehabilitation officials who were often its target.

Title I of the Rehabilitation Act of 1973 requires state rehabilitation agencies to solicit and respond to the views of the people they serve. ACCD applied for and was awarded a grant from the Rehabilitation Services Administration (RSA) to study how various states were carrying out this mandate and how consumer involvement policies could be improved.

A frequent complaint of rehabilitation professionals has been that there are too many disabled leaders and not enough consensus among their groups. Some disabled activists, in turn, have argued that professionals use this charge as a smokescreen to avoid responding to criticism. ACCD did not expect to resolve this conflict for all time. Yet ACCD did believe there was a need for an in-depth examination of factors promoting and inhibiting cooperation among disability groups. Studying state coalition building, therefore, was one of the goals of the project.

After the grant was awarded and information about the project was sent to each state rehabilitation agency, four agencies volunteered to participate in the study: Massachusetts, Michigan, New Jersey, and Virginia. Each assigned an agency official to work with us and serve as liaison between our project and the director of the agency. We began by reviewing the consumer involvement plans of each state. We also interviewed state officials, attended meetings of the consumer advisory committees established by the state agencies, and interviewed consumers who served on the committees. Many of the disabled people on these committees were active in disability rights groups. Some had been vocal critics of agency policies and were named to the committees precisely because they were well known in the disabled community. Because public policy and pressure-group politics often intertwine, we realized from the outset that in order to understand consumer involvement, we had to look not only at what the agencies were doing but at what was going on within the disabled community itself.

Because the project spanned three years, we were able not only to explore advocacy issues as they emerged but to carry out follow-up investigations once passions had cooled. The results and recommendations from the project have been reported in several publications. We developed, for example, a Model State Plan for Consumer Involvement in Rehabilitation (Varela, 1980b), which offered guidelines on how to select consumer advisors, how to write a state plan, and how to facilitate better communication between organizations throughout the state.

Yet, important as how-to guidelines are to any consumer

movement, we knew that our project had achieved another landmark as well. We had retrieved a missing page in the history of the American social reform movement in the sense that we had undoubtedly kept better records on the four-state project than most disabled activists keep on their own efforts (Varela, 1979, 1980a). Through the project we had collected material on the organizing activities of disability rights leaders at the state and local levels. These activists had contributed so much to the dynamism and drama of the project that we wanted to give them the last word; and we did. In 1980, the final year of the project, we held an evaluation conference attended by many of those who had participated in the project. We brought over sixty activists to Cherry Hill, New Jersey, and, during training sessions and lectures, eavesdropped as they talked about their work. Their deliberations, objective correlatives of the research data we had been gathering, are reported in the following pages.

We begin with a look at what had been happening in each state during the three-year project.

Coalition: The View from the States

Massachusetts. Massachusetts, a pioneer in many areas, was the first state to establish a coalition of organizations run by disabled people. Leaders of that group, the Massachusetts Council of Organizations of the Handicapped (MCOH), helped to establish ACCD in the early 1970s. By 1978, however, activists were charging that MCOH was losing both membership and political clout.

These critics began organizing a new group, to be called the Massachusetts Coalition of Citizens with Disabilities (MCCD). The challenge infuriated some MCOH people and won the endorsement of others. The dissidents' first major controversy involved the issue of membership criteria. Was MCCD to be an organization of organizations, with each member group electing representatives to the new coalition? If so, how should voting powers be allocated between local groups and local chapters of statewide organizations? Would individual disabled activists not affiliated with any organization also have a vote? If individual membership was allowed, what was to stop members of a single group from demanding the right to vote as individuals?

MCOH leaders felt that only a coalition of organizations (such as MCOH) could fairly represent all groups. MCCD leaders felt that the MCOH idea worked on paper but not in fact. The conflict was settled through a truce, not a compromise. MCCD's by-laws designated MCCD as a coalition of individuals, and its leaders formally recognized MCOH as an organization of organizations.

Underlying these controversies was a rivalry between MCOH and MCCD over style. MCCD people saw themselves as younger and more radical, while MCOH people saw themselves as keepers of a political tradition that worked the political game from the inside. The rivalry mattered because both factions were large and included the most committed disability rights activists in Massachusetts.

Michigan. Coalitions are not a new idea in Michigan. Between 1970 and 1978, most legislative objectives were achieved through ad hoc coalitions of consumers, service providers, and public officials. However, these coalitions disbanded after each battle.

On a wintry afternoon in March 1978, I traveled to the Handicapped Affairs Center in Lansing, Michigan, for a meeting of movement leaders and agency officials. This center, like many others, offers peer support services, a meeting place, and a place from which to organize. During the meeting, there was a long discussion of coalition building. But group leaders did not want just a definition. If they were going to form a coalition, they wanted to know who would head it, who would be in charge of public relations, who would set the agenda for meetings, and what would happen if a member organization disagreed with the majority view on a particular issue. The people in that room had overcome many obstacles and had attained recognition and respect among their peers by becoming leaders of disability rights groups. Not all were willing to give up prominent positions in established, though small, organizations for the prospect of a statewide coalition, particularly since Michigan coalitions had been tried before. At the same time, participants did feel a need for better communication and cooperation among disability groups. There was a strong consensus on one point: They were not comfortable with the term *coalition building*. Michigan activists preferred the term *networking*.

At the close of the meeting, the group elected a steering committee to design a mechanism that would enable activists throughout Michigan to learn what other activists were doing. The work of the steering committee, announced and discussed at a series of meetings following the one in March, led to the formation of an organization called Michigan PEOPLE (People Educating Other People for Lifestyle Equity). PEOPLE's principal objective was to exchange information.

New Jersey. When the study began, virtually the first group we contacted was New Jersey's Disabled in Action (DIA). DIA, with chapters in New York, New Jersey, Pennsylvania, and other states, was synonymous with militancy in disability rights advocacy. Interviews with DIA leaders and attendance at DIA meetings gave us an intimate view of grassroots activism. That view formed the basis of the hypothetical group meeting described in Chapter Two of *Self-Help Groups in Rehabilitation* (Varela, 1979).

New Jersey's DIA mirrored the disabled community. Its members included lawyers, teachers, psychologists, office workers, and too many friends who were unemployed. Its leaders knew their strengths and were proud of them. DIA people cared about one another and had very strong, supportive bonds. Theirs was an organization with a track record and a reputation for being able to mobilize large numbers of disabled people when key issues were at stake. They also knew their weaknesses. Since most had been together a long time and knew one another's flaws, DIA had a "play it safe" management style in which a handful of people did most of the work. Far more time and energy were devoted to the needs of current members than, say, to recruiting within other groups or expanding the financial base of the organization. Our interview with DIA leaders was a major factor leading to our decision to hold a consumer involvement conference in each of the four states during the second year of the project. Preconference outreach, phone calls, and mailings became the focal point of the second year as we sought to demonstrate the importance of making direct contact with all the individuals and interest groups (professional and voluntary) who make up the disabled community.

Participants in New Jersey's consumer involvement conference established a committee to form a statewide organization, the New Jersey Coalition of Citizens with Disabilities (NJCCD). Some on the committee were DIA members, others represented various disability associations, and still others were new to the movement.

NJCCD's structure falls somewhere between that of a tightly knit organization and that of a loose network of activists. NJCCD maintains an active recruitment and public awareness campaign, has applied for several grants, and sponsors statewide conferences and board meetings. Yet a number of its leaders also head long-established, community-based organizations (some of which are, increasingly, providing independent living and peer support services).

Virginia. Disabled leaders have worked hard to build Handicaps Unlimited of Virginia (HUVA) into a powerful statewide umbrella organization of disability-related groups. Yet they place equal emphasis on strengthening local member groups.

The statewide organization began with the alliance of three self-advocacy groups: Mobility on Wheels; the Association of Handicapped Persons in the Tri-City Area; and Handicaps Unlimited of the Peninsula. Forging the alliance was not simple, involving, for example, controversies over where to hold meetings and what to name the organization. Strategic disputes also ied. One camp felt that the best way to serve disabled people was to direct all energy to the top, that is, toward swaying public officials. Although the other camp agreed that disabled leaders must serve on councils and task forces, they were equally concerned for the viability and competence of grassroots groups.

This second camp became HUVA's organizing vanguard. Its leaders travelled across the state speaking before small groups and established agencies alike. They tried to stay in contact with all these organizations, even those that did not join

HUVA, and to help them raise funds or resolve local problems. As a result, local leaders came not only to rely on HUVA people but also to see themselves as HUVA people.

This emphasis on strengthening each link in the chain continues. When HUVA talks about itself it often talks about money—about getting grants, large and small, and about helping local groups. HUVA has received various grants, including, most significantly, one from Virginia's Department of Rehabilitative Services to operate an independent living center.

Conference: The View from Cherry Hill

The differences that emerged among the states are as fascinating as the similarities. The Massachusetts experience draws attention to an issue which recurs often but which few people discuss openly; namely, what is the difference between a coalition and an organization? Michigan's activists raised a similar question; namely, what is the difference between an organization and groups of people working toward kindred goals? In New Jersey the issue emerged as the old guard versus the new. Subsumed in this issue is the problem of outreach: What is the best method of developing a new leadership class? In Virginia, HUVA's objectives were similar to those of NJCCD; namely, leadership training and encouragement of members at the grassroots level.

These issues emerged repeatedly, at times dramatically, when over 60 leaders from the four states were billeted in Cherry Hill, New Jersey, for two and a half days of workshops on constituency building.

At the conferences that had been held in each state, we had asked conferees to designate a consumer to serve as a liaison to the project. Thus, in each state we had an agency liaison, appointed by the director of the state rehabilitation agency, and a consumer liaison, elected by disabled people. In planning the Cherry Hill conference, which was to serve as the hallmark of the third and final year of the project, we convened an advisory group consisting of the consumer and agency liaisons from all four states. They knew beforehand that they would be not only setting the agenda but selecting the participants who would be invited to Cherry Hill.

At the advisory meeting these leaders talked about mobilizing disabled people, lobbying, and providing leadership training to local groups. Interestingly, they talked about politics in much the same way as Max Weber had when he addressed students at the University of Munich in 1918: "Politics ... means striving to share power or striving to influence the distribution of power, either among [nation] states or among groups within a [nation] state. ... When a question is said to be a 'political' question, when a cabinet minister or an official is said be a 'political' official, or when a decision is said to be 'politically' determined, what is always meant is that interests in the distribution, maintenance or transfer of power are decisive for answering the questions and determining the decision or the official's sphere of activity" (Gerth and Mills, 1946, p. 78).

Though committee members shared much of Weber's outlook on politics, they came to the planning meeting with the priorities of practitioners, less interested in defining power than in examining methods for wielding it most effectively. In discussions of grassroots organizing, for example, they worried not only about combating apathy but about keeping mailing lists up to date. Reflecting this dual concern with theory and practice, the conference agenda included sessions on community organizing and management, and one on the Cleveland Amendment, an important congressional battle facing disabled people in 1980.

At the conference, membership emerged as one of the most controversial issues. Why should membership criteria provoke such conflict? As Bill Scott, one of the conferees from New Jersey, told the group, "Membership is the first 'distribution of power' issue facing a new group. Membership criteria dictate who votes and how many votes they get."

The controversy emerges early on, when organizers are trying to recruit allies while preserving their original vision of the group's purpose and structure. Those asked to join will have their own visions; if they are group leaders, they also have their own set of responsibilities. Getting involved in a new group takes a physical and emotional toll. Would-be allies want to know what kind of people they will be dealing with and what the rewards will be.

These early skirmishes illustrate the two main aspects of group life: the personal and the programmatic. Social psychologists hold that groups express two types of human needs. Personal needs include the desire for companionship, recognition, respect, and support. Programmatic needs refer to the goals, tasks, and direction of a group. Group conflicts arise when either personal needs are frustrated or programmatic commitments ignored. So-called personality clashes can be as divisive as ideological ones; often it is difficult to distinguish between them. (See Olmsted, 1959, for an overview of theories of group behavior.)

At the conference, members of one group told us that they had relied on example to help them solve the problem. They reviewed copies of membership criteria used by other groups. Then, at least, the arguments involved words written by people whom they didn't know, and the debates became a bit less personal. This approach took them just so far, however, and then negotiation had to be used to finish the process. Another group decided to appoint a committee and let them fight it out. Although the admission drew some laughter, the conferees knew that setting up a committee is a very traditional way of handling conflict.

Some analysts warn that this strategy can become a form of task avoidance. They offer a number of clues for judging individual cases. For example, are committee members serious enough to meet and, if necessary, continue meeting until they develop a report? If they fail to meet or to develop options, what is the response of the group? *Must* every controversy be settled? Membership criteria are so central to the operation of an organization that viability generally hinges on establishing them. Other controversies, however, may not be. Does the group follow the recommendations of the committee? Does it choose one of the options presented or is the ensuing discussion so heated that the issue is tabled? This situation could indicate either that the issue was sent to committee prematurely, cutting off debate before it should have been, or that the group was not serious about negotiating its way out of that particular deadlock.

Unresolved conflicts can delay or hinder the work for which an organization was created. Ira Resnick, a professional community organizer, warned the conferees, "When you focus on internal stuff you tear each other up. You've got to have an enemy" (Varela, 1980a, p. 31).

What makes people march and struggle? Resnick, who conducted a training session on organizing during the conference, had pinpointed at least part of the answer: precipitating issues. Events, sometimes totally unexpected, sometimes the consequences of ongoing situations, can spark mass action. In his training session, Resnick singled out the assassination of Martin Luther King, Jr., as an example of an incident that sparked riots in various American cities. The conferees found examples of incendiary issues in the history of their own movement as well, most notably the struggle to make former HEW Secretary Joseph Califano sign regulations implementing section 504 of the Rehabilitation Act of 1973. By 1977, over three years after the legislation had become law, the regulations for section 504 remained unsigned and mired in controversy. When ACCD learned that President Carter's administration was being pressured to rewrite and weaken the proposed regulations, ACCD's national office coordinated a series of demonstrations in Washington, D.C., New York, California, and cities throughout the country (Bowe, Jacobi, and Wiseman, 1978).

Sociologist Neil J. Smelser (1962) has studied the factors that must be present in order for a movement to succeed. According to Smelser, incendiary issues—those major events that suddenly seize the attention of the public—constitute only one facet of collective behavior. Social conduciveness is also a key ingredient. Social conduciveness refers to the opportunity for people to interact and to determine what is happening to them. Professional groups such as a union or a trade association allow people with similar interests to exchange views. Black churches in the South have traditionally served as centers of spiritual, social, and political life for people barred from other forums. As Resnick discussed the role of churches in community action,

the conferees could readily draw parallels from their own movement. Social conduciveness was, indeed, an organizational imperative. Many of today's disability rights leader-activists once
belonged to peer groups organized primarily around sports and
recreational activities.

Still, the concept of precipitating factors has a particular
attraction, for it implies that there exist issues that can ignite
even the most passive and oppressed people. This premise
formed the crux of Ira Resnick's presentation at the conference.
Ira Resnick worked as a community organizer for an archdiocese in New Jersey made up primarily of inner-city, multiracial
neighborhoods. Though he had had virtually no contact with
the disability rights movement, he agreed to come to Cherry
Hill and conduct a training session on recruitment. Our planning
committee wanted someone from outside the disability rights
field. They felt conferees should know more about the civil
rights movements of other disenfranchized groups.

Resnick discussed the issue of catalysts at his training session. It was during one of the open forums, however, that the
most dynamic exchange occurred. Conferees had been engaged
in a long debate over membership and organizational structure
when Resnick asked what section 504 was and who the government official responsible for implementing it was. Many people
spoke up, answering his questions with an impressive display of
insider's information. Someone explained that throughout 1979,
the federal Department of Justice had assigned only three or
four people to work full-time on section 504 cases and on cases
involving the rights of handicapped children to public education. Resnick stated that he thought this was an outrage and
went on to inquire how much of a case backlog there was at the
Department of Justice. He was told that there was probably
none, that all of the backlog was at the Office of Civil Rights in
the Education Department. The Office of Civil Rights doesn't
like to give up its cases, it was explained, and so it never refers
them to the Department of Justice. Yet only the Department of
Justice has the authority to prosecute such cases.

Here, said Resnick, was the information he had been
missing. He charged that the conferees were too intellectual. He

said that throughout the weekend, all anyone seemed to talk about was legislation and court cases—matters that people in blue-collar neighborhoods of New Jersey were not likely to get excited about. Resnick insisted that issues had to be personalized. He pointed out that people who wouldn't blink an eye over volumes of statistics would rise up in arms over "a story about one bureaucrat in Washington keeping disabled people from getting a fair deal" (Varela, 1980a, p. 32).

Resnick contended that one of the main jobs of a community organizer was to present problems, statistics, and abstract injustice in terms of the precipitating factors that make people fight city hall. Ethan Ellis of New Jersey remarked on the liveliness of the discussion. He told Resnick: "Last night I disagreed with you about the importance of personalizing issues, but you proved your point today. Once we started talking about the Justice Department we stopped arguing among ourselves about organizational structure" (Varela, 1980a, p. 33).

During one of the dinner breaks, Barbara Oswald of Massachusetts gave another example of personalizing an issue. She discussed a case in Seattle, where she had once worked as a community organizer. The city had ordered that a certain building be torn down. Under pressure from local activists, officials promised that debris from the building would be either hauled away or broken into pieces no larger than two feet by three feet so that mobility-impaired people would not face new barriers. However, the construction crew routinely ignored the agreement and the city ignored the resulting complaints. Finally, activists hired a truck and loaded it with a half-ton slab from the construction site. They painted the inscription "two feet by three feet" on the slab and delivered it to the mayor, who then apologized to the group and took appropriate steps to fulfill his pledge.

It is possible to overemphasize the importance of precipitating factors; after all, they are just one facet of collective behavior. As John Chappell of Virginia put it: "What happens in between the big battles? Sure, everybody likes to get involved in the glamorous stuff, but after a bill is signed or a court case is won you have to have people around to watch what's going on and let others know if their rights are in jeopardy" (Varela, 1980a, p. 34). This was the problem examined in our lab session on the Cleveland Amendment.

Section 504 of the Rehabilitation Act of 1973 states that no otherwise qualified disabled person can, solely by virtue of his or her handicap, be denied the services or benefits of any program or agency that uses federal funds. Every law has loopholes; however, in simplest form, section 504 says that if someone is getting federal money for doing something, handicapped people must have the same sort of relationship to that activity as nonhandicapped people do. If that someone is a hospital, disabled people should be able to get into the building. If it is a fire department, a deaf homeowner should have some way of getting help in case of fire; either the fire department or the police department should have a TTY and be trained to receive and respond to calls from deaf citizens.

Although the law was enacted in 1973, disability rights groups had to wage a four-year struggle to persuade the Secretary of HEW to sign the regulations implementing the law. Regulations describe how the government expects a law to be followed and what exceptions, if any, will be allowed. The regulatory process is often long and arduous. It begins when a government agency publishes proposed regulations in the *Federal Register,* followed by a period of thirty to ninety days during which the public may comment. Sometimes the government also schedules public hearings in major cities as an added vehicle for public comment. Serious compliance efforts rarely get underway until this process is completed.

Disabled people were not the only ones who felt strongly about the regulations that would implement section 504. Had they been, there would have been no delay and no controversy —because there would have been no countervailing political forces to exert pressure on the Secretary of HEW.

The civil rights guarantees of section 504 affected a very wide range of activities, programs, and vested interests, resulting in a struggle that had to be waged on many fronts. The battle pitted the disability rights movement, largely an ill-financed, volunteer army, against lobbyists from General Motors and the transportation industry. Armed with volumes of industry-financed cost studies, the transportation industry mounted an aggressive, heavily financed campaign against section 504 in the courts, in Congress, and in the press. Seizing on the public's anti-Washington mood, they portrayed the issue as a confrontation between distant federal bureaucrats and oppressed local officials and steadfastly denied that they were trying to block policies designed to meet the transportation needs of disabled and elderly people (Cannon and Rainbow, 1980).

In 1980, several congressmen introduced legislation that threatened to weaken section 504. The early version of one of these bills (the so-called Cleveland Amendment), introduced by Representative James C. Cleveland (R.-N.H.) would have given local authorities so much discretion in responding to the transportation problems of disabled people that section 504 might well have become meaningless. The Cleveland Amendment was introduced without much fanfare. In fact, it was sneaked into the hopper. As disability organizations such as ACCD, the Paralyzed Veterans of America, and Berkeley's Center for Independent Living began hearing about the amendment, their first strategy was to delay consideration of the bill and alert other movement groups as quickly as possible. ACCD distributed press releases and fact sheets throughout the country. But printed material cannot equal dialogue as an organizing tool. Most of the organizing went on by phone. Local activists are always busy trying to keep promises they've already made, and they cannot be ordered to set their priorities aside. They must be persuaded.

At our lab session on the Cleveland Amendment, Peter Myette discussed the struggle from the vantage point of an ACCD staff person assigned to section 504 issues, and Steve Janick of New Jersey discussed it from the perspective of an activist at the state level. Steve Janick's first reaction to the Cleveland Amendment was an interesting one. After he started hearing rumors and found he couldn't get information quickly enough, he realized that whatever was going on was tremendously important. Janick did not consider himself a state leader at the time (although others do now), yet he seemed to be at the center of the year's most critical disability rights issue. What placed him at the center of the action was time and a telephone.

Janick had been working with the group that was organizing the New Jersey Coalition of Citizens with Disabilities. When he began hearing about the Cleveland Amendment, he didn't want to be the only one with that kind of information and he called other leaders in New Jersey. They asked him to keep on it and keep them informed. The more information he received, the more he had to process and pass on, and the more time he took away from the issues he had been dealing with previously. Janick was the man who reported at small meetings, Janick was the man with the most information, and Janick, therefore, was the man in New Jersey most closely identified with transportation. As a result, Janick was the man people looked to when the time came to decide whether to ratify the compromises hammered out in the long, divisive battle.

The disability rights movement is a microcosm of political life. The themes that surfaced at the Cherry Hill conference have been with us for hundreds of years. Conferees talked about personality clashes, but they also talked about bonds strong enough to overcome transportation barriers, public neglect, and political ghettoization. They talked about the need to personalize issues together with the need to understand them: Not everything can be won on a picket line. They talked about how the success of a group depends not just on fervor but on the ability to write newsletters, keep mailings lists, find a bookkeeper, and help coordinate transportation so homebound people can get to meetings. In fact, over the three years of the project we noticed an increasing interest in peer support and in the management skills that are needed when a self-advocacy group that began in someone's living room becomes a self-help organization with an office, a staff, and clients.

Affection, belief, and the technical aspect of organizational life were what we talked about at Cherry Hill—very old issues indeed. These themes fascinated Max Weber as well. His work brims with illustrations from every age and culture—a symphony of the mind that did not always follow the rules set by today's behavioralists. He spoke about the loyalty of peasants for a prophet; the role of ideology in history; and the importance of administrative control and regularity to pharaohs, to kings, and to party bosses. Affection, belief, the technical aspect of organizational life. The Four-State people understood politics better than they know.

18

The Future
of Independent Living

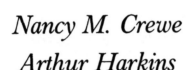

Nancy M. Crewe
Arthur Harkins

The Independent Living Movement is so new that most of its history has been written in the brief span of a decade. With roots in the civil rights, deinstitutionalization, and consumer movements of the 1960s and 1970s, it has grown to become a significant force in opening new opportunities to severely disabled citizens.

Some of its achievements have been tangible, for example, the removal of architectural barriers in many public buildings; the development of accessible transportation systems in a few cities; the construction of accessible housing; and the creation of some reimbursement mechanisms for attendant care services.

Other achievements involve changes in the consciousness of both disabled and able-bodied people. Coalitions have sprung up to press for support services and an end to discrimination, and disabled individuals have become more visible on the streets and in the media.

What might the future hold for this movement, which has accomplished so much in a few short years? The purpose of this chapter is not to make predictions but rather to examine possibilities. The goals of the IL movement, as described earlier in this book, are likely to endure. Control over decisions about one's life and freedom to participate fully in the community have been and will continue to be the essence of IL. What may change is the speed of progress toward those goals and the methods available to achieve them.

Given the importance of public financial support for IL services, it is tempting to view the future of IL primarily in terms of legislation and appropriations. Within that framework, however, events in the early 1980s would point to a rather dismal prediction. The promise of the 1978 Amendments to the Rehabilitation Act and subsequent funding authorizations seems vitiated by miniscule appropriations and the larger problems of a troubled economy.

Nevertheless, a broader perspective requires us to go beyond the question of how present IL services will continue to be provided and explore how the society as a whole is likely to change during the next twenty years and what implications those changes will have for independent living.

In a strict sense, none of us living today in Western society is entirely independent. We receive continual help from other people, from machines, and from systems. The simple fact of wearing clothing, for example, involves the manufacture of fabric, thread, buttons, and zippers; design and assembly of garments; merchandising of either fabric or completed garments; and selection and maintenance by the user. Some people need help with all these tasks, and others need help with only some of them, but everyone has a place somewhere on the continuum between complete dependence and complete independence.

A small and declining number of people make their own clothes, and those who are incapable of doing so are not thought to lack independence. Most people do dress themselves, however, and so the inability to perform this task becomes an IL issue. In the near future, technological innovations are likely to change the way most tasks are carried out—both those that are currently considered relevant to IL and those that are not. The future of independent living cannot be separated from the future of daily living for all.

Toffler (1980) has described the myriad of societal changes that are occurring as we shift from a "second wave" industrial society to a "third wave" technological civilization. Although the transformation began twenty or more years ago, our present hospitals, schools, and corporations are still relics of the earlier age. By and large, so is IL as it is presently envisioned. Despite the development of technology described in this book, our conception of IL is fairly primitive. With regard to transportation, for example, IL still means using automobiles with hand controls, buses with lifts, or other vehicles to move the disabled person. In the realm of attendant care, it primarily means making funding available so that a disabled individual has the resources to hire another person to bathe, dress, feed, and toilet him or her.

To date, the IL movement has mainly focused on the removal of physical barriers, the person-to-person transmission of information and support, the provision of human assistance with personal care tasks, and assistance from dumb (that is, not self-programmable) devices or information systems. Most of these services are labor-intensive and, consequently, expensive. At best, they only permit the disabled person to approximate the efficiency of an able-bodied person.

Within a very few years, however, we may come to see great differences in the kinds of IL services that are available and in the ways in which they will be provided. The basis for this expectation is the accelerating rate at which knowledge is increasing. At the beginning of human history, knowledge doubled only with the passage of millennia. Later, the interval was reduced to hundreds of years, and now it is about three to five years. Before the end of the century, it is conceivable that knowledge will be doubling in a matter of weeks.

The prospect of such rapid change is anticipated with feelings that are best described as mixed. Our cultural myths reveal a pervasive mistrust of technology and of robots in particular. Dr. Frankenstein's wonderful creation became a monster, as did Hal, the computer, in *2001: A Space Odyssey.*

Despite our reservations, however, we are rushing into development of a remarkable new field that promises to demolish the present limitations on our capabilities and blur our definition of the boundaries between human and machine. That field is ethnotronics, the science and technology of developing inorganic electronic devices that have interactive cultural capabilities shared both with people and with other systems.

Until recently, there has been little basis for disputing the assertion that people alone are the builders, carriers, and transmitters of human culture. No comparable process has been documented on other planets, and although some animals have been found to possess forms of culture, these are so primitive in comparison to human standards that qualitatively they fall into a separate category.

Machines have been created to carry out many tasks, from the brute labor of a bulldozer to the dazzling calculations of a mainframe computer. With a few, very recent exceptions, however, they have been able to perform only the specific functions that they were designed to perform. Furthermore, they are unable to learn new skills as they gain experience. They simply continue to carry on their prescribed functions until they wear out. So important is this inability that even the most complex computers have been described as stupid because they are utterly unable to do anything that they were not precisely programmed to do.

Recent laboratory and commercial work has led to the development of a number of low-complexity, non-biological systems that possess the capacity to receive programmed cultural information and selectively act on it, learning new material as they function. Although these ethnotronic devices are still at very early stages of evolution, they have already had significant impact on people, and throughout the 1980s their influence will grow exponentially. Systems are already being marketed that allow ordinary people to carry with them low-cost data and information appliances in the form of calculators, language translators, timepieces, memory devices, music synthesizers, and electronic games. Larger systems are also becoming available; these include home microcomputers, programmable ovens and television recorders, and "convivial" intruder alert and discouragement systems. (Convivial devices are able to interact with people in ways that are helpful or enjoyable, unlike ordinary devices, which are simply acted on. A convivial intruder alert system will "recognize" the occupants of the home, perhaps even greet them as they enter, but will bar others and call the police if they force entry.) Automobiles are also becoming ethnotronic systems as they are designed to have greater self-diagnosis and fail-safe capability. Convivial, accident-avoiding cars may not be far off.

In the future, appliances or robots will be created with more and more human capabilities, including seeing, hearing, learning, and communicating. They will respond to people and will also be able to initiate conversations with the people they serve and with other appliances. Intelligent or purposive ethnotronic systems of the future will allow for the amplification of conviviality beyond the bounds of present imagination, both between and among humans and machines. The task of encoding cultural information into silicon chips and wafers has just begun. At present, silicon chips—the ganglia of present computers and the forerunners of brains in probable future computers—are less capable than human intelligence, but they may equal or exceed human ability in the future. Furthermore, they can stand great acceleration and other stresses better than higher-order biological systems. They weigh less and essentially "live" forever. Humans now share the earth with the early versions of these systems. Whether in the future they are seen as machines, pets, or even members of the family, these and their "children" are part of our evolution.

As machines become more and more like people, human beings will depend increasingly on mechanical implants and prostheses to maintain their health, extend their lives, and amplify their abilities. In such devices, we can already observe the early stages of hybrid ethnobiological or ethnotronic systems.

These technological developments will lead to many societal changes, probably including the following:

- Increased diversity among people, resulting from more individualized education and media
- Easier access to all kinds of information
- Decreased routine and physical labor
- Shift from reliance on mass production of goods to the availability of custom-made goods
- Improved communication, resulting in reduced need for physical transportation
- Decreased emphasis on large buildings and institutions, with proportionately greater reliance on the home as the place for education and work.

Each of these trends, directly and indirectly, will influence the future of independent living. Their impact will become apparent as we consider each of the major areas of IL service. The IL systems presently in operation are described elsewhere in this book. Most commonly, people who want assistance go to an IL center, program, or agency where a counselor helps them find the information or services needed. If future consumers are able to establish satisfactory communication through video screens and obtain up-to-the-minute information from their home computer systems, the need for physical centers could be much reduced. The following sections speculate about the kinds of services these future consumers may be able to receive.

Information and Referral

The provision of information is clearly relevant to the ṭ.echnological revolution discussed above. Technology for computerized information and referral systems is already available; all that is still needed is the development of appropriate software to match the distribution of hardware.

Both the independent living center and the home computer terminal of the future should be equipped with an up-to-date memory bank of information about matters of concern to disabled people. Information about eligibility for various benefit programs, for example, would allow a printer to produce an application form on the spot. Better yet would be an interactive capability that would allow the person to apply directly through the terminal and receive immediate information about the disposition of the request.

Other types of information that could be offered to a disabled consumer include:

- Video catalogues of adaptive equipment, cross-referenced by function and manufacturer, together with consumer ratings of quality, cost, and specific indications and contraindications for use.
- Information about organizations, service providers, and meetings.
- Accessibility information about public buildings in the community.
- Information about college, university, and community education classes, including location, prerequisites, and costs.
- Information about existing and pending legislation relevant to citizens with disabilities.

One stumbling block to the development of such a system has been concern about the cost and labor involved in keeping it complete and up-to-date. One possible solution is represented by the projected increase in occupations involving the manipulation of numbers and symbols. This increase would offer a natural employment opportunity for many disabled people. Another possibility is that disabled people could contribute their time and knowledge to the creation and maintenance of the system in exchange for access to it.

Peer Education and Counseling

The IL movement has emphasized the importance of peer counseling for people who are seeking ways to live in the community. Peers are in an excellent position to provide information, support, and practical assistance. For the purposes of this discussion, the term *peer counselor* will refer to those individuals who are qualified to provide help to disabled consumers primarily because of their own life experiences. They may have had some training, and they may operate under some supervision, but their primary credential is *having been there.* Professional counselors, by contrast, are those who have completed full training and certification; they may or may not be disabled.

Counseling has traditionally been conducted by bringing together a professional helper and a seeking client. The limitations inherent in that arrangement are much the same as those involved with personal appointments for any purpose. Counseling sessions are labor-intensive, are available only at certain times and on a prearranged basis, and involve transportation, usually on the part of the person who is seeking assistance.

Several changes have been apparent during recent years including the growth of group counseling, telephone counseling, and peer counseling. Each of these forms relieves some, but not all, of the problems identified in the traditional model. In the future, substantially different alternatives are likely to become available as supplements to, if not replacements for, traditional counseling.

Both peer and professional counseling and education services could be programmed and made available to consumers through ethnotronic devices whenever and wherever they are needed. Eventually, programs could be written to cover any problem area, and access could be provided in whatever form the person would find most congenial. Voice recognition by computers is in its infancy, but its development will make possible faster and easier interaction, eventually approaching or (for some people) surpassing the ease of face-to-face communication. A telephone, microphone, or video screen representing the counselor might, for example, initiate a conversation with a person who had been sleeping an excessive number of hours or who had not been going out of the house, inquiring about the reasons for the behavior.

To allow the person being counseled relatively unrestricted choice of responses, programming would have to take a different form than the familiar linear or branched programs. A simulation approach would involve incorporating key suppositions and vocabulary into the program, which would be able to act on links between the vocabulary and concepts of the counseling theory and the usual vocabulary of the person.

Simulations have been used by the military, for example, to train pilots. They have also become available for certain kinds of medical training. For example, a mannikin may be diagnosed as having had a heart attack. If the proper care is provided quickly enough, the "patient" recovers. Otherwise, it "survives" for varying periods of time, developing additional symptoms, before expiring.

Counseling programs could be created following the same basic patterns. It might seem that medical treatment would be more amenable to simulation programming because it is easier to determine which actions are correct and which ineffective or harmful. In the realm of counseling, personal values and feelings seem to defy classification as right or wrong. Nevertheless, counselors do rely on problem-solving models that apply regardless of the particular content being considered. If the consumer were to specify his or her particular goals, it would not be an overwhelming task to write a program that would guide the person toward achievement of the desired goal.

A more difficult (and perhaps impossible) task is to simulate the relationship that develops between two human beings engaged in the counseling process. Carl Rogers (1961) and many others consider the relationship to be the critical factor that frees clients to change and grow. In the future we may be able to develop relationships with convivial ethnotronic devices, but what part these ties would play in counseling is an unanswerable question. Ethnotronic counseling may more closely resemble self-care than counseling. If so, its development would not be inconsistent with the philosophy of independent living.

The simulation process would also have implications for the training of counselors. Rather than learning at the expense of real counselees with problems, novice counselors could develop their listening and communications skills on models that could not be harmed by the process.

It should not be assumed that the advent of computerized counseling will eliminate face-to-face interviews, but even traditional counseling may be delivered in substantially new ways. Counseling via videophone would represent a relatively small change. The interaction would occur as usual between two human beings, but communication would take place through a telephone with a video screen. The individuals could see as well as hear each other, although they might be hundreds or thousands of miles apart. Groups might be established using this mechanism, allowing people with extremely rare conditions to converse with others who had the same problem. Peer support or counseling groups created in this way would allow for greater selectivity in terms of interests, age, disability-related problems, or any relevant characteristic.

Technology may also prove useful to counselors in providing data that would improve their performance during interviews. For example, devices with visual and computing ability might be able to analyze body posture, motion, and other nonverbal information that few counselors are able to pick up. Nonverbal signals comprise a significant portion of human communication, and recognizing them might lead to better understanding of the emotional aspects of problems. The same devices could also analyze the verbal and nonverbal content of the interview, synthesize it, and inform the counselor about topics that might be fruitful to explore. While the counselor would be free to override the suggestions, he or she would still command much more information and many more choices than are now available to any but the most experienced of traditional therapists. Peer counselors with minimal training will thus be able to deal with a wider variety of problems with skill and confidence.

Education and Learning

Although education is not ordinarily thought of as one of the key independent living services, the areas are at least closely related. Many IL consumers are students in colleges or vocational schools, and other potential consumers are still in high school. Learning is a central activity of daily living for all of them. Beyond the sphere of formal education, the more general subject of learning is relevant to everyone.

The future will bring about a shift in the definition and location of education. No longer will it be seen as an activity that happens to young people within formal institutions (schools and universities) but rather as a continual pursuit of people, young and old, who seek answers to their own questions. The greater part of education will take place in the home rather than in classrooms. Clearly, this will entail changes in teaching methods. Shifts in content should be expected as well.

Traditionally, the goal of education has been to load students with the accumulated knowledge of the past in the hope that they will be able to draw on it to solve the problems of the future. Teaching methods reflect this strategy: lectures and reading assignments followed by examinations that emphasize names, dates, and facts.

Moreover, the content of education is taught over and over again, year after year, by hundreds of thousands of elementary, secondary, and college teachers. Whether the content is letters of the alphabet or cultural characteristics of Pacific Island peoples, instructors pour it into the waiting receptacles of their students' minds and then look for it to reappear, virtually unchanged, in response to oral or written test questions.

The statistics on retention are so overwhelmingly negative that the only explanation for the continuance of this approach to education is that no one has created a better alternative. Listeners forget almost 90 percent of what they hear in a lecture within a few hours, and after several days, only about 2 percent of the information remains. Furthermore, the costs are enormous in terms of both time and money. Little opportunity is left for students to raise their own questions and pursue the answers.

Ideally, in the future, those priorities will be reversed. Students will spend most of their time and energy engaging in research and development, and their mastery of basic skills such as reading, writing, and mathematics will emerge as byproducts of the search for knowledge. The emphasis on memory work will be virtually eliminated as computers provide universal and immediate retrieval of information whenever it is needed.

The decreased emphasis on rote learning may also have positive implications for some of the students who currently find school very difficult. Those with learning disabilities or mental retardation may be able to cope with a wider range of material if it is presented using teaching methods that allow almost unlimited opportunity for repetition and reformulation. Students may be able to emphasize input of the kind that best suits them, whether visual, auditory, or tactile, and to choose similar modes to demonstrate their achievements. Some may focus on verbal tasks and others on graphics; individual differences will be more easily accommodated and even encouraged.

The trend toward home-based education and work will reduce problems for students with mobility impairments, who now have difficulty with transportation and architectural barriers. At the same time, it raises the specter of even greater isolation than is currently experienced by many disabled people. This is not a prospect to be dismissed lightly, but some loss of face-to-face contact may be counterbalanced by increased opportunities for multisensory communication with acquaintances around the city and even around the globe.

Housing

Although predictions about housing of the future have been interesting and varied, some of the once-popular scenarios have now faded from sight. For example, few visionaries now await the ascendance of disposable housing and furniture, built to last for a few months or years and then discarded by a hypermobile society. Our awakening to the fact that global resources are limited has made such a practice seem not only economically unsound but even immoral.

Many of these prognostications are strongly at variance with one another. Mason (1978) predicted that by the year 2000, with increasing population density, we will see the development of huge, self-contained structures including residential, service, and commercial facilities. People could literally spend their whole lives inside such a building and never face the necessity of traveling outside. The space shuttle, populated by a busy colony of earthlings, represents an exotic version of this idea. Although the prospect of spending a lifetime within a single megastructure probably sounds less than attractive to people who are used to traveling outdoors every day, this sort of lifestyle would certainly reduce, if not eliminate, many problems for people with severe mobility impairments. Such intense concentration of homes and services would go far toward answering the concerns Phillips raised in his chapter on appropriate location of buildings frequented by the disabled.

However, there are indications that we may be moving away from high-rise buildings and toward more moderately sized and geographically dispersed buildings. Toffler (1980) argued that decentralization will be a feature of the "third wave" society, affecting both residential and commercial architecture. In his chapter on special housing for the disabled, Wiggins provided evidence to support that view. He noted that government subsidies which once encouraged the construction of large buildings are now available only to support smaller units.

Whatever their size, homes of the future seem destined to become the locus for an increasing proportion of our daily activities. Wired with powerful computing and communications devices, these "electronic cottages" will enable people to work at home rather than commuting daily to large offices. Students, too, will carry out much of their work at home rather than in classrooms. The economic pressures behind these trends are obvious. The costs of land and construction have skyrocketed and may soon become prohibitive for smaller businesses and for services provided by the public sector. Commuting is likewise extremely expensive, both in terms of time and of the costs required to build and fuel vehicles. The development of modern technology increasingly obviates the need to herd people under a single roof for productive activity.

Electronic information and communication systems will also make it possible for people who are ill or disabled to receive care at home, perhaps delivered by a robot that is capable not only of seeing and hearing but also of gently touching, moving, and lifting. Similarly, individuals who have formerly required care in nursing homes or extended-care facilities might more comfortably and economically be kept in their own homes with intermittent or continuous monitoring by family members or service providers.

In addition to comfort, security will be increased in the home of the future. Security has long been a serious concern of people with disabilities. With limited mobility and capacity to defend themselves, they have been frequent targets of assault and robbery. Because of difficulty handling small items such as keys or heavy ones such as doors, their dwellings are often left unlocked. Their vulnerability has been further increased by the need to hire attendants who, when they leave, take with them house keys and intimate knowledge of the dwelling and its occupants.

The technology of the future will make possible radically different, convivial intruder alert systems. Individuals will be fitted with devices that are literally electronic signatures. Buildings will be programmed to give access only to individuals with the correct signatures.

Attendant Care

Attendant care, as DeJong and Wenker showed in their chapter, is probably the central IL service. Prospects for change in this area are therefore extremely important. Elsewhere in this book, Zola argues that because personal care is, by definition, a human function, services provided by machines or animals tend to dehumanize the recipient. In this connection, he notes that psychological rejection may occur when a person is fitted with artificial prostheses or implants. Like most people today, he perceives a sharp line of demarcation between what is human and nonhuman, and predicts that significant problems can be expected if human services are replaced.

The purpose of this chapter, however, has been to show that together with accelerating technological innovations we can anticipate concomitant changes in attitudes towards our creations. As convivial, interactive robots become an indispensable part of households everywhere, they will be recognized increasingly as helpers, companions, and even friends.

Robots are already important contributors to Japanese industry, and they are quickly becoming more numerous in America and elsewhere. Currently, they bear little resemblance to living beings, and they are being used to carry out repetitive tasks, sometimes in hazardous settings. By the early 1990s, they will be more flexible and much more widely available. They will be used in homes to perform disagreeable or time-consuming tasks, such as cleaning. Cameras, lasers, or a sonar system may provide them with vision, and they will be capable of voice input and speech. By the time they reach this stage of development, they will be able to carry out many of the tasks that are presently provided by attendants and housekeepers. However, further advances will be required to produce touch-sensitive automatic arms that would be capable of lifting or moving a person.

At the present time, one of the most difficult problems in IL is how to care for persons with disabilities such as head trauma. Where the primary need is for monitoring and supervision rather than physical care, such help is not reimbursable under the usual medical provisions. As a result, most of these persons live with their parents, in nursing homes, or in homes for the mentally retarded. In some cases, these arrangements are satisfactory, but in other cases they are destructive to the person or to the family and are accepted simply because no alternative can be found.

For many individuals with psychiatric disabilities or with limited intellectual ability, the main barrier to independent living is simply the availability of help with planning, decision making, and appropriate behavior. Sophisticated telecommunications technology will also be useful in monitoring and supervising these people at home. The person whose ability to take initiative is impaired, for example, might use a mechanical tutor to instruct him or her on when to get up, what to wear, what bus to take, and where to be at various times during the day. A small, wearable device could even be programmed to supply appropriate "thoughts" to persons whose own thought processes tended to get them into trouble. For example, it could help to counteract impulsiveness by instructing the person to stop and think, or prevent the escalation of disputes by reminding him or her of calming thoughts and behaviors.

Transportation

Transportation will probably become less essential as an IL service during the coming decades. The reason for this is simply that the movement of light and sound waves will increasingly replace the transport of heavy, bulky cargo such as human bodies. Although travel will not cease, people will be provided with more and better alternatives to transportation. The rising incidence of home-based employment and education will dramatically reduce the amount of daily commuting that is necessary. Over longer distances, satellite teleconferences and person-to-person communication via videophone will become common for both business and other purposes.

The addition of visual output to our usual auditory telephone systems is still fairly rare, but no longer revolutionary. Dramatic changes are in store, however, when five-sense simulations become possible. The transmission of multisensory signals around the globe could make it possible for an individual to experience events thousands of miles away without the investment involved in physical travel. While usable by any person, this option will have special implications for anyone whose physical limitations make travel risky or impossible. Suppose, for example, that one wished to attend the winter Olympics. One could rent a robot on site and connect oneself to it via satellite, receiving sensory information of such diversity and precision that one would enjoy the experience of actually being there. One would be able to control the actions of the robot, directing it to move from place to place or engage in conversation with human beings or other robots. The languages being spoken would present no barriers, as they could be instantly translated.

Great distances are not the only reason that an individual might choose to converse, work, or play through a robot rather than in person. A severely disabled individual, homebound as the result of mobility impairment, restrictive personal care needs, allergies, or disfigurement, might find that the robot provided an avenue for both social intercourse and productive activity.

Assistive Devices and Health

Assistive devices are not new, but their number and variety have always been limited. Elsewhere in this book, Newman, Schatzlein, and Sparks attribute the scarcity of devices primarily to market forces. Products manufactured by traditional processes are profitable only when they can be sold to a mass market. However, because of the idiosyncrasies of individual physiques, impairments, and functions, assistive devices have to be custom-made in many cases. New methods of production should make it possible to produce small-run or custom-made items as profitably as items are mass-produced today. This is because the machinery of production will not have to be replaced when a different item is desired. Instead, it will be modified by computer to produce items according to unique specifications.

Another problem has been the limited dissemination of knowledge about available assistive devices. Creation of an electronic catalogue that will provide up-to-date information about all types of devices will help to reduce costs and improve equipment selection.

Changes in health care will probably be more profound and extensive than changes in any other area discussed in this chapter. Already, publications are filled with accounts of research in the areas of genetic engineering, tissue regeneration, organ replacement, and innovative surgical procedures. Perhaps the time will come when disabilities that are presently accepted as incurable can be cured, when missing or defective parts can be replaced, when a new body can be created to house a functioning central nervous system. Until that time, independent living will remain a subject of critical importance to people with disabilities.

19

Toward Independent Living: Goals and Dilemmas

Irving Kenneth Zola

Every rehabilitation conference I attend has at least one session devoted to consumer involvement. During the 1980s, this issue will require the same level of discussion and implementation as the issue of physical accessibility did during the early 1970s. Then, the emphasis was on passing legislation to assure physical accessibility for the millions who had previously been excluded. It was, of course, but a first step. Since then, this effort has largely been stalled in the name of economic constraints. Like black people before us, however, we have come to realize that the causes of such gradualism go much deeper.

While the old battle goes on, new ones emerge. Currently, we are working through legislative channels to gain access to the decision-making process—in other words, to assure a voice, a role, and more important, a vote in areas where others make decisions about what is best for us. But this legislation can do only so much: the battle will not be over when people with disabilities serve on all the important committees. That will only solve the problem of physical isolation of the disabled from the nondisabled. The conceptual gap will then emerge as of most importance. My task in this chapter is to discuss some of the beliefs, values, and theoretical models that divide the rehabilitation world from its potential clients.

We can start by examining a strongly held American value: our traditional emphasis on independence and self-reliance. Our political leaders need only mention our dependence on foreign energy sources and the public rises in indignation. Similarly, the desire for independence is a hallmark of rehabilitation literature. But I would claim that as unreal as complete independence is in the field of energy, so, too, is it in the life of many a disabled person. The key seems to be *who* defines *what* independence is. In my own life, the issue has most clearly surfaced in regard to wheelchair use. Most people with mobility problems have had to face the increased physical difficulty in doing things that once were easy. In order to use our muscles, we have had to overcome reluctance, fear, and even pain—not to mention the rebellion of arms, legs, and head. And once we had attained certain physical goals—taken those steps, climbed those stairs, scaled that hill—we were told explicitly that we must continue to do those things in order to maintain our strength and independence. This may be true, but let us also look at the consequences of this advice. I was always told to push myself to the maximum of my physical capability. I was never given any advice as to what to do when my capability had reached its limits. In my case, this meant traveling just like everyone else. I would park my car where the others parked and walk the full distance to wherever it was that I wanted to go—even in winter on icy sidewalks. No matter that it took me five times as long to get there, or that I slipped along the way, or that I arrived at my destination cramped and exhausted. The important thing was that I got there under my own steam: physically independent and mainstreamed. But was I really independent? The answer is a resounding "No!" After a while, fewer and fewer people wished to walk at my pace. Thus, either through my embarrassment or through theirs, I eventually went earlier, or alone, or not at all. In the middle period of my life (until my late thirties) this meant that I omitted many activities that required considerable walking or where my slowness impeded the activity. Specifically, I stopped going on tours, visiting museums, or attending large public events. I occasionally mentioned this to my orthopedists and prosthetists. They, in turn, only shook their heads in sad acknowledgment. None of them ever suggested that I use a wheelchair. Only a change in my consciousness permitted this, and then only very reluctantly, and only in the last eight years.

The point is clear: In living in accord with someone else's definition of physical independence, I, for far too long, contributed to the demise of my own social and psychological independence. The dilemma is even more immediate for people who only use wheelchairs, particularly those who are forced to use physical means to propel themselves when electronic means are available. I would argue that there is literally no physical circumstance in which the *increased* physical independence is worth the *decreased* social and psychological independence. In the rare circumstance where physical exercise is essential, I am sure other forms can be discovered. In the rare circumstance when a substitute cannot be found, why not have at least two wheelchairs—one electric and one hand-propelled?

At times, the issue of independence seems to resolve into the question of *who* is to control our dependence. A great fuss is made over dependence on personal care attendants, over letting the client control the money, and over the fact that attendant fees may range from $3 to as high as $10 per hour. In contrast, there seems to be little argument about our costly dependence on kidney dialysis machines. One can only wonder whether this is in any way related to the fact that such dialysis treatments are profitable, medically dominated, and technologically fascinating. Efforts to make us independent of in-clinic dialysis machines are greatly resisted. Thus, attempts at in-home and self-dialysis seem to vary with geographical location rather than physical condition—ranging from under 15 percent in the Northeast to over 50 percent in the Northwest (Kolata, 1980a, 1980b). Indeed, since the introduction of complete insurance coverage, the percentage of patients dialyzing at home has steadily declined from 44 percent in 1972 to 14 percent in 1980 (Bingaman, 1981). The impact of this trend on independent living can be measured by the fact that Kutner and Brogan (1982) report that the more likely individuals are to use in-clinic hemodialysis, the less likely they are to feel in control of their lives. Thus does high-technology medicine pursued in a questionable manner contribute to the greater dependence of those it seeks to help.

The Independent Living Movement crystallized around the issue of independence. We in the movement would argue that independence cannot be measured by the mundane physical tasks we can do but by the personal and economic decisions we make. It is not the quantity of tasks we can perform without assistance that matters but the quality of life we can live with help (DeJong, 1979). To retain the old physicalist criteria of independence only contributes to the very isolation and dependence we seek to avoid.

Assumptions about disability are not always so obvious as in the matter of independence. Sometimes they are buried in more pragmatic matters such as the way rehabilitation programs assess an individual's physical and mental capabilities. That such assessments may be unduly influenced by time and space consideration was illustrated to me by an experience I had when living at Het Dorp.

For those of you unfamiliar with this place, let it suffice to say it is a village in the Netherlands, created specifically to house people with severe physical difficulties. Aside from the medical criteria that residents had to satisfy in order to live there, they were not admitted unless they had no other place to go. This was not a medical center. It was a village, and no rehabilitation was done here. For all intents and purposes, residents of Het Dorp were there because nothing more could be done for them. Yet, not merely did many residents live a more viable existence than otherwise possible, some actually improved sufficiently to leave the village. Some critics have attributed this to a faulty selection policy, but I don't think the matter was so simple. Many residents, uninhibited by external standards and time-tables, were simply able to experiment with new ways of doing things, at no cost to themselves. They were able to fail—and when they did, they could try again. Often, they eventually succeeded. I am not talking about miracles of returned functioning but about improved functioning. One implication of this observation is that many programs not only give up too early in the rehabilitation process but also have no systematic way of assessing long-term progress and capability. In fact, most of us with disabilities are never given a chance to improve, a chance to be reassessed, or even a chance to learn about new devices.

Here again it is easy to be very concrete. For I am an excellent example—a well-educated, well-informed individual, with good health insurance, interested in prevention, enrolled in a health maintenance organization, a staff member of several local hospitals, and a friend and colleague of many physicians. Now let me add these facts. It has been thirty years since my polio and twenty-six since my accident—which together left me with considerable right-side weakness. I thus wear a long leg brace and a back support, I limp, and I use a cane. Now, in the over twenty-five years since my rehabilitation was completed, I have never been called in by any of my orthopedists or prosthetists for a check-up or to discuss new ways I could do things or new devices I could use. I do not mean, of course, that I have not seen these people, but rather that I did so only when something particular went wrong, and then, quite naturally, we all focused on the trouble. Anything new that I do or use today, I learned from friends or journals. I would argue that this kind of haphazard rehabilitation is a dead end in that it consigns me and many like me to the "we have done all we could" category. I am not claiming callousness, but I am claiming that the rehabilitation system is built on certain assumptions that prevent rehabilitation professionals from ever really knowing whether they have done all they can.

The implications of this are, of course, more tragic when children rather than adults are affected. Because children have no other resource, and because they are involved in rehabilitation so early in life, the damage may be permanent. The same effect may occur in a more insidious way when it is a question of mental functioning. For years I have argued about the detrimen-

tal consequences of maintaining a single-minded concept of nor-
mality and development. As a sociologist, I have long been
aware of how time and culture-bound are our ideas of good and
evil. Since then, it has become apparent that this is also true of
the concepts *crazy* and *sane,* and also of *healthy* and *ill* (Zola,
1966, 1972, 1975). More recently, it has taken political developments, such as the civil rights movement, to show that this
was true even of things we thought were genetically determined
biological givens—I refer specifically to IQ. We have come to
realize not only that some of the basic questions on IQ tests are
biased against certain populations but also that the very dimensions traditionally assumed to be the essence of intelligence are
so biased.

Westerners grow up in a setting that demands the acquisition of logical, analytic, and, especially, verbal abilities. As
McBroom has aptly noted: "The minds that blossom in this
environment are highly adept at categorizing the world into
many discrete bits of information and organizing this material
into abstract systems of knowledge. This kind of mind concep-
tualizes, theorizes, and explains, and in so doing it gains a high
level of control over the physical environment. Such abilities
yield high scores on IQ tests" (1980, p. 168). People not committed to the Western and urban style of living generally have
no need to develop the cognitive skills we value so highly. Anyone who does not need these skills will simply not devote much
effort to obtaining them. As a result, it is argued that what is
measured on IQ tests is less genetic factors than cultural prerequisites. One can, of course, argue that to succeed in *our* world,
one needs the appropriate abilities. But *our* world is not the
only world people live in. At the very least, such reasoning
means that a test does *not* measure someone's given, unchanging
ability to succeed in our world; rather, it merely measures the
person's current inability to do so.

John Gleidman has recently claimed that the same disparity in cognitive styles may be seen in the standards by which
handicapped children are assessed. During the 1960s, a professor of psychology at the University of Montreal, Thérèse Govin-
Décarie, studied children born with deformities to mothers who

had taken the drug thalidomide. In particular, she was struck by how little light conventional psychological theories shed on the children's development (Gleidman, 1979). A psychoanalyst, André Lussier, came to quite similar conclusions in his work with a child born with severe limb deformities. He continually found that behavior he "first interpreted as pathological and harmful to the child's development frequently turned out to be an essential ingredient in the child's conquests of his physical limitations. For example, when the child boasted that he could learn to play the trumpet, Lussier interpreted it as un-realistic fantasy—until the boy actually succeeded in doing it. All manner of actions that seemed pathological when assessed by the norms of standard psychoanalytic theory turned out to have a different functional meaning in the disabled child's life" (Gleidman, 1979, p. 101). Such data led Gleidman to the following conclusion:

> Because of the stigmata of disability, for example, handicapped people often move through a different social world from the one the rest of us inhabit; many of them do so in bodies that place important constraints on the way they obtain information about the world around them. Researchers frequently appear to assume that the developmental theories proposed by Piaget and others, elaborated from observations of able-bodied children, will work for the handicapped. But it may be that the cognitive and emotional growth of handicapped children follows its own health logic. A disabled child who is physically dependent may be putting his most sophisticated cognitive skills into learning how to charm, manipulate, or otherwise enlist the help of others; to keep safe from harm; to deal with the split between his social worlds: the home, where he is loved and respected, and the street, where he is viewed as a biological fact. The able-bodied child of the same age may be spending the same energy on working free of his dependence on parents and building his sense of competence by developing skills [p. 99].

In other words, while persons with profound physical difficulties may be deficient in some cognitive abilities, they may also have highly developed and underappreciated abilities of their own. Some of the old truisms about the extraordinary development of other senses in those who are visually or hearing-impaired thus deserve closer examination. Moreover, I suspect that the same phenomenon occurs in other people as well, albeit more subtly.

To use myself again as an example: I have both a highly developed sense of time and an extraordinary analytic ability to break tasks down into their smallest and most common components. I think both of these talents are related to two periods of total confinement of nearly a year apiece (once paralyzed and once in a body cast), during which I became extraordinarily concerned with time and with how to conserve my energy as well as with how to keep myself busy and sane. I am not raising these observations to note the special blessings of being handicapped. I am arguing that as we physically learn to compensate one muscle for another, so too we may well engage in a similar compensatory process both cognitively and psychologically. When we have little enough to be rewarded for, that alone may be reason enough to acknowledge such new traits. More important, such abilities may well be the essential building blocks of the rehabilitated self.

In the context of such global considerations, I want to examine the effect of similar assumptions on the application of rehabilitation technology. An issue of great concern in the design of programs and devices for those with handicaps is safety: the protection of the individual from unnecessary harm. (This entire section owes an intellectual debt to the work of Perlik, 1980.) While the wish to protect vulnerable people from danger is a worthy goal, it is often achieved at too great a cost. Loring Mandel (1971) wrote of this in a play, *Do Not Go Gently into This Good Night*. Melvyn Douglas portrayed a retired cabinetmaker who was placed in a nursing home "for his own good." His breaking point occurred when the staff refused to allow him to use the available woodworking machinery because it was too dangerous. He rebelled; he claimed that he had the right as a human being to run the risk of injuring or losing his finger. Since they disagreed, he quit the home. Most of us are not so fortunate: we do not have the power to quit, and we have no place to go.

This kind of treatment is most commonly given to people

with mental handicaps—those labelled retarded. The norm was set early in this century. I can do little better than let the age speak for itself: "Self-control and independent life are not for mental defectives, either in their own best interests, or in the best interests of the family, the community, and the nation. Common sense forbids it. In the nature of things it cannot be. Mental defectives may be nearly or quite self-supporting; they can never be self-controlling or self-directing except in a childish way, and they can never be the masters of their own fate except at the cost of disaster and ruin to themselves and others —disaster that affects future generations as well as the present generation, and that tends to undermine as far as it goes, the security of the homes and the nation concerned. Mental defectives are permanent children" (MacMurchy, 1917). It took over sixty years to begin to change the attitudes represented in this statement and to question what was social fact and what self-fulfilling prophecy. Though many had speculated about what overprotection might do to such children (see, for example, Levy, 1943), it was not until the early 1970s that empirical study gave form to this fear.

In a study of mildly retarded children, Sharlin and Polansky (1972) reported that the more overprotective and controlling the mother was, the more likely the child was to suffer a decrease in IQ score and to experience poor muscle coordination. In short, many became "permanent children" when they need not have.

There is a body of psychological literature that argues that risk-taking is essential to the growth and development of all individuals (Viscott, 1977). Aaron Wildavsky (1979), the political scientist, has even claimed that it is essential to the growth and development of society itself. When it is absent, society stagnates and dies. Robert Perske summed up the argument well: "The world in which we live is not always safe, secure, and predictable. It does not always say 'please' or 'excuse me.' Every day there is a possibility of being thrown up against a situation where we may have to risk everything, even our lives. This is the REAL world. We must work to develop every human resource within us in order to prepare for these days. To deny any retarded person his fair share of risk experiences is to further cripple him for healthy living" (1972, p. 26).

I recently spent time with a paraplegic who races autos and before that with a quadriplegic who was learning how to ski. These are high-risk sports that I would not have engaged in even before I got polio. With full recognition of the skill and courage involved in auto racing and skiing, I think that another important aspect of these individuals' achievement is putting risk back into their lives. I realize that in my own life, risk defiance takes the form of a continual neglect of seat belts and an almost congenital inability to keep to the fifty-five-mile-an-hour speed limit. So far, the main consequence is that I'm on the way to collecting a speeding ticket in every state in the union.

The real significance of these examples, large and small, seems to be that if society tries to eliminate normal risk from our lives, many of us will go to extreme lengths to reestablish it. An environment or device that prevents any kind of risk produces not a real life but a mirage of one. There is human dignity in risk. There can be dehumanizing indignity in safety.

Technology also can do too much for those of us with disabilities. The machines or devices technology creates may achieve such completeness that they rob us of our integrity by making us feel useless. A prime example of this kind of effect comes from the commercial world. Some years ago, when the convenience food business was in its most expansive phase, manufacturers discovered that where cake mixes were concerned they had gone too far. Early in their marketing, all ingredients were included in a mix. All one needed to do was to add water and stir—the same formula that had worked so successfully with soups. But these mixes met with resistance. Sales faltered. It was discovered that cake-making differed in important ways from soup preparation. Baking had more intimate connotations associated with being fresh and special. Manufacturers quickly altered their strategy. They not only instructed the customer to add fresh eggs, but they also gave hints on how to improve the recipe—how to make it more special, more one's own.

A similar phenomenon occurs among users of prosthetic

devices. I have come across many cases in which disabled persons have invented an addition to their appliance or altered its use to suit their purposes. For years I thought this was merely our way of correcting the faults of our prostheses. But now I think something more is at stake. My own leg brace has not fit properly for the past fifteen years. No matter what is done to it, there is always one place where within twenty-four hours a pressure sore will be produced. However, I have solved this problem by creating a special patch, which I place over the spot every day. I have a certain pride in having solved a problem no one else could. But I have also done something else: I have made the brace more a part of me because I have given it my own unique stamp. I am not arguing that rehabilitation specialists should stop inventing devices that we need, particularly when we ask for them. But I am arguing that, whatever the device, it need not do everything. Moreover, we should encourage ourselves not only to create things that serve us better but to make them more our own.

There are other, more subtle instances in which the use of technology may have gone too far. For example, we have very limited understanding of what happens when bodily parts and functions are replaced by equipment. In the case of transplants and skin grafts, the physiological body often rejects the alien parts. So, too, may the psyche reject those aspects of the self that it feels are alien. No one who thinks of himself as independent wants to use even a cane or crutches. When he does have to, he will often try to avoid it in public or simply get angry, as Barry Goldwater did in his 1980 speech before the Republican National Convention. I, for one, am more subtle—I manage to misplace my cane at least once a day. Moreover, the problems escalate with the degree of dependence on the appliance and its proximity to the user's body. The adjustment may even produce a kind of psychosis when we become *internally* attached to, and thus dependent on, machines—whether through insertion of a pacemaker or attachment to a kidney dialysis machine. A warning note was sounded thirty years ago, when Francis MacGregor (1951) studied the effects of plastic surgery on people with major facial disfigurements. Unprepared for what their new faces would look like, patients experienced profound feelings of distrust, anger, depression, and even suicide, instead of relief and gratitude. I am not, of course, arguing for the elimination of all such mechanical devices but merely arguing that those who use them may be neither as proud nor as grateful as the inventors think they should be. One can only conclude that certain appliances may alter the sense of self so profoundly as to make a life not worth living.

The overtechnicalization of care, exemplified by the invention of robots or the training of chimpanzees to service, dress, and feed quadriplegics, raises similar questions. While it might well be cute when one's favorite pet brings in the newspaper, it is considerably less cute when more intimate tasks are involved. Part of the appeal of machines and animals is that it may be easier to share intimacy with them than with humans. But this short-term gain conceals a long-term loss. I did not accidentally use the term *care* when I introduced this thought. According to the dictionary, care involves "painstaking or watchful attention," "regard coming from desire or esteem," and "a person that is an object of attention, anxiety, or solicitude." My point is a simple one—that care is not merely a technical task. On the contrary, it involves quite personal aspects. To objectify care as a technical service, to replace the human element with a mechanical or an animal one, can only lead to the objectification of the individual receiving that service. It is true that traditional health care for disabled persons has frequently been patronizing or infantilizing. But as bad as such qualities are, they are at least human ones. They reinforce the humanity of the individuals involved. To be handled by a machine or animal, where once I was handled by a person, can only invalidate me.

We must expand the concept of independence to include both physical and intellectual achievements. Independence should take into account not only quantity of physical tasks but also quality of life. Our idea of human integrity must recognize the importance of taking risks. Rehabilitation personnel must change their model of service so that it focuses less on doing something *to* someone and more on planning and creating services *with* someone. In short, unless the rehabilitation world frees itself from some of its culture-bound and time-limited standards and philosophy, we may one day find ourselves in the position of Walt Kelly's Pogo, who once exclaimed: "We have met the enemy and he is us."

Epilogue

Freedom for Disabled People: The Right to Choose

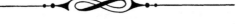

Nancy M. Crewe

What is freedom? Freedom is the right to choose: the right to create for yourself the alternatives of choice. Without the possibility of choice and the exercise of choice a man is not a man but a member, an instrument, a thing.

—Archibald MacLeish

Freedom. The very name of the Independent Living Movement heralds freedom as the central issue. The concept of freedom is older than the Republic and so dear to its heart and mythology that for years many of us believed that freedom had, in fact, been fully achieved. The great civil rights struggles of the sixties shook the country, however, and made the mainstream aware at last that deep and persistent inequities still existed.

Until that point, freedom had been assumed primarily because formal barriers to basic rights had been abolished. The vote was generally available, as were the rights to hold office, own property, worship, attend school, and work. Yet our society was forced to go further and recognize that "separate" facilities were inherently "unequal," and that even an open door to an institution riddled with attitudinal and cultural barriers did not guarantee equal opportunity to benefits.

Likewise, simply announcing that all applicants for jobs, housing, schools, and services would be given identical consideration did not automatically free disadvantaged people to participate equally in society. Equal treatment did not necessarily .n equal opportunity. As Purtilo (1981) pointed out, cert..in other societal changes were necessary before disadvantaged groups would be in a position to utilize the freedom which was presumably already theirs.

For people with disabilities, the need for institutional change as a precursor to freedom is especially clear. No laws forbid people in wheelchairs to ride public buses or to enter public buildings, for example, but the steps at their entrances serve as more effective barricades than laws. That they were built in ignorance rather than malice does nothing to mitigate their effect and may actually make their removal more difficult to accomplish.

Our usual environment and our ordinary policies are accepted by most people as functionally normal. When able-bodied people are made aware of the ways in which the "usual" and the "ordinary" can and do limit citizens with disabilities, the reaction is often surprise and regret, but the onus remains on the disabled person to amend the situation—to request some "special" accommodations.

The Rehabilitation Act of 1973, particularly section 504, came closer than anything before it to admitting societal responsibility for the integration of people with disabilities. It prohibited programs that received federal funding from discriminating on the basis of handicap. Then the 1978 Amendments to the Rehabilitation Act, for the first time, mandated independent living services for people with severe disabilities. The words were clear, and a commitment was made. Even this, however, did not succeed in fully shifting the opportunity for independent living from the category of special favors to that of a right. The proof is the lack of appropriations to implement the programs. Small amounts of seed money have been provided for demonstration IL centers, but support for widespread services has been withheld. Furthermore, the federal government, which has often taken the initiative to impel a more equitable distribution of resources among the populace, is in the process of handing responsibility for many social programs back to state and local governments. Along with that transfer looms the likelihood of weakening in the regulations that are used to implement the Rehabilitation Act.

Today the IL movement appears to stand at a crossroads. In a society that is changing at an ever-accelerating pace, commitments can flash and fade like fireworks on the Fourth of July. Could it be that IL is already an idea whose time has passed? Perhaps vigorous enforcement will be deemed too costly, and in the name of fiscal responsibility and deregulation we will retreat, leaving the rhetoric almost untouched but sucking out most of the wherewithal for action.

It is impossible to deny either the power of economic realities or the consistency with which disabled people have emerged at the bottom of the heap after battles over priorities. But the IL movement has given hope and experience to a cadre of people for whom the issue of independence has become literally a matter of life and death. They cannot and will not resign themselves to incarceration in institutions, however benevolent, yet they cannot exist without adequate housing and attendant care services. For them it is critical that the movement survive. Even for others who could manage to live without it, the IL movement means the difference between a life of emptiness and isolation and one of satisfying involvement with others.

The message of the experience to date is apparent. America means well. We have taken a public stand against discrimination, and we want to believe that a disabled citizen, like anyone else, has access to the American dream. It is in the difficult business of implementing the philosophy that the other lesson emerges: to the extent that freedom calls for social and environmental changes—changes that cost money and directly or indirectly subtract from the resources available to other groups—it will not be offered up to disabled people without a struggle.

In exchange for passivity and quiet endurance, society will voluntarily provide a bit of charity in much the same spirit as food baskets are dispensed to the needy at Thanksgiving. But full equality, with all its consequences, must be desired, claimed, and demanded by disabled people themselves.

It would be naive to assume that all disabled persons even want such freedom. Obtaining and maintaining it involve risks, and like others many disabled people prefer the security of being cared for. Others vainly wish for the delights of both security and freedom without the dangers and inconvenience of either. These people will be of little help in the fight for independent living.

On the other hand, the movement could reach out to encompass millions of others who have a stake in the outcome but who have been involved minimally, if at all, until now. People with hidden and chronic disabilities, those with hearing, visual, and other sensory impairments, individuals with heart disease, cancer, stroke, and other chronic diseases, and that burgeoning population identified as elderly, all grapple with the frustrations of attitudinal and environmental barriers to participation in their communities. However, they may resist identification with the movement because they mentally cling to their former position in the mainstream. Even more, many are loathe to militancy because of almost-repressed feelings of guilt and shame that make them fear that they deserve whatever treatment they may receive. Such is the legacy of generations of discrimination and separation. Nor is the antidote easy to specify. What slogan could do the unifying job of "Black is Beautiful" or "Gay Pride"? People with disabilities are as diverse as the human race, united only by an impairment in some area of functioning and common, though often unacknowledged, social disenfranchisement. For the most part they live with, work with, and love people who are classified as able-bodied. Unity is difficult to establish, and to the extent it has been achieved at all, it has usually occurred within narrower categories such as paraplegia, cerebral palsy, or muscular dystrophy. The majority of disabled

persons are poor and therefore disadvantaged, and such fragmentation ensures that as a group they will remain powerless,
while the rest of the world remains "temporarily able-bodied,"
denying that "*it*"—be it aging, chronic disease, or disability—
will ever happen to them.

Perhaps the pivotal reason that disability has been the last
of the civil rights movements is the extent to which it threatens
the values of the society at large. As a nation we have made
progress in recognizing that prejudice based upon race, creed,
sex, or class is inappropriate, but it still seems justifiable to
judge a person on the basis of what he or she can do. The IL
movement insists on the equality of all people regardless of
their capabilities or limitations. Beauty, health, youth, vigor,
employability, communication, and even the ability to control
one's own body are discarded as criteria for classifying some
people as worthy of independence and others as unfit. IL asks
only about the individual's choice and willingness to accept responsibility for the consequences. Exterior characteristics are
insignificant—only human dignity matters.

The IL movement is fighting an uphill battle. Compared
with the nuclear arms race, the bankruptcy of gigantic corporations, environmental pollution, and unemployment, its plight
commands little public attention. What will be the consequences
if it is defeated by inertia, the budget squeezers, fragmentation,
the aesthetic sensibilities of the beautiful people, or by a refusal
of the powerful to release the underprivileged minority beneath
them? Surely the greatest price will be paid by all the current
and future generations of severely disabled persons whose very
lives depend upon the ability to be free. But who can doubt
that we will all be poorer for having sold our ideals short and
for having cut off the potential contributions of millions of our
fellow Americans. What we do to the disabled today, we will
have done to ourselves for tomorrow.

References

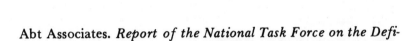

Abt Associates. *Report of the National Task Force on the Definition of Developmental Disabilities.* Cambridge, Mass.: Abt Associates, 1977.

Allport, G. *Becoming.* New Haven, Conn.: Yale University Press, 1955.

American Public Works Association. *American Public Works Association Guidelines for Design and Construction of Curb Ramps for the Physically Handicapped.* Los Angeles: Institute for Municipal Engineering of the American Public Works Association, 1977.

Arkansas Research and Training Center. *Peer Counseling as a Rehabilitation Resource.* Eighth Institute on Rehabilitation Issues, Rehabilitation Research and Training Center, University of Arkansas, 1981.

Arter, E. C., Baugh, C. W., and Elias, J. W. "A Peer Advisory Consumer Program for the Elderly." *The Personnel and Guidance Journal,* 1979, *58,* 106.

Ayers, W. R. "Application of Technology to Handicapping Conditions and for Handicapped Individuals." Washington, D.C.: White House Conference on Handicapped Individuals, 1977.

Babbie, E. R. *The Practice of Social Research.* (2nd ed.) Belmont, California: Wadsworth, 1979.

Back, K. W., and Taylor, R. C. "Self-Help Groups: Tool or Symbol." *Journal of Applied Behavioral Science*, 1976, *12*, 295–306.

Bandura, A. "Behavioral Modification Through Modeling Procedures." In L. Krasner and L. Ullman (Eds.), *Research in Behavior Modification*. New York: Holt, Rinehart and Winston, 1966.

Bank-Mikkelsen, N. E. *Rehabilitation in Denmark*. Copenhagen, Denmark: Government Publication, 1977.

Bank-Mikkelsen, N. E. "Legislative and Administrative Integration of Services for Handicapped People in Denmark." Paper presented at the World Congress of Rehabilitation International, Winnipeg, Canada, 1980.

Beale, C. L. *Rural and Small Town Population Change, 1970–80*. Washington, D.C.: Economics and Statistics Services, U.S. Department of Agriculture, February 1981.

Bell, T. E. *Technologies for the Handicapped and the Aged*. Report prepared for the House Select Committee on Aging and the House Committee on Science and Technology. Washington, D.C.: National Aeronautics and Space Administration, Office of Space and Terrestrial Applications, Technology Transfer Division, 1979.

Betnun, S. *Housing Finance Agencies: A Comparison Between States and H.U.D.* New York: Praeger, 1976.

Bingaman, C. "Reimbursement Policies: A Question of Too Much Profit." *Contemporary Dialysis*, 1981, *2*, 12–13, 21–24.

Blauner, R. "Death and Social Structure." *Psychiatry*, 1966, *29*, 378–394.

Blommestijn, R. J. "Implementation and Administration of Legislation Concerning the Handicapped." Paper presented at the Second International Conference on Legislation Concerning the Disabled, Manila, Philippines, 1978.

Board, M. A., Frieden, L., and Cole, J. *Peer Counseling*. Houston, Tex.: Institute for Rehabilitation and Research, 1982.

Board, M. A., and others. *Independent Living with Attendant Care (A Guide for the Person with a Disability, A Guide for the Personal Care Attendant, A Guide for the Parents of*

Handicapped Youth). Houston, Tex.: Institute for Rehabilitation and Research, 1980.

Bolton, B. "Factor Analysis in Rehabilitation Research: III." *Rehabilitation Counseling Bulletin,* 1978, *22,* 446-462.

Boston Women's Health Book Collective. *Our Bodies, Ourselves.* New York: Simon & Schuster, 1979.

Bowe, F. G. *Handicapping America: Barriers to Disabled People.* New York: Harper and Row, 1978.

Bowe, F. G. *Rehabilitating America.* New York: Harper and Row, 1980.

Bowe, F. G., Jacobi, J. E., and Wiseman, L. D. *Coalition Building.* Washington, D.C.: American Coalition of Citizens with Disabilities, 1978.

Bradley, V. J. "Deinstitutionalization: Social Justice or Political Expedient?" *Amicus,* 1980, *5,* 82-87.

Brattgard, S. O. "Integration in Society." *Handikappforskningen.* [*Research in the Field of Disability*] Sweden: University of Göteberg, 1973.

Brolin, D. E. *Life-Centered Career Education: A Competency-Based Approach.* Reston, Va.: Council for Exceptional Children, 1980.

Brolin, D. E., and Kokaska, C. J. *Career Education for Handicapped Children and Youth.* Columbus, Ohio: Merrill, 1979.

Brooks, N. A., and Hartman, J. J. "The Urban Residential Center: Report of a Sociological Investigation." Unpublished manuscript, Department of Sociology, Wichita State University, 1979.

Brown, B. M. "Second Generation: West Coast." *American Rehabilitation,* 1978, *3,* 23-30.

California State Benefits and Advisory Board. *In-Home Supportive Services.* Sacramento: California State Health and Welfare Agency, 1977.

Campbell, D. T., and Stanley, J. C. *Experimental and Quasi-Experimental Designs for Research.* Chicago: Rand McNally, 1963.

Canada Mortgage and Housing Corporation. *Housing the Handicapped.* Ottawa: Canada Mortgage and Housing Corporation, 1977.

Cannon, D., and Rainbow, F. *Full Mobility: Counting the Costs of the Alternatives.* Washington, D.C.: American Coalition of Citizens with Disabilities, 1980.

Carkhuff, R. R. *The Art of Helping.* Amherst, Mass.: Human Resources Development Press, 1973.

Carnes, G. D. "Social Justice Through Handicapped Power: Perspectives from England and Sweden." Unpublished manuscript, Columbia: University of Missouri, 1981.

Center on Environment for the Handicapped. "Visit to SHAD—Design for Special Needs." *Journal of the Center on Environment for the Handicapped,* 1980, *21.*

Chandler, G. "Peer Counseling." Unpublished correspondence, March 1979.

Chizmadia, G. R. Statement on the 1978 Amendments to the Rehabilitation Act, given at the hearings before the Subcommittee on the Handicapped, Senate Committee on Human Resources, Washington, D.C., March 10 and 14, 1978, 318–359.

Clark, G. M., and White, W. J. *Career Education for the Handicapped: Current Perspectives for Teachers.* Boothwyn, Pa: Educational Resources Center, 1980.

Cleland, M., and Elisburg, D. Statements for the oversight hearing on the Architectural and Transportation Barriers Compliance Board, given before the Subcommittee on Select Education, House Committee on Education and Labor, Washington, D.C., June 31, 1981, 2-22, 88-114.

Cole, J. A. "What's New About Independent Living?" *Archives of Physical Medicine and Rehabilitation,* 1979, *60,* 458-462.

Cole, J. A., and others. *New Options.* Houston, Tex.: Institute for Rehabilitation and Research, 1979a.

Cole, J. A., and others. *New Options Training Manual.* Houston, Tex.: Institute for Rehabilitation and Research, 1979b.

Conrad, P., and Schneider, J. *Deviance and Medicalization: From Badness to Sickness.* St. Louis, Mo.: Mosby, 1980.

Cooper, C. "House as Symbol of Self." In J. Lang, and others (Eds.), *Design for Human Behavior: Architecture and the Behavioral Sciences.* Stroudsburg, Pa: Dowden, Hutchinson and Ross, 1974.

Corcoran, P. *Annual Progress Report. Medical Rehabilitation Research and Training Center.* Boston: Tufts-New England Medical Center, 1978, 60-70.

Corcoran, P., Bartels, E., and McHugh, R. *The BCIL Report.* Boston: Rehabilitation Institute, Tufts-New England Medical Center, 1977.

Corn, R. *Aiding Adjustment to Physical Limitation: A Handbook for Peer Counselors.* Columbia, Md.: Howard Community College, 1977.

Council for Exceptional Children. "Full Educational Opportunities for Handicapped Individuals." Washington, D.C.: White House Conference on Handicapped Individuals, 1977.

Counts, R. *Independent Living Rehabilitation for Severely Handicapped People.* Washington, D.C.: The Urban Institute, 1978.

Crewe, N. M., and Athelstan, G. T. *Functional Assessment Inventory.* Minneapolis: Department of Physical Medicine and Rehabilitation, University of Minnesota, 1978.

Crosby, T. "Mass Transportation's Emotional Blockbuster." *Washington Star,* September 14, 1978, A1.

DeJong, G. *Need for Personal Care Services by Severely Physically Disabled Citizens of Massachusetts.* Personal Care and Disability Study, Report No. 1. Waltham, Mass.: Levinson Policy Institute of Brandeis University, 1977a.

DeJong, G. *Meeting the Personal Care Needs of Severely Disabled Citizens in Massachusetts.* Personal Care and Disability Study, Report No. 2. Waltham, Mass.: Levinson Policy Institute of Brandeis University, 1977b.

DeJong, G. "Independent Living: From Social Movement to Analytic Paradigm." *Archives of Physical Medicine and Rehabilitation,* 1979, *60,* 435-446.

DeJong, G. "The Historical and Current Reality of Independent Living: Implications for Administrative Planning." *Proceedings of the Policy Planning and Development in Independent Living.* East Lansing: University Center for International Rehabilitation, Michigan State University, 1980.

Dembo, T. "The Utilization of Psychological Knowledge in Rehabilitation." In J. Stubbins (Ed.), *Social and Psychological*

Aspects of Disability: A Handbook for Practitioners. Baltimore: University Park Press, 1977, 13–23.

Doyle, P. B. "The Role of Vocational Rehabilitation in Independent Living." Report presented to the Fifth Institute on
Rehabilitation Issues, Omaha, Nebr., May 23–25, 1978.

Dubos, R. *The Mirage of Health.* Garden City, N.Y.: Anchor,
1961.

Durman, E. C. "The Role of Self-Help in Service Provision."
Journal of Applied Behavioral Science, 1976, *12,* 433–443.

Dybwad, G. *Is Normalization a Feasible Principle of Rehabilitation? Models of Service for the Multihandicapped Adult.* New
York: United Cerebral Palsy of New York City, 1973.

Dyssegaard, B. *Role of Special Education in an Overall Rehabilitation Program.* New York: World Rehabilitation Fund,
1981.

Edgerton, R. B., and Langness, L. L. "Observing Mentally Retarded Persons in Community Settings: An Anthropological
Perspective." In G. P. Sackett (Ed.), *Observing Behavior, Theory and Applications in Mental Retardation.* Vol. 1. Baltimore: University Park Press, 1978, 335–348.

Egan, G. *The Skilled Helper: A Model for Systematic Helping
and Interpersonal Relating.* Monterey, Calif.: Brooks/Cole,
1975.

Eggert, G. "Postrehabilitation Experience of a Population of
Spinal Cord Injured Veterans." Unpublished doctoral dissertation, Florence Heller Graduate School for Advanced Studies
in Social Welfare, Brandeis University, 1973.

Erikson, E. H. *Insight and Responsibility.* New York: Norton,
1964.

Ettarp, L. *Vocational Rehabilitation During a Recession.* Stockholm, Sweden: Ministry of Labour Report, 1980.

Falta, P. "Freedom to Live and 'Integrated Living' in Action."
Habitat, 1975, *8,* 26–32.

Falta, P. "Integration in the Community—Community and Residential Housing in Canada." Paper presented at the World
Congress of Rehabilitation International, Winnipeg, Canada,
1980.

Fichter, J. H., and Kolb, W. L. "Ethical Limitations in Sociological Reporting." In W. J. Filstead (Ed.), *Qualitative Methodology: Firsthand Involvement with the Social World.* Chicago: Markham, 1970, 261-270.

Filstead, W. J. (Ed.). *Qualitative Methodology: Firsthand Involvement with the Social World.* Chicago: Markham, 1970.

Fox, R. C. "Illness." In D. Sills (Ed.), *International Encyclopedia of Social Science.* New York: Free Press, 1968, *7*, 90-96.

Fox, R. C. "The Medicalization and Demedicalization of American Society." In J. Knowles (Ed.), *Doing Better and Feeling Worse: Health in the United States.* New York: Norton, 1977, 9-22.

Freidson, E. *Profession of Medicine: A Study of the Sociology of Applied Knowledge.* New York: Dodd, Mead, 1970.

Frieden, L. "IL: Movement and Programs." *American Rehabilitation,* 1978, *3*, 6-9.

Frieden, L. "Adapting IWRP's to Independent Living." Paper presented at conference sponsored by the Independent Living Research Utilization Project, Houston, Tex., Sept. 1980a.

Frieden, L. "Independent Living Program Models." *Rehabilitation Literature,* 1980b, *41*, 169-173.

Frieden, L., and Frieden, J. "Observations of the Lifestyles of Disabled People in Sweden and the Netherlands." In J. A. Cole (Ed.), *Living Independently: Three Views of the European Experience with Implications for the United States.* New York: World Rehabilitation Fund, 1981.

Frieden, L., and Sharp, D. *Peer Counseling Program Models: Report of the Eighth Institute of Rehabilitation Issues.* Hot Springs: Arkansas Rehabilitation and Research Center, 1982.

Frieden, L., and Widmer, M. L. *Registry of Independent Living Programs in the United States.* Houston, Tex.: Institute for Rehabilitation and Research, 1982.

Frieden, L., and others. *ILRU Source Book: A Technical Assistance Manual on Independent Living.* Houston, Tex.: Institute for Rehabilitation and Research, 1979.

Gans, H. J. *The Urban Villagers.* New York: Free Press, 1962.

Gardeström, L. "The Swedish Handicap Movement." *Current Sweden,* 1978, *203*, 1-12.

Gartner, A., and Riessman, F. "Lots of Helping Hands." *New York Times,* February 19, 1980.

Gerth, H. H., and Mills, C. W. (Eds.). *From Max Weber: Essays in Sociology.* New York: Oxford University Press, 1946.

Gillette, P. *Career Education for the Handicapped.* Salt Lake City, Utah: Olympus, 1981.

Glaser, B. G., and Strauss, A. L. *The Discovery of Grounded Theory: Strategies for Qualitative Research.* Hawthorne, N.Y.: Aldine, 1967.

Glazer, M. *The Research Adventure: Promises and Problems of Fieldwork.* New York: Random House, 1972.

Glazer, N., and Moynihan, D. P. *Beyond the Melting Pot.* Cambridge, Mass.: M.I.T. Press, 1963.

Gleidman, J. "The Wheelchair Rebellion." *Psychology Today,* 1979, *12,* 99-103.

Goffman, E. "Characteristics of Total Institutions." In M. R. Stein, A. J. Vidich, and D. M. White (Eds.), *Identity and Anxiety: Survival of the Person in Mass Society.* New York: Free Press, 1960.

Goffman, E. *Stigma: Notes on the Management of Spoiled Identity.* Englewood Cliffs, N.J.: Prentice-Hall, 1963.

Goldsmith, S. *Designing for the Disabled.* (3rd ed.) London: Royal Institute of British Architects, 1976.

Goodman, M. E. *The Individual and Culture.* Homewood, Ill.: Dorsey Press, 1967.

Gordon, G. *Role Theory and Illness: A Sociological Perspective.* New Haven, Conn.: College and University Press, 1966.

Greendale, A., and Knock, S. F., Jr. (Eds.). *Housing Costs and Housing Needs.* New York: Praeger, 1976.

Greenstein, D., and Leonard, E. "No One At Home: A Brief Review of Housing for Handicapped Persons in Some European Countries." *Rehabilitation Literature,* 1976, *37,* 2-9.

Griffin, L., and Martin, W. "Peer Counseling: Process and Goal." Paper presented at the 1979 National Spinal Cord Injury Foundation Convention, 31st Annual Convention, Denver, Colo., August 5-9, 1979.

Handlin, O. (Ed.). *Immigration as a Factor in American History.* Englewood Cliffs, N.J.: Prentice-Hall, 1959.

Hansen, J. "Can You Hear Me?" *Science Digest*, 1979, *85*, 42–45.

Harrington, M. *The Other America: Poverty in the United States*. New York: Macmillan, 1962.

Harrison, D. K., Garnett, J. M., and Watson, A. L. *Client Assessment Measures in Rehabilitation*. Ann Arbor: Rehabilitation Research Institute, University of Michigan, 1981.

Health Policy Advisory Committee (Ed.). *American Health Empire: Power, Profits, Politics*. New York: Random House, 1971.

Heihle, G. *Measuring Independent Living Program Effectiveness: A Working Paper*. Sacramento: California State Department of Rehabilitation, 1981.

Helsel, E. D. "Residential Services." In J. Wortis (Ed.), *Mental Retardation and Developmental Disabilities*. Vol. 3. New York: Grune & Stratton, 1971, 76–101.

Heumann, J. Personal communication concerning the Center for Independent Living. Berkeley, Calif. July 1979.

Hoffman, M. O. "A Statewide Service Delivery System: Independent Living Services Program." *Innovations in Rehabilitation*, 1979, *1*, 25–29.

Hostetter, C. D. "Oklahoma Social and Rehabilitative Services." In *Tooling Up for Accessibility (Seminar): A Report of the Proceedings*. Washington, D.C.: National Center for a Barrier Free Environment, 1978, 18–19.

Hurvitz, N. "Origins of the Peer Self-Help Psychotherapy Group Movement." *Journal of Applied Behavioral Science*, 1976, *12*, 283–294.

Illich, I. *Medical Nemesis: The Expropriation of Health*. New York: Pantheon, 1976.

Institute for Information Studies. *Rehabilitation Engineering Sourcebook*. Falls Church, Va.: Institute for Information Studies, 1979.

Jackins, H. *Fundamentals of Co-Counseling Manual*. Seattle, Wash.: Rational Island Publishers, 1970.

Jones, H. "An Overview of the Canadian Mosaic (Legislation)." *Rehabilitation Digest*, 1979, *10*, 5–7, 21.

Jorgensen, I. S. (Ed.). *Special Education in Denmark*. Danish In-

formation Handbook Series. Copenhagen: Det Danske Sel-
skab, 1979.

Jorgensen, I. S. *Independent Living in Denmark.* East Lansing:
University Center for International Rehabilitation, Michigan
State University, 1981.

Juhr, G., and others. *Barriers to the Development and Applica-
tion of Technological Aids for Handicapped Persons.* East
Lansing: University Center for International Rehabilitation,
Michigan State University, 1979.

Kalish, R. A. "The Aged and the Dying Process: The Inevitable
Decision." *Journal of Social Issues,* 1965, *21,* 87–96.

Kallman, P. O. *Nationwide Transportation Service: A Swedish
Experiment.* East Lansing: University Center for International Rehabilitation, Michigan State University, 1981.

Katz, A. H., and Bender, E. I. "Self-Help Groups in Western Society, History and Prospects." *Journal of Applied Behavioral
Science,* 1976, *12,* 265–282.

King's Fund Center. *Stress and the Caring Relative—Crossroads
Care Attendant Schemes.* Report of two meetings held at the
King's Fund Center for the King Edward's Hospital Fund for
England, London, 1980.

Kleck, R., Hiroshi, O., and Hastort, A. "The Effects of Physical
Deviance upon Face-To-Face Interaction." *Human Relations,*
1966, *19,* 425–436.

Kolata, G. B. "NMC Thrives Selling Dialysis." *Science,* 1980a,
208, 379–382.

Kolata, G. B. "Dialysis After Nearly a Decade." *Science,* 1980b,
208, 473–476.

Kornbluh, M. "Summary of Congressional Workshop Entitled
'Application of Technology to Handicapped Individuals:
Progress and Issues.'" In Institute of Electrical and Electronics Engineers, *Application of Personal Computing to Aid
the Handicapped.* New York: Institute of Electrical and Electronic Engineers, 1980.

Kuhn, T. *The Structure of Scientific Revolutions.* Chicago: University of Chicago, 1970.

Kutner, N. G., and Brogan, D. R. "Disability Labelling versus
Self-Help Ideology in Services for the Chronically Ill." Un-

published paper, Department of Rehabilitation Medicine, Emory University, 1982.

Labovitz, S. and Hagedorn, R. *Introduction to Social Research.* New York: McGraw-Hill, 1971.

LaRocca, J. *Peer Counseling in Rehabilitation.* Washington, D.C.: The Urban Institute, 1981.

LaRocca, J., and Turem, J. S. *The Application of Technological Development to Physically Disabled People.* Washington, D.C.: The Urban Institute, 1978.

Laurie, G. *Housing and Home Services for the Disabled.* New York: Harper and Row, 1977.

Laurie, G. "Relationships Between American and European Concepts of Independent Living." In J. A. Cole (Ed.), *Living Independently: Three Views of the European Experience with Implications for the United States.* New York: World Rehabilitation Fund, 1981.

Levin, L. "Self-Care: An International Perspective." *Social Policy,* 1976, *7,* 70–75.

Levy, D. *Maternal Overprotection.* New York: Columbia University Press, 1943.

Levy, L. H. "Self-Help Groups: Types and Psychological Processes." *Journal of Applied Behavioral Science,* 1976, *12,* 310–322.

Liebow, E. *Tally's Corner: A Study of Negro Streetcorner Men.* Boston: Little, Brown, 1967.

Lifchez, R., and Winslow, B. *Design for Independent Living: The Environment and Physically Disabled People.* New York: Whitney Library of Design, 1979.

Lofland, J. *Analyzing Social Settings: A Guide to Qualitative Observation and Analysis.* Belmont, Calif.: Wadsworth, 1971.

Lowman, E., and Klinger, J. L. *Aids to Independent Living: Self-Help for the Handicapped.* New York: McGraw-Hill, 1969.

McBroom, P. *Behavioral Genetics.* Science Monographs No. 2. Washington, D.C.: U.S. Department of Health, Education and Welfare, 1980.

Mace, R. L. "Architectural Accessibility." *Awareness Papers.* Washington, D.C.: White House Conference on Handicapped Individuals, 1977, 147–166.

MacGregor, F. C. "Some Psychosocial Problems Associated with Facial Deformities." *American Sociological Review,* 1951, *16,* 629-638.

MacMurchy, H. "The Personality of the Mentally Defective." *Journal of Psycho-Asthenics,* 1917, *22,* 89-93.

Mager, R. F. *Preparing Instructional Objectives.* Belmont, Calif.: Fearon, 1975.

Mallik, K., and Sablowsky, R. "Model for Placement—Job Laboratory Approach." *Journal of Rehabilitation,* 1975, *41,* 14-20.

..del, L. *Do Not Go Gently Into This Good Night.* In R. Averson and D. M. White (Eds.), *Electronic Drama: Television Plays of the Sixties.* Boston: Beacon Press, 1971.

Mann, T. *The Magic Mountain.* New York: Random House, 1927.

Mason, R. "Architecture Beyond 2000." In *1999: The World of Tomorrow.* Washington, D.C.: World Future Society, 1978.

Mechanic, D. "Health and Illness in Technological Societies." *Hastings Center Studies,* 1973, *1,* 7-18.

Michigan State Housing Development Authority. *Special Group Housing for Adults Development Process.* Lansing: Michigan State Housing Development Authority, 1978.

Ministry of Local Government. *Local Government in Sweden.* (Government report.) Stockholm: 1978.

Ministry of National Health and Welfare. *Disabled Persons in Canada.* (Government report.) Canada, 1980.

Minnesota Department of Public Welfare. *Personal Care Services.* St. Paul: State of Minnesota, 1978.

Moyer, J. J. "Technology Aids for Blind People." In Institute of Electrical and Electronics Engineers, *Application of Personal Computing to Aid the Handicapped.* New York: Institute of Electrical and Electronics Engineers, 1980.

Nagi, S. Z. *R & D Disability Policies and Programs: An Analysis of Organizations, Clinics, and Decision-Making.* Columbus: Mershon Center of Ohio State University, 1973.

Nagi, S. Z. *An Epidemiology of Disability Among Adults in the United States.* Columbus: Mershon Center of Ohio State University, 1975.

National Center for Health Statistics. *Home Care for Persons 55 and Over, United States, July 1966-June 1968.* Vital and Health Statistics, Series 10, No. 73. Washington, D.C.: U.S. Department of Health, Education and Welfare, 1972.

National Center for Health Statistics. *Health Characteristics of Persons with Chronic Activity Limitations, United States, 1974.* Vital and Health Statistics Series 10, No. 112. Washington, D.C.: U.S. Department of Health, Education and Welfare, October, 1976.

National Labour Market Board. "Vocational Rehabilitation in Sweden." *AMS.* Solna, Sweden: 1978.

National Rehabilitation Information Center. *Request for Continuation.* Submitted by the School of Library and Information Science, Catholic University of America, to the National Institute of Handicapped Research, Washington, D.C., 1981.

National Research Council of National Academy of Sciences. *Science and Technology in the Service of the Physically Handicapped.* Vol. 1. Springfield, Va.: National Technical Information Service, 1976.

Nebraska Division of Rehabilitation Services. *For the Disabled: Annual Report, 1972.* Lincoln: Nebraska State Department of Education, 1972.

Neimark, S. Statement on the 1978 Amendments to the Rehabilitation Act, presented at hearings before the Subcommittee on the Handicapped, Senate Committee on Human Resources, Washington, D.C., March 10 and 14, 1978, 185-198.

Oberman, C. E. *A History of Vocational Rehabilitation in America.* Minneapolis, Minn.: Denison, 1965.

Olmsted, M. *The Small Group.* New York: Random House, 1959.

O'Mara, P. *Residential Development Handbook.* Washington, D.C.: Urban Land Institute, 1978.

Pankowski, J., and others. *Peer Counseling as a Rehabilitation Resource.* Hot Springs, Ark.: Institute on Rehabilitation Issues, Arkansas Rehabilitation Research and Training Center, 1981.

Parmenter, T. R. *Vocational Training for Independent Living.* New York: World Rehabilitation Fund, 1980.

Parrish, K. (Ed.). *Knowledge in Motion.* Washington, D.C.: American Coalition of Citizens with Disabilities, 1981.

Parsons, M. C., and Counts, R. "Historical Development of the Independent Living Movement." (Mimeographed.) Omaha, Nebr.: May 1978, 1-6.

Parsons, M. C. and Rappaport, M. W. "Rehabilitation Engineering." Washington, D.C.: White House Conference on Handicapped Individuals, 1977.

Parsons, T. *The Social System.* Glencoe, Ill.: The Free Press, 1951, 428-479.

Perkinson, M. A. "Alternate Roles for the Elderly: An Example from a Midwestern Retirement Community." *Human Organization,* 1980, *39,* 219-226.

Perlik, S. "Risk Taking and Its Implications for the Mentally Retarded." Unpublished paper, Florence Heller School for Advanced Studies in Social Welfare, Brandeis University, 1980.

Perske, R. "The Dignity of Risk and The Mentally Retarded." *Mental Retardation,* 1972, *10,* 24-27.

Pflueger, S. *Independent Living.* Washington, D.C.: Institute for Research Utilization, 1977.

Phillips, J. M. "Measurement of the Effectiveness of the Location of Existing Projects Used by Physically Disabled People." Unpublished report, for the Province of Alberta, Ministry of Housing and Public Works, Edmonton, Canada, 1981.

Pierce, N. "The Great Wheelchair Flap." *Washington Post,* December 28, 1978.

Pitts, J. "Social Control." *International Encyclopedia of Social Science.* New York: Free Press, 1968.

Posner, I. *Functional Capacity Limitations and Disability.* Social Security Disability Survey, Report No. 2. Washington, D.C.: U.S. Department of Health, Education and Welfare, 1972.

President's Committee on Employment of the Handicapped. *Getting Through College with a Disability: A Summary of Services Available on 500 Campuses for Students with Handicapped Conditions.* Washington, D.C.: President's Committee on Employment of the Handicapped, 1977.

Prewitt, K. "Usefulness of the Social Sciences." *Science*, 1981, *211*, 659.

Purtilo, R. *Justice, Liberty Compassion—"Humane" Health Care and Rehabilitation in the U.S.: Some Lessons from Sweden.* New York: World Rehabilitation Fund, 1981.

"PVArchives." *Paraplegia News*, 1981, *35* (2), 51.

Reagan, A. *Grove Road House Scheme.* Sutton-in-Ashford, England, 1980.

Rehabilitation Services Administration. *Proceedings of the Workshop on Research Utilization Specialist Model.* Rehabilitation Services Administration: Pasadena, Calif., 1975.

Reswick, J. B. "Rehabilitation Engineering." In E. L. Pan, T. E. Backer, and C. L. Vash (Eds.), *Annual Review of Rehabilitation.* New York: Springer, 1980.

Rice, B. D., and Roessler, R. T. *Introduction to Independent Living Rehabilitation Services.* Arkansas Rehabilitation Research and Training Center, Fayetteville: University of Arkansas, 1980.

Riessman, F. "How Does Self-Help Work?" *Social Policy*, 1976, *7*, 41–48.

Rogers, C. *On Becoming a Person.* Boston: Houghton-Mifflin, 1961.

Rude, C. D. (Ed.). *Citizen Advocacy Resources.* Lubbock: Research and Training Center in Mental Retardation, Texas Tech University, 1979.

Sale, R. T. "Employment." Washington, D.C.: White House Conference on Handicapped Individuals, 1977.

Sanders, C. "Rope Burns: Impediments to the Achievement of Basic Comfort in the Field Research Experience." In W. B. Shaffir, R. A. Stebbins, and A. Turowetz (Eds.), *Fieldwork Experience: Qualitative Approaches to Social Research.* New York: St. Martin's Press, 1980.

Saxton, M. "A Peer Counseling Training Program for Disabled Women." *Journal of Sociology and Social Welfare*, 1981, *8*, 334–346.

Schatzlein, J. E. "Spinal Cord Injury and Peer Counseling/Peer Education." Unpublished paper, Regional Spinal Cord Injury Center, Department of Physical Medicine and Rehabilitation, University of Minnesota Hospital, 1978.

Schwartz, H., and Jacobs, J. *Qualitative Sociology: A Method to the Madness.* New York: Free Press, 1979.

Shaffir, W. B., Stebbins, R. A., and Turowetz, A. (Eds.). *Field-work Experience: Qualitative Approaches to Social Research.* New York: St. Martin's Press, 1980.

Sharlin, S. A., and Polansky, N. A. "The Process of Infantilization." *American Journal of Orthopsychiatry,* 1972, *42,* 92–102.

Sharp, D. C. *Evaluation of Independent Living Skills of the New Options Participants.* Unpublished master's thesis, School of Social Work, University of Houston, 1980.

Sidel, V. W., and Sidel, R. "Beyond Groping." *Social Policy,* 1976, *7,* 67–69.

Siegler, M., and Osmond, H. "The Sick Role Revisited." *Hastings Center Studies,* 1973, *1,* 41–58.

Sigelman, C. K., and Parham, J. D. *Independent Living and Mentally Retarded Persons.* Houston, Tex.: Institute for Rehabilitation and Research, 1981.

Smelser, N. J. *Theory of Collective Behavior.* New York: Free Press, 1962.

Smith, D., and Canada House of Commons. *Obstacles.* Report of the Special Committee on the Disabled and the Handicapped. Canada House of Commons, Ottawa, 1981.

Smith, P. *Housing for Disabled People—Recent Initiatives in Britain.* London, England: Centre on Environment for the Handicapped, 1980.

Spaniol, L. "A Comprehensive Study of the Service Needs of Individuals with Combined Severe Physical and Psychiatric Disability." Boston: Center for Rehabilitation Research and Training in Mental Health, Boston University Sargent College of Allied Health Professionals, 1981.

Special Office for the Handicapped. *Accessible Housing.* Raleigh, N.C.: Special Office for the Handicapped, Insurance Commissioner's Office, 1980.

Speier, M. *How to Observe Face-to-Face Communication: A Sociological Introduction.* Pacific Palisades, Calif.: Goodyear, 1973.

Spivak, M. "Archetypal Places." *Architectural Forum,* 1973, *140,* 43-48.

Stack, C. B. *All Our Kin: Strategies for Survival in a Black Community.* New York: Harper and Row, 1974.

Star, R. *Housing and the Money Market.* New York: Basic Books, 1975.

Steinman, R., and Traunstein, D. M. "Redefining Deviance: The Self-Help Challenge to the Human Services." *Journal of Applied Behavioral Science,* 1976, *12,* 347-361.

Stock, D. D., and Cole, J. A. *A Cooperative Self-Support System for Severely Physically Disabled Young Adults: A Final Project Report.* Houston: Texas Institute for Rehabilitation, 1971.

Stoddard, S. "Independent Living: Concept and Programs." *American Rehabilitation,* 1978, *3,* 2-5.

Stoddard, S., and Brown, B. "Evaluating California's Independent Living Centers." *American Rehabilitation,* 1980, *5,* 18-23.

Stoddard, S., Katsuranis, F., Toms, L., and Finnegan, P. *Evaluation Report on the State's Independent Living Centers Funded by AB 204: Final Report.* Berkeley, Calif.: Berkeley Planning Associates, 1980.

Stubbins, J. (Ed.). *Social and Psychological Aspects of Disability: A Handbook for Practitioners.* Baltimore: University Park Press, 1977.

Study Group on Rehabilitation Engineering. *Rehabilitation Engineering: A Counselor's Guide.* Menomonie, Wis.: Study Group on Rehabilitation Engineering, Stout Vocational Rehabilitation Institute, Research and Training Center, 1979.

Swaczy, B. *Getting People Together in Rural America.* Helena, Mont.: Northern Rockies Action Group, 1979.

Swedish Government Commission on Long-Term Employment Policy. *Employment for Handicapped Persons.* Summary of the commission's report of January 1978 and of five research projects. Stockholm: Swedish Ministry of Labour, 1978.

Swedish Institute for the Handicapped. *Rehabilitation in Sweden.* Bromma: Swedish Institute for the Handicapped, 1979.

Swedish Institute for the Handicapped. *Support for the Handicapped in Sweden.* (Fact sheet on Sweden.) Stockholm: Swedish Institute for the Handicapped, 1980.

Switzer, M. E. "Foreword," *VRA R & D Grant Program,* 1965. Quoted in *Proceedings of the Workshop on Research Utilization Specialist Model.* Pasadena, Calif.: Rehabilitation Services Administration, 1975.

Symington, D. C., and others. *Independence Through Environmental Control Systems.* Toronto: Canadian Rehabilitation Council for the Disabled, 1980.

Tate, D., Jarvis, R., and Juhr, G. "International Efforts in Independent Living." *Archives of Physical Medicine and Rehabilitation,* 1979, *60,* 462–465.

Tax, S. "Self-Help Groups: Thoughts on Public Policy." *Journal of Applied Behavioral Science,* 1976, *12,* 448–454.

Telesensory Systems, Inc. *Recommendations Regarding Rehabilitation Technology: Increasing the Effectiveness of Federal Government Involvement in the Development and Dissemination of Technological Aids for People with Disabilities.* A position paper prepared by Telesensory Systems, Inc., Palo Alto, Calif., November 1979.

Thomas, L. "The Technology of Medicine." *New England Journal of Medicine,* 1971, *285,* 1366–1368.

Tocqueville, A. de. *Democracy in America.* (R. D. Heffner, ed.) New York: New American Library, 1961. (Originally published in two vols., 1835 and 1840.)

Toffler, A. *The Third Wave.* New York: Morrow, 1980.

Trieschmann, R. B. *Spinal Cord Injury: Psychological, Social and Vocational Adjustment.* Elmsford, N.Y.: Pergamon Press, 1980.

Turner, R. "The Theme of Contemporary Social Movements." *British Journal of Sociology,* 1969, *20,* 321.

Twaddle, A. C. "Illness and Deviance." *Social Science and Medicine,* 1973, *7,* 751–762.

U.S. Congress. House. Committee on Science and Technology. Subcommittee on Science, Research and Technology. Senate. Committee on Labor and Human Resources. Subcommittee on the Handicapped. *Application of Technology to*

Handicapped Individuals: Process, Problems and Progress. 96th Cong., 2d sess., 1980. Joint Committee Print.

U.S. Department of Agriculture. *1980 Handbook of Agriculture Charts.* Washington, D.C.: U.S. Department of Agriculture, 1980.

U.S. Department of Health, Education and Welfare. *Work Disability in the United States.* Washington, D.C.: Social Security Administration, 1978a.

U.S. Department of Health, Education and Welfare. *From Simple Idea to Complex Execution, Home Health Services Under Titles XVIII, XIX, and XX.* Washington, D.C.: Government Printing Office, 1978b.

U.S. Department of Housing and Urban Development. *Section 202 Direct Loan Program for Housing for the Elderly or Handicapped: Processing Handbook.* Washington, D.C.: U.S. Department of Housing and Urban Development, 1978.

U.S. Department of Housing and Urban Development. *Federal Register.* Part III. Washington, D.C.: Office of Assistant Secretary for Housing, Federal Housing Commissioner, 1979.

University of Virginia Rehabilitation Engineering Center (Ed.). *Rehabilitation Engineering: A Plan for Continued Progress, II.* Washington, D.C.: joint publication of Rehabilitation Services Administration, Office of Human Development Services, Department of Health, Education and Welfare; and Veterans Administration, 1977.

The Urban Institute. *Report of the Comprehensive Needs Study.* Washington, D.C.: Department of Health, Education and Welfare, 1975.

Van Soest, E., and staff of the Sioux Vocational School. *Independent Living Evaluation-Training Program.* Menomonie: Stout Vocational Rehabilitation Institute, University of Wisconsin-Stout, 1979.

Varela, R. A. "Self-Advocacy and Changing Attitudes." In Richman and Trohanis (Eds.), *Public Awareness Viewpoints.* Chapel Hill, N.C.: Developmental Disabilities Technical Assistance System, 1978, 27–36.

Varela, R. A. *Self-Help Groups in Rehabilitation.* Washington, D.C.: American Coalition of Citizens with Disabilities, 1979.

Varela, R. A. "Consumer and Advocate Involvement in Federal and State Vocational Rehabilitation Program Planning." Washington, D.C.: National Institute of Handicapped Research, Department of Education, 1980a.

Varela, R. A. *Participating Citizens.* Washington, D.C.: American Coalition of Citizens with Disabilities, 1980b.

VIA Rail. "VIA Acts to Help Passengers with Special Needs." *Rehabilitation Digest,* 1980, *11* (4), 9, 10, 15.

Viscott, D. *Risking.* New York: Bantam, 1977.

Walls, R. T., Zane, T., and Thredt, J. E. *The Independent Living Behavior Checklist.* Morgantown: West Virginia Rehabilitation Research and Training Center, West Virginia University, 1979.

Walter, F. *An Introduction to Domestic Design for the Disabled.* London, England: Swan Press, 1969.

Whyte, W. F. *Street-Corner Society: The Social Structure of an Italian Slum.* Chicago: University of Chicago Press, 1943.

Wildavsky, A. "No Risk Is the Highest Risk of All." *American Scientist,* 1979, *67,* 32–37.

Wilner, M., Pease, J. A., and Wallgren, R. S. (Eds.). *Planning and Financing Facilities for the Elderly.* Washington, D.C.: American Association of Homes for the Aging, 1978.

Withorn, A. "To Serve the People: An Inquiry Into the Success of Service Delivery as a Social Movement Strategy." Unpublished dissertation, Florence Heller School for Advanced Studies in Social Welfare, Brandeis University, 1977.

Wolfensberger, W. "The Origin and Nature of Our Institutional Models." In R. B. Kugel and W. Wolfensberger (Eds.), *Changing Patterns in Residential Services for the Mentally Retarded.* Washington, D.C.: President's Committee on Mental Retardation, January 1969, 59–172.

Wolfensberger, W. *The Principle of Normalization in Human Services.* Toronto, Canada: National Institute on Mental Retardation, 1972.

Zelditch, M., Jr. "Some Methodological Problems of Field Studies." In B. J. Franklin and H. W. Osborne (Eds.), *Research Methods: Issues and Insights.* Belmont, Calif.: Wadsworth, 1971.

Zola, I. K. "Culture and Symptoms—An Analysis of Patients' Presenting Complaints." *American Sociological Review*, 1966, *31*, 615-630.

Zola, I. K. "Medicine as an Institution of Social Control." *Sociological Review*, 1972, *20*, 487-504.

Zola, I. K. "In the Name of Health and Illness: On Some Socio-Political Consequences of Medical Influence." *Social Science and Medicine*, 1975, *9*, 83-87.

Zola, I. K. "Healthism and Disabling Medicalization." In I. Illich, and others, *Disabling Professions*. London: Calder & Boyars, 1977.

Zola, I. K. "Communication Barriers Between 'The Able-Bodied' and 'The Handicapped.' " *Archives of Physical Medicine and Rehabilitation*, 1981, *62*, 356-359.

Zola, I. K. *Missing Pieces: A Chronicle of Living with a Disability*. Philadelphia: Temple University Press, 1982a.

Zola, I. K. "Socio-Cultural Disincentives to Independent Living." *Archives of Physical Medicine and Rehabilitation*, 1982b, *63*, 394-397.

Name Index

385

Subject Index

E

F

For information about submitting manuscripts
for the People with Disabilities Press, please write:
Stanley D. Klein, Ph.D. People with Disabilities
Press P. O. Box 470715 Brookline, MA 02445